Preventing Low Birthweight

Committee to Study the
Prevention of Low Birthweight
Division of Health Promotion and
Disease Prevention
INSTITUTE OF MEDICINE

NATIONAL ACADEMY PRESS
Washington, D.C. 1985

NATIONAL ACADEMY PRESS **2101 Constitution Avenue, NW** **Washington, DC 20418**

NOTICE: The project that is the subject of this report was approved by the Governing Board of the National Research Council, whose members are drawn from the councils of the National Academy of Sciences, the National Academy of Engineering, and the Institute of Medicine. The members of the committee responsible for the report were chosen for their special competences and with regard for appropriate balance.

This report has been reviewed by a group other than the authors according to the procedures approved by a Report Review Committee consisting of members of the National Academy of Sciences, the National Academy of Engineering, and the Institute of Medicine.

The Institute of Medicine was chartered in 1970 by the National Academy of Sciences to enlist distinguished members of the appropriate professions in the examination of policy matters pertaining to the health of the public. In this, the Institute acts under both the Academy's 1863 congressional charter responsibility to be an adviser to the federal government and its own initiative in identifying issues of medical care, research, and education.

A digest of this volume is available from the National Academy Press at the address above. Please inquire for price and quantity discounts.

Library of Congress Catalog Card Number 84-62849

International Standard Book Number 0-309-03530-9

First Printing, January 1985
Second Printing, July 1987
Third Printing, August 1988
Fourth Printing, November 1988
Fifth Printing, August 1989

Cover photo by Susie Fitzhugh for Children's Hospital National Medical Center, Washington, D.C.

Printed in the United States of America

Committee to Study the Prevention of Low Birthweight

RICHARD E. BEHRMAN, *Chairman,* Committee to Study the Prevention of Low Birthweight, Institute of Medicine, and Dean, School of Medicine, Case Western Reserve University, Cleveland, Ohio

JEFFREY E. HARRIS, Associate Professor, Department of Economics, Massachusetts Institute of Technology, Cambridge, Massachusetts, and Clinical Associate, Massachusetts General Hospital, Boston, Massachusetts

CALVIN J. HOBEL, Professor of Obstetrics, Gynecology and Pediatrics, School of Medicine, University of California at Los Angeles, and Director, Maternal-Fetal Medicine, Cedars Sinai Medical Center, Los Angeles, California

JEROME O. KLEIN, Professor of Pediatrics, Boston University School of Medicine, and Director, Division of Pediatric Infectious Diseases, Boston City Hospital, Boston, Massachusetts

LUELLA KLEIN, President, American College of Obstetricians and Gynecologists, and Professor of Gynecology and Obstetrics, Emory University School of Medicine, Atlanta, Georgia

MARIE C. MCCORMICK, Assistant Professor of Pediatrics, University of Pennsylvania School of Medicine, Philadelphia, Pennsylvania

JAMES METCALFE, Professor of Medicine, Oregon Health Sciences University, Portland, Oregon

C. ARDEN MILLER, Professor and Chairman, Department of Maternal and Child Health, School of Public Health, University of North Carolina at Chapel Hill, Chapel Hill, North Carolina

JOHN T. QUEENAN, Professor and Chairman, Department of Obstetrics and Gynecology, Georgetown University Hospital, Washington, D.C.

JULIUS B. RICHMOND, Director, Division of Health Policy Research and Education, and John D. MacArthur Professor of Health Policy and Management, Harvard University, Boston, Massachusetts

JUDITH P. ROOKS, President, American College of Nurse-Midwives, Portland, Oregon

SAM SHAPIRO, Professor of Health Policy and Management, and Past Director, Health Services Research and Development Center, School of Hygiene and Public Health, Johns Hopkins University, Baltimore, Maryland

Study Staff

SARAH S. BROWN, *Study Director*, Committee to Study the Prevention of Low Birthweight

ENRIQUETA C. BOND, *Director*, Division of Health Promotion and Disease Prevention

STEPHANIE C. BRUGLER, *Research Assistant*, Division of Health Promotion and Disease Prevention

EVE K. NICHOLS, *Editor*, Division of Health Promotion and Disease Prevention

WALLACE K. WATERFALL, *Editor*, Institute of Medicine

LINDA DEPUGH, *Administrative Secretary*, Division of Health Promotion and Disease Prevention

NAOMI HUDSON, *Administrative Secretary*, Division of Health Sciences Policy

Consultant

LORRAINE KLERMAN, Professor of Public Health and Head, Division of Health Services Administration, Department of Epidemiology and Public Health, School of Medicine, Yale University, New Haven, Connecticut

Commissioned Papers

ROBERT GOLDENBERG, Professor of Obstetrics and Gynecology, Department of Obstetrics and Gynecology, The University of Alabama, Birmingham, Alabama

VILMA HUNT, Professor of Public Health, Pennsylvania State University, University Park, Pennsylvania

LORRAINE KLERMAN, Professor of Public Health and Head, Division of Health Services Administration, Department of Epidemiology and Public Health, School of Medicine, Yale University, New Haven, Connecticut

CAROL C. KORENBROT, Research Specialist, Center for Population and Reproductive Health Policy, Institute of Health Policy Studies, University of California, San Francisco, California

JOAN MAXWELL, Senior Associate, Greater Washington Research Center, Washington, D.C.

MARGARET A. MCMANUS, Health Policy Consultant, Washington, D.C.

MARIE MEGLEN, Director, Bureau of Maternal and Child Health, South Carolina Department of Health and Environmental Control, Columbia, South Carolina

MARY PEOPLES, Assistant Professor, Department of Maternal and Child Health, School of Public Health, University of North Carolina at Chapel Hill, Chapel Hill, North Carolina

BEATRICE J. SELWYN, Research Assistant Professor in Epidemiology, School of Public Health, University of Texas, Houston, Texas

JOE LEIGH SIMPSON, Professor of Obstetrics and Gynecology and Head, Section of Human Genetics, Prentice Women's Hospital and Maternity Center, Northwestern University Medical Center, Chicago, Illinois

STEVEN SMOOKLER, Assistant Dean for Special Programs, School of Medicine, Case Western Reserve University, Cleveland, Ohio

SUSAN WILNER, Pew Fellow, Institute of Health Policy Studies, University of California at San Francisco, San Francisco, California

Contributed Papers

HEINZ W. BERENDES, Director, Epidemiology and Biometry Research Program, National Institute of Child Health and Human Development, Bethesda, Maryland

NAOMI BRESLAU, Associate Professor of Epidemiology and Community Health, School of Medicine, Case Western Reserve University, Cleveland, Ohio

AMY FINE, Project Director, Child Health Outcomes Project of the University of North Carolina, Washington, D.C.

STEPHEN G. GABBE, Professor of Obstetrics, Gynecology and Pediatrics, and Director, Jerrold R. Golding Division of Fetal Medicine, University of Pennsylvania, Philadelphia, Pennsylvania

KENNETH G. JOHNSON, Director, Health Services Research Center, The Kingston Hospital, Kingston, New York

SAMUEL S. KESSEL, Chief, Research and Training Branch, Division of Maternal and Child Health, Department of Health and Human Services, Washington, D.C.

MARK KLEBANOFF, Medical Staff Fellow, Epidemiology and Biometry Research Program, National Institute of Child Health and Human Development, Bethesda, Maryland

MILTON KOTELCHUCK, Assistant Professor of Health Policy, Department of Social Medicine and Health Policy, Harvard Medical School, Boston, Massachusetts

MORTON LEBOW, Administrator for Public Affairs, American College of Obstetricians and Gynecologists, Washington, D.C.

DAVID SALKEVER, Professor of Health Policy and Management, School of Hygiene and Public Health, Johns Hopkins University, Baltimore, Maryland

JOHN SINCLAIR, Professor of Pediatrics, Department of Pediatrics, McMasters University, Hamilton, Ontario

LEON SPEROFF, Professor and Chairman, Department of Obstetrics and Gynecology, Case Western Reserve University, and Director, McDonald Hospital for Women, Cleveland, Ohio

Preface

The future of the nation depends on the well-being of its children. To explore how the nation might best invest its resources to promote child health and development, the Institute of Medicine convened a planning group in 1982, with the support of The Commonwealth Fund. The planning group evaluated numerous areas for further study by the Institute and then recommended an investigation of the potential for the prevention of low birthweight in the United States.

The birth of infants who have not attained their normal intrauterine growth and development is a major determinant of neonatal and infant mortality and contributes to childhood morbidity, which imposes major social and economic burdens. The issue of low birthweight is especially salient in the United States, because the low birthweight rate has not followed the recent decline in infant mortality. In addition, the rates of both low birthweight (2,500 grams or less) and very low birthweight (1,500 grams or less) deliveries are known to be higher in the United States than in at least 12 other developed countries (Table 1) and are quite likely higher than those of several additional countries whose infant mortality rates are lower than those of the United States.

To determine if promising opportunities exist for reducing the incidence of low birthweight, the Institute of Medicine established an interdisciplinary committee to study the complex problems of prematurity and intrauterine growth retardation, the twin contributors to low birthweight. The committee was asked to review available measures for preventing or reducing the occurrence of low birthweight in infants; to define those interventions likely to be effective and to consider their costs in relation to the continuing incidence of low birthweight. As background to such an analysis, the group also was asked to assess the relationship of low birthweight to mortality and morbidity; to review existing information on the etiology of low birthweight and the risk factors associated with it; and to examine trends over time.

In meeting this charge, the committee has developed a report in two parts. Part I defines and describes the significance of low birthweight, the data on etiology and risk factors, and recent state and national trends in the incidence of low birthweight among various groups. Part II describes the preventive approaches found most desirable and considers their costs. The committee based its study on a combination of existing information and several new analyses of selected vital statistics. With a few important exceptions, the committee confined its literature reviews to research and evaluation studies conducted and published in the United States. This limitation was dictated by constraints of time and resources and by the committee's belief that, particularly in the area of maternity care, the demographic, cultural and socioeconomic differences between the

TABLE 1. Percentage of Very Low Birthweight (VLBW) and Low Birthweight (LBW) Live Births in Selected Developed Countries, 1980

Country	VLBW[a]	LBW[b]
Austria	0.80	5.68
Canada[c]	0.84	6.10
Denmark	0.72	6.00
Federal Republic of Germany	0.71	5.51
German Democratic Republic	0.55[d]	6.19
Israel	0.99	7.16
Italy	0.83	6.71
Japan	0.39	5.18
New Zealand	0.65	5.27
Norway	0.59	3.25
Sweden[e]	0.49	4.03
Switzerland	0.49	5.14
United Kingdom		
England and Wales[f]	0.77	6.79
Scotland[g]	0.96	6.73
United States	1.15	6.84

[a]1,500 grams or less. May represent underestimates if infants weighing less than 500 grams are excluded.

[b]2,500 grams or less.

[c]Data for 1979.

[d]Probably an underestimate due to a nonstandard definition of live births and late fetal deaths.

[e]Data for 1978.

[f]Macfarlane A and Mugford M: Birth Counts, Statistics of Pregnancy and Childbirth, p. 14. London: Her Majesty's Stationary Office, 1984.

[g]McIlwaine GM, Dunn F, Howat RCL, Smalls M, Wyllie MM, and MacNaughton MC: Perinatal Mortality Survey, Scotland, 1977-1981. Glasgow: University of Glasgow, 1983.

SOURCE: United Nations: Demographic Yearbook 1981. New York, 1983.

United States and other countries often limit the applicability of data collected abroad to the United States.

Acknowledgments

Funding was provided principally by the Commonwealth Fund, with additional support from the Ford Foundation, the March of Dimes Birth Defects Foundation, the National Institute of Child Health and Human Development, and the National Research Council Fund. The support of these funding sources is gratefully acknowledged.

In my role as chairman of the committee that developed this report, I also wish to express my gratitude to the many individuals who contributed so much to our deliberations. In particular, it was a privilege to be associated with such a hardworking and dedicated committee, whose members gave so generously and unreservedly of their time and energies. Similarly, the committee joins me in acknowledging our great appreciation and indebtedness to the staff of this study, especially the study's director, Sarah Brown. Without her support and exceptional efforts in our behalf, the work could not have been so successfully completed. The many contributions of Lorraine Klerman, a consultant to the study and the author of several papers for the project, are also gratefully acknowledged. And particular thanks go to Eve Nichols, the report editor, for her tireless attention to countless details of both form and substance.

We were also fortunate in benefitting from the substantial help and stimulation provided by a number of thoughtful commissioned and contributed papers, the authors of which are listed at the beginning of the report. These authors also provided useful personal insights for which we are thankful. Several components of the Department of Health and Human Services provided valuable assistance in data analysis, in locating various materials needed by the committee, and in providing helpful commentary. We extend particular thanks to Vince Hutchins and Samuel Kessel within the Division of Maternal and Child Health; Joel Kleinman, Jacob Feldman, Paul Placek, Selma Taffel, Robert Hartford, and Mary Grace Kovar of the National Center for Health Statistics; and Heinz Berendes, Mark Klebanoff, Sumner Yaffe, Wendy Baldwin, and Charles Lowe of the National Institute of Child Health and Human Development.

Many other individuals played an important role in the committee's deliberations by providing information, critical analysis, advice, and reviews of draft material. In particular, we gratefully recognize the help provided by Robert Bragonier, Alexander Burnett, John Carl, Frederick Frigoletto, Phyllis Freeman, Steven Gortmaker, Asta Kenney, Mary Lou Moore, Merry-K Moos, Elena Nightingale, Anthony Robbins, Sara Rosenbaum, Anne Rosewater, Lisbeth Schorr, Steven Warsof, and Ronald Williams.

RICHARD E. BEHRMAN, M.D.
Chairman

Contents

Summary and Recommendations

Low birthweight is a major determinant of infant mortality in the United States. Most infant deaths occur in the first 4 weeks of life, the neonatal period, and most are a consequence of inadequate fetal growth, as indicated by low birthweight (2,500 grams--about 5.5 pounds--or less). Inadequate fetal growth may result from prematurity (duration of pregnancy less than 37 weeks from the last menstrual period), poor fetal weight gain for a given duration of pregnancy (intrauterine growth retardation), or both. The risk of mortality increases as birthweight decreases; very low birthweight infants (1,500 grams or less) are at greatest risk.

The proportion of low-weight births not only is a major determinant of the overall neonatal mortality rate for a population, but also is an important factor in the differences in neonatal mortality rates among various groups in the population. Thus, the higher neonatal mortality rates seen for nonwhite mothers, teenage mothers, and mothers of low educational attainment are explained largely by higher proportions of low birthweight infants among these groups.

In addition to increasing the risk of mortality, low birthweight also increases the risk of illness. Although low birthweight is not a major determinant of the total burden of morbidity among infants and children, the relative risk of morbidity among low birthweight infants is high. The association of neurodevelopmental handicaps and congenital anomalies with low birthweight has been well established; low birthweight infants also may be susceptible to a wide range of other conditions, such as lower respiratory tract infections, learning disorders, behavior problems, and complications of neonatal intensive care interventions. Moreover, a low-weight birth and the infant's subsequent problems may place substantial emotional and financial stress on a young family.

Although the neonatal mortality rate in the United States has dropped greatly over the past 15 years, there has not been a comparable decrease in the incidence of low-weight births. Instead, the mortality decline has been accomplished primarily by improving the survival of low birthweight infants, largely through neonatal intensive care. The proportion of infants born at low birthweight has changed only modestly since the late 1960s, and little change, if any, has been seen in the proportion of infants born at very low birthweight. The current statistics suggest that further reductions in neonatal mortality and decreases in the differentials between high- and low-mortality subgroups will require a reduction in the rate of low birthweight.

Etiology and Risk Factors

Despite steady advances in the science of obstetrics, our understanding of the basic causes of preterm labor and intrauterine growth retardation is limited. In the absence of adequate information about etiology, a large body of information has developed about factors associated with low birthweight, often termed "risk factors" because their presence in an individual woman indicates an increased chance, or risk, of bearing a low birthweight infant. These factors include demographic characteristics, such as low socioeconomic status, low level of education, nonwhite race (particularly black), childbearing at extremes of the reproductive age span, and being unmarried; medical risks that can be identified before pregnancy, such as a poor obstetric history, certain diseases and conditions, and poor nutritional status; problems that are detected during pregnancy, such as poor weight gain, bacteriuria, toxemia/preeclampsia, short interpregnancy interval, and multiple pregnancy; behavioral and environmental risks, such as smoking, alcohol and other substance abuse, and exposure to various toxic substances; and the health care risks of absent or inadequate prenatal care and iatrogenic prematurity. Newer hypotheses suggest that another group of factors also may place a woman at risk of low birthweight, particularly preterm labor: stress, uterine irritability, certain cervical changes detected before the onset of labor, some infections, inadequate plasma volume expansion, and progesterone deficiency.

By grouping the factors as summarized above, the committee observed that many risks for low birthweight can be identified before pregnancy occurs; detection and possible intervention need not always wait until the prenatal period. Smoking is perhaps the best example of this perspective. The grouping also helps to highlight the importance of behavioral and environmental risks and the need for interventions that go beyond medical care. The demographic measures can help to define target populations. The cluster of health care risks highlights the fact that not all risks for low birthweight derive from characteristics of women themselves. And finally, the category of evolving concepts of risk suggests some important research areas. These themes appear throughout the report.

The committee concluded that a variety of factors are clearly and consistently linked to low birthweight. These factors should be used to help define high-risk groups and to develop and target interventions. It is also apparent, however, that the importance of each factor for an individual or a group cannot be calculated easily; that the risks for low birthweight are widely distributed throughout the population; and that a substantial incidence of low birthweight deliveries will continue to occur outside of groups currently defined as high risk. These circumstances highlight the need for greater understanding of risk and causation, but should not be used to minimize the value of using existing risk information for targeting interventions.

More research is needed on risk factors, not only those somewhat speculative but also those firmly linked to low birthweight. For some factors, such as race, research is needed to understand how the factor exerts its effect. For others, such as alcohol, the magnitude of risk at various levels of consumption should be better defined. And for both definite and less certain risk factors, efforts should be made to distinguish risks for very low birthweight (1,500 grams or less) from risks for moderately low birthweight (1,501 to 2,500 grams) at various gestational ages, because the sequelae and incidence trends of these two classes of low birthweight differ.

The committee's review of risk assessment instruments indicates that they are helpful in distinguishing between high- and low-risk pregnancies. The not infrequent occurrence of low birthweight deliveries in low-risk women, however, suggests that additional research is needed to improve the predictive capability of these systems. It also indicates that clinicians must be alert to the possibility of low birthweight even in pregnant women judged to be at low risk of such an outcome.

Trends in Low Birthweight

The committee investigated trends in the rate of low birthweight and the composition of low-weight births in the United States as a whole and in five selected states (California, Massachusetts, Michigan, North Carolina, and Oregon) during the past 10 to 15 years. For the nation, the proportion of low-weight births declined from 7.6 percent of live births in 1971 to 6.8 percent of live births in 1981.

The decline in rates was confined to the moderately low birthweight group. No decline, or perhaps a slight increase, was observed in the very low birthweight group. Although birth certificate data on gestational age are incomplete and of uncertain quality, the observed decline in low birthweight was apparently concentrated mostly in the full-term low birthweight group.

Both white and black low birthweight rates have declined, but blacks remain at increased risk of low birthweight compared with whites. The data show no closing of the gap, although quantifying the white-black differential in low birthweight rates depends on the index used to measure the gap. White and black low birthweight rates vary appreciably among the states studied.

Teenage mothers and those 35 years of age or older have higher rates of low birthweight than mothers in their twenties or early thirties. Teenage mothers have the highest relative risk of low birthweight, especially among whites. Childbearing by teenagers is more prevalent among blacks, however. The risks of low birthweight among teenagers probably derive more from other factors associated with teenage childbearing (such as low socioeconomic status and poor utilization of prenatal care) than from young age itself.

For both races, the risk of low birthweight declines sharply among mothers with at least 12 years of education. The relationship between education and low birthweight is independent of maternal age and race. The gap in low birthweight rates among mothers with disparate educational attainment is not closing, and may be widening. Because educational attainment of mothers generally has increased during the past 10 to 15 years, the finding of a widening gap in low birthweight rates among mothers with disparate education suggests that the poorly educated may constitute an increasingly high-risk group.

Unmarried mothers have consistently higher rates of low birthweight. The elevated risk is not attributable to differences in age or race. The proportion of unmarried mothers appears to be increasing; among blacks, 56 percent of mothers were unmarried in 1981.

No clear change has occurred in the relationship between parity and the risk of low birthweight. High-parity births continue to have a slightly greater risk of low birthweight, and termination of the last pregnancy in a fetal death increases the risk of low birthweight in the subsequent pregnancy. Among mothers with a previous live birth, an interpregnancy interval of less than 6 months enhances the subsequent risk of low birthweight.

The risk of low birthweight is reduced among mothers who initiate prenatal care during the first 3 months of pregnancy. The proportion of mothers with early prenatal care has increased during the past 10 to 15 years. This has been accompanied by a decline in low birthweight rates among mothers in the early care group.

The committee performed a multivariate tabulation of single live births in the United States during 1981 according to educational attainment, marital status, age/birth order category, and the timing and quantity of prenatal care. With all other factors controlled, a change in timing of initiation of prenatal care was associated with a minor reduction in the risk of low birthweight. The estimated contribution of prenatal care to a reduction in the low birthweight rate was more marked, however, when care was gauged by an index of "adequacy" that reflected both the start of care in the first trimester and number of visits. The tabulation suggests that the analyzed risk factors might account together for as much as 30 percent of the risk of low birthweight in both races. Moreover, the sensitivity of the estimated contribution of prenatal care to the method of measuring such care suggests that the pattern of care may have an important influence on the risk of low birthweight.

An Overview of Preventive Approaches

The committee concluded that, although there are many unanswered questions about the causes of and risks for low birthweight, policymakers and health professionals know enough at present to intervene more vigorously to reduce the incidence of low birthweight in infants. Methods already available have demonstrated their value in reducing low birthweight. These and a few new measures merit additional support. No single approach will solve the low birthweight problem. Instead, several types of programs should be undertaken simultaneously. These range from specific medical procedures to broad-scale public health and educational efforts.

Because of a lack of data, the committee was not able to calculate the precise impact of the recommended interventions on the incidence of low birthweight. Based on the information that is available, however, the committee believes that if the recommended interventions were implemented, the nation would be able to meet the goal set by the U.S. Surgeon General for 1990--that low birthweight babies should constitute no more than 5 percent of all live births, and that no county or racial/ethnic subpopulation should have a rate of low birthweight that exceeds 9 percent of all live births.

The committee was not able to calculate the cost or cost-effectiveness of most of the recommended interventions because of problems in the quality and uniformity of available cost data, difficulties in delineating the services received, and uncertainties about target populations. The committee found, however, that it could perform a straightforward analysis of some of the financial implications involved in the provision of prenatal services to pregnant women. A description of this analysis is presented at the end of this summary.

Moving ahead in the directions advocated by the committee will require that the problem of low birthweight become more widely understood and recognized as an important national issue. Low birthweight and its consequences merit the attention of Congress, state governments, professional groups, business and labor organizations, church and women's groups, schools, and the information media. The federal government, particularly the executive branch, is uniquely positioned to play a leadership role in stimulating necessary discussion and action. The committee recommends that the Department of Health and Human Services define and pursue a variety of activities designed to focus attention on low birthweight--its importance, its causes and associated risks, and pathways for its prevention. Such leadership must include an increased commitment of resources to the problem of low birthweight through approaches such as those outlined in this report.

Throughout the report, and in relation to each of the interventions advocated, the committee emphasizes the need for research on a wide variety of issues. It also highlights the importance of more adequate data systems and better techniques to monitor the impact of various programs on low birthweight and on pregnancy outcome generally.

Planning for Pregnancy

Numerous opportunities exist before pregnancy to reduce the incidence of low birthweight, yet these are often overlooked in favor of interventions during pregnancy. In a fundamental sense, healthy pregnancies begin before conception. The committee emphasizes, therefore, the importance of prepregnancy risk identification, counseling, and reduction; health education related to pregnancy outcome generally, and low birthweight in particular; and the full availability of family planning services, especially for low-income women and adolescents.

Among the risk factors that can be recognized and dealt with before pregnancy are certain maternal chronic illnesses, smoking, moderate to heavy alcohol use and substance abuse, inadequate weight for height, poor nutritional status, susceptibility to rubella and other infectious agents, age (under 17 and over 34), the possibility of a very short interval between pregnancies, and high parity. For some of these factors, reducing the risk before conception may offer more protection than doing so once pregnancy has been established.

Prepregnancy counseling is especially important for women who already have had a low birthweight delivery because the risk of repeating a poor outcome is high. Health care professionals should pay special attention to risk factor identification and reduction in these women.

Realizing the benefits of prepregnancy risk identification will require:

• further discussion by the relevant professional groups of the content and timing of counseling, with particular attention to data on the risks associated with low birthweight (and other poor pregnancy outcomes) that can be modified before conception;

• incorporation of such consultations into a wide variety of settings to reach as many women as possible;

• development of appropriate written materials for women and the professionals who counsel them;

• health services research to monitor the costs and results of prepregnancy consultations;

• willingness of third-party payers to reimburse such services, once defined and evaluated;

• education of health care providers and other professionals in touch with women of reproductive age about these concepts;

• determination of the adequacy of health services resources in a given setting to manage problems that are identified through prepregnancy assessment; and

• additional research on how best to influence the health-related behavior of individuals, particularly teenagers.

A second strategy for the period before pregnancy involves health education related to reproduction. Education about reproduction, contraception, pregnancy, and associated topics already is provided in a variety of ways: by public information campaigns; in school-based classes, group sessions, lectures, and related printed materials; and in various health care settings. To increase the impact of these education programs on the problem of low birthweight, they should be expanded to include the following six topics:

• the major factors that place a woman at risk of poor pregnancy outcome, including low birthweight;

• the general concept of reducing specific risks before conception and the advisability of preconception counseling to identify and reduce risks associated with low birthweight;

- the importance of early pregnancy diagnosis and of early, regular prenatal care (including how to obtain such services);
- the importance of immunizing against rubella and of identifying other infection-related risks to the fetus;
- the value of altering behavior to reduce a range of risks associated with low birthweight, including smoking, poor nutrition, and moderate to heavy alcohol consumption; and
- the heightened vulnerability of the fetus to environmental and behavioral dangers in the early weeks of pregnancy, often before pregnancy is suspected or diagnosed, and therefore the need to avoid x-rays, alcohol and drug use, selected toxic substances, and similar threats in the first trimester.

The committee believes that health education should be an important component of low birthweight prevention. It should be provided in a variety of settings, particularly in family planning clinics and schools, and should be strengthened in the private sector as well. This education should focus on the role of men as well as women in choices about reproduction; family planning should be a shared responsibility, and education about pregnancy should not be confined to women.

Family planning services also should be an integral part of overall strategies to reduce the incidence of low birthweight. Several studies suggest that family planning has contributed to reducing the rate of low birthweight in the United States over the past 20 years, probably by reducing the rate of childbearing among high-risk women, by increasing interpregnancy intervals, and by other means.

The large number of unintended pregnancies in the United States, the percentage of women at risk of unintended pregnancy who do not use contraception, and the number of abortions indicate that existing family planning strategies do not meet the need for services. The reasons for this problem range from service inadequacies to the knowledge, attitudes, and practices of women themselves.

The unmet need appears to be largest among two groups at high risk of low birthweight, the poor and the young. For this reason, the committee emphasizes the importance of Title X of the Public Health Service Act. Title X authorizes project grants to public and private nonprofit organizations for the provision of family planning services to all who need and want them, including sexually active teenagers, but with priority given to low-income persons. The committee urges that federal funds be made generously available to meet documented needs for family planning. The Title X program and family planning services should be regarded as important parts of the public effort to prevent low birthweight.

Ensuring Access to Prenatal Care

Efforts to reduce the nation's incidence of low birthweight must include a commitment to enrolling all pregnant women in prenatal care. Many of the women who now receive inadequate prenatal care are those at greater than average risk of a low birthweight delivery. Moreover, participation in a system of prenatal care is a prerequisite for many individual interventions that help reduce the risk of low birthweight.

In reaching this conclusion, the committee reviewed carefully the data documenting the effectiveness of prenatal care and concluded that, although a few studies have not been able to demonstrate a positive effect of prenatal care, the overwhelming weight of the evidence indicates that prenatal care reduces low birthweight and that the effect is greatest among high-risk women. This finding is strong enough to support a broad national commitment to ensuring that all pregnant women, especially those at socioeconomic or medical risk, receive high-quality prenatal care.

National, state, and local data indicate that the proportion of mothers beginning prenatal care in the first trimester increased steadily from 1969 until 1980, but that this trend has leveled off or possibly reversed since 1981. The committee views with deep concern the possibility that the nation's progress in extending prenatal benefits to all women has been disrupted.

In developing the major recommendation that all pregnant women should receive early and regular prenatal care, the report describes the population of women who receive little or no prenatal care; the reasons why such women receive insufficient care; and several ways to remove important barriers. Principal barriers discussed in the report include:

1. Financial constraints: These may result from absent or inadequate private insurance to cover prenatal care, lack of public funds for prenatal care, or lack of support for public agencies that provide maternity services. In its recommendations, the committee chose to focus on Medicaid because it is the largest public program financing prenatal care. Support of the Medicaid program, which helps finance care for many high-risk women, should be part of a comprehensive effort to reduce the nation's incidence of low birthweight. Changes in the program, a topic of considerable controversy both in federal and state governments, should be dedicated to enrolling more eligible women and to providing them with early and regular, high-quality prenatal care.

The Health Care Financing Administration (HCFA), in collaboration with the Division of Maternal and Child Health (DMCH), should establish a set of generous eligibility standards that maximize the possibility that poor women will qualify for Medicaid coverage, and thus be able to obtain prenatal care. All Medicaid programs should be required to use such standards.

Medicaid policies and reimbursement rates also should reflect the high-risk nature of the Medicaid-eligible population. Program policies should not set a limit on the number of prenatal visits, because pregnant women enrolled in the Medicaid program may require more frequent visits and more specialized care than more affluent, low-risk women. DMCH should develop a model of prenatal care for use in publicly financed facilities, and the guidelines incorporated into this model should be adopted by all Medicaid programs. HCFA and appropriate state agencies should monitor adherence to this standard of care.

2. Lack of maternity care providers: The number of private physicians providing prenatal care is inadequate in many parts of the country. Of particular concern is the evidence that the participation of obstetrician/gynecologists in Medicaid is relatively low and may be decreasing, thereby limiting the number of private practitioners available to care for high-risk, low-income women. To overcome this problem, the committee recommends that HCFA develop a series of demonstration/evaluation projects aimed at increasing the participation of obstetrician/gynecologists in Medicaid. Approaches should include reducing delays in reimbursement, increasing reimbursement rates, and increasing the number of prenatal visits reimbursed by Medicaid. The results of these projects should be vigorously disseminated to policy leaders.

To the extent that provider attitudes are found to impede Medicaid participation, local and national professional societies, including the American College of Obstetricians and Gynecologists, should undertake appropriate education to encourage members to increase their Medicaid patient loads.

The increased risk of a poor pregnancy outcome among high-risk women creates an additional disincentive to caring for these groups. Poor outcomes raise the possibility of a malpractice suit, and the threat of malpractice has emerged as a barrier to expanding obstetric care to women at risk of low birthweight and related problems. In response to increasing malpractice insurance premiums and other factors, obstetrician-gynecologists are decreasing their obstetric case loads and decreasing the number of high-risk patients in their practices. Because prevention of low birthweight requires fully available prenatal care and, more important, specialized care for high-risk women, these findings are of major concern.

A partial solution to the problem of access would be to place greater reliance on certified nurse-midwives and nurse practitioners, who have been shown to be particularly effective in managing the care of pregnant women at high risk of low birthweight because of social and economic factors. Maternity programs designed to serve high-risk mothers should increase their use of these providers; and state laws should be supportive of nurse-midwifery practice and of collaborations between physicians and nurse-midwives/nurse practitioners.

3. The possibility that there are insufficient prenatal care services in sites routinely used by high-risk populations, such as Community Health Centers, Maternity and Infant Care Projects, hospital outpatient departments, and health departments: The committee emphasizes the importance of these organized facilities, especially local health departments, in the effort to increase access to prenatal care. Health departments are highlighted in the report because almost every person in the United States lives in an area that is served by one, because they are known to be active providers of prenatal care, and because their comprehensive programs often are especially suitable for low-income women at high risk for pregnancy problems. National and state data indicate that reliance on health departments for maternity care has increased in the 1980s.

To address unmet needs for prenatal care, health departments should be given increased resources. Every community is different, however, and in some it may be more appropriate to provide additional support for Community Health Centers, Maternity and Infant Care Projects, hospital outpatient departments, or related settings.

4. Factors that make women disinclined to seek prenatal care: Access to prenatal care is affected by a pregnant woman's perceptions of whether care is useful, supportive, and pleasant; by her general knowledge about prenatal care; and by her cultural values and beliefs.

Two major strategies exist to overcome barriers related to these factors: i.e., general education about prenatal care and the development of a personal, caring environment in which such services are provided, especially for socioeconomically disadvantaged women. Among the attributes that should be built into this environment are accessibility, including easy access for telephone consultations; responsiveness to the concerns that are most salient to women in early pregnancy, such as relief of first trimester nausea and recognition of the need for emotional support and acceptance; and flexibility in the package of services offered so that providers are encouraged to help women obtain nonmedical benefits. Other attributes are described in the full report.

5. Inadequate transportation and child care services: Provision of child care and transportation should be viewed as an integral part of prenatal care services for socioeconomically disadvantaged populations. Distance and difficulty in arranging babysitting for other children can lead women to put off seeking care unless an emergency occurs.

6. Lack of systems to recruit hard-to-reach women into care: Sometimes health care programs must do more than provide an open door. They must take the initiative to find and educate women about the importance of care. Two methods are the use of outreach personnel and the establishment of referral relationships with other service systems, such as the Special Supplemental Food Program for Women, Infants and Children (WIC).

The committee believes that the use of outreach workers is an effective way to improve access to care for difficult-to-reach populations. More research is needed, however, on the comparative advantages of different case-finding approaches, the costs of different outreach systems and their effectiveness, and the types of personnel best suited to various program goals and target groups.

A System of Accountability

The committee believes that although many different factors contribute to the problem of inadequate access to prenatal care, an underlying cause is the nation's patchwork, nonsystematic approach to making prenatal services available. Numerous programs have been developed in the past to extend prenatal care to more women, but no institution bears responsibility for ensuring that such services are available to those who need them. Without a structure of accountability, gaps in care will remain, and efforts to expand prenatal services will continue to face major organizational and administrative difficulties.

The federal government, which has long supported prenatal care and urged that all women secure such care early in pregnancy, is uniquely positioned to play a leadership role in the effort to ensure access to prenatal services. The committee recommends that the federal government, through the Department of Health and Human Services, increase its commitment to these goals by:

- providing sufficient funds to state and local agencies to remove financial barriers to prenatal care (through channels such as the Maternal and Child Health Services Block Grants, Medicaid, health departments, Community Health Centers, and related systems);
- providing prompt, high-quality technical consultation to the states on clinical, administrative, and organizational problems that can impede the extension of prenatal care;
- defining a model of prenatal services for use in public facilities providing maternity care; and
- funding demonstration and evaluation programs and supporting training and research in these areas.

States should take a complementary role in extending prenatal services. This could be accomplished by designating one organization--probably the state health department--as responsible for ensuring that prenatal services are available and accessible in every community. Through such an organization, each state should:

- assess unmet needs for prenatal care;
- serve as a broker to contract with private providers to fill gaps in services; and
- if necessary, provide prenatal services directly through facilities such as Community Health Centers and health department clinics.

In addition, each state should designate a local organization in each community--probably the local health department--to be the "residual guarantor" of services and to arrange care for pregnant women who still remain outside of the prenatal care system.

To begin the development of a functioning system of responsibility and accountability, the committee recommends that the Secretary of the Department of Health and Human Services convene a task force charged with defining a system for making prenatal services available to all pregnant women. Such a group should include representatives from Congress, the Public Health Service, HCFA, state governments and health authorities, maternity care providers, and consumers.

This task force should focus on at least four specific issues: (1) how to bring together the knowledge and goals of maternal and child health programs with the "financial power" of the Medicaid program; (2) how to build on the strength of existing experience with the regionalization of perinatal services to combat the problem of low birthweight; (3) how to improve the capacity of state and national data systems to assess unmet need for prenatal services; and (4) how to ensure that prenatal care is financed adequately in times of cost containment, when preventive services often lose the competition for dollars.

Improving the Content of Prenatal Care

Participation in conventional prenatal care programs is associated with a reduced incidence of low birthweight. The committee believes, however, that enhancing the content of prenatal care could increase its contribution to the development of healthy infants.

The committee has identified seven components of prenatal care that merit increased emphasis in the effort to prevent low birthweight.

1. Establishing explicit goals: Explicit goals can help focus the attention of the patient on the purposes of prenatal visits and help the provider structure appropriate interventions. Examples of goals include reducing the risks of preterm delivery and intrauterine growth retardation, prevention of fetal anomalies and perinatal mortality, and preparation for labor and delivery. Defining the prevention of low birthweight as a major goal of prenatal care will require a variety of adjustments in clinical practice. For example, current prenatal care seems particularly oriented toward the prevention, detection, and treatment of problems that are manifested in the third trimester. By contrast, may of the risks associated with low birthweight, including smoking and poor nutritional status, require attention early in pregnancy. These issues suggest a different schedule of visits from that currently followed, putting additional emphasis on care and education in the first and second trimesters of pregnancy.

2. Using formal risk assessment systems: Prenatal care should include formal assessments of risk, initiated at the first visit and repeated throughout pregnancy to identify developing problems.

3. Increasing the accuracy of pregnancy dating: Accurate dating of pregnancy is a cornerstone of good prenatal care. Without it, the clinician is less able to detect intrauterine growth retardation, to determine if labor is premature and the extent of the prematurity, or to avoid iatrogenic prematurity caused by labor induction or an elective cesarean section.

4. Expanding the appropriate use of ultrasound imaging: A federal consensus development conference in 1984, sponsored jointly by the National Institutes of Health and the Food and Drug Administration, concluded that available data do not support routine ultrasound examination of all pregnancies, but identified almost 30 specific

situations in which ultrasound is warranted. Among these are many indications relevant to the prevention of low birthweight.

5. Increasing the detection and management of behavioral risks: Prenatal care should include explicit attention to detecting behavioral risks associated with low birthweight, especially smoking, nutritional inadequacies, moderate to heavy alcohol use, and substance abuse.

6. Expanding prenatal education: Health education for women who are pregnant or contemplating pregnancy should be expanded to include greater emphasis on behavioral risks in pregnancy; early signs and symptoms of pregnancy complications such as preterm labor; and the role that prenatal care plays in improving the outcome of pregnancy.

Childbirth education classes could play an expanded role in the prevention of low-weight births. To do so, these classes should begin earlier, place greater emphasis on the prenatal period and the risk factors described above, and make a greater effort to enroll women from lower socioeconomic groups.

7. Recognizing the importance of health care system factors: Prenatal care providers need to organize their programs to manage a wider variety of patient problems and risk factors. For example, nutritional counseling, psychosocial counseling, strategies to modify smoking and other health compromising behaviors, and related services should be provided directly or through a well-organized referral system.

Information on the causes of low birthweight and the risk factors associated with it has led to the development of several innovative programs designed to prevent preterm delivery. Preliminary data from these programs suggest several approaches that could be added to basic prenatal care to decrease the chance of a preterm delivery among high-risk women. These approaches stress repeated risk assessments, expanded patient education, and enriched provider education.

Efforts to arrest preterm labor hinge on its early detection and prompt management. Women at elevated risk of this problem should be taught to identify and lessen events in their daily lives that can trigger uterine contractions, which may in turn lead to preterm labor; the importance of early detection of the symptoms of preterm labor, such as bleeding and periodic contractions; how to differentiate normal contractions that occur throughout pregnancy from those signaling early labor; and what to do when the signs and symptoms of preterm labor occur.

To complement patient education, provider education should include increased emphasis on the importance of being receptive to patients' complaints, some of which may indicate early signs of preterm labor; the need for prompt identification of preterm labor and the uses of hospitalization for observation and possible treatment of women with suspected preterm labor; and the various approaches available for arresting true preterm labor, such as tocolysis.

Many of the risk factors linked to preterm labor also are associated with intrauterine growth retardation (IUGR); thus, some of the prenatal care interventions designed to avoid one component of low birthweight also may help prevent the other. For example, careful risk assessment is as important for IUGR detection and treatment as it is for prevention of prematurity. The literature suggests that in caring for women at elevated risk of IUGR, prenatal care providers should place extra emphasis on reduction of behavioral risks such as smoking and alcohol use, nutritional surveillance and counseling, and early diagnosis and effective management of IUGR through accurate assessment of gestational age and fetal growth and maturity. Ultrasonography can help establish gestational age when uterine size/date discrepancies occur.

Programs Complementary to Prenatal Care

Because many of the risks associated with low birthweight have a behavioral basis, the committee examined selected interventions designed to reduce these risks, including smoking reduction strategies and nutritional intervention programs such as the Special Supplemental Food Program for Women, Infants and Children (WIC).

The committee urges that efforts to help women stop or reduce smoking in pregnancy become a major concern of obstetric care providers. Several attributes of successful programs drawn from the literature on smoking intervention programs are described in the report.

The committee also recommends that nutritional supplementation programs such as WIC be part of a comprehensive strategy to reduce the incidence of low birthweight among high-risk women and that such programs be closely linked to prenatal care.

The committee also evaluated stress and fatigue abatement approaches, although the evidence that these factors contribute to low birthweight is controversial. A variety of programs have been organized to reduce the levels of stress experienced by pregnant women. Some are concerned primarily with physical stress and fatigue, others more with psychosocial and emotional stress.

One potentially important stress-reducing intervention is maternity leave. The patchwork arrangement in this country of sick leave, disability leave, leave without pay, and other leave categories are not adequate to provide job security for pregnant women and new mothers who participate in the labor force. The committee recognizes that revision of maternity policies is a complicated issue, but suggests that more adequate maternity leave, particularly for certain high-risk women, could contribute to a reduction in low birthweight. At a minimum, labor unions, women's groups, and health professionals should explore this issue.

Encouraging Change in Prenatal Care

To encourage the provision of improved, more flexible prenatal care services, particularly for women at elevated risk of low birthweight, the committee recommends several specific strategies, two of which are that:

- the professional societies representing the principal maternity care providers should carefully review the suggestions made by the committee regarding prenatal care to determine whether their general guidelines for clinical practice should be revised and enriched accordingly; and
- the Division of Maternal and Child Health (DMCH), in collaboration with both consumer and professional groups, should define a model of prenatal services to be used in publicly financed facilities that provide care to pregnant women. This model should be updated and revised frequently to incorporate new knowledge and experience and should not be used in a way that discourages research on improved approaches to prenatal care.

Research Needs

Major progress in reducing low birthweight will require a far more sophisticated understanding of prenatal care content than now exists. Thus, research on the content of prenatal care should be a high funding priority for foundations, public agencies, and institutions concerned with improving maternal and child health. This research should focus on three major areas: (1) description and analysis of the current composition of prenatal care; (2) assessment of the efficacy and safety of numerous individual components of prenatal care; and (3) evaluation of certain well-defined combinations of prenatal care interventions designed to meet the widely varied needs and risks among pregnant women.

The Assistant Secretary for Health should take the lead in organizing activities to collect information on current prenatal care practices. Existing surveys conducted by the National Center for Health Statistics should include special emphasis on prenatal care content. Consumer experience with prenatal care should be analyzed, and the professional societies of the major maternity care providers should be consulted about ways to survey their members regarding various content issues. In some instances, direct studies of provider practices may be necessary.

Both public and private institutions should support studies to assess the effectiveness of well-defined combinations of prenatal interventions in reducing low birthweight and improving infant health generally. In particular, these studies should assess the merits of different prenatal care strategies for women at elevated risk of prematurity or IUGR.

Too often, research on prenatal care has been oriented toward the broad question of whether it improves pregnancy outcome. The appropriate goal now is to identify the components and combinations of prenatal services that are effective in preventing various poor pregnancy outcomes in well-defined groups of women.

A Public Information Program

The committee believes that a carefully designed public information program could contribute to the prevention of low birthweight. Such a program would help create a climate in which change and progress are possible and also convey specific types of information.

The committee sketched the broad outlines of a plan incorporating two major objectives. The first is to call the problem of low birthweight to the public's attention and to reinforce its importance with the nation's leaders. The second is to help reduce low birthweight by conveying a set of ideas to the public about avoidance of important risk factors.

Public awareness of the low birthweight problem is fostered through discussions of the topic in reports by a variety of public and private organizations interested in maternal and child health. Thus, the committee recommends that the Office of the Assistant Secretary for Health develop and publicize a report every 3 years on the nation's progress in reducing low birthweight. Also, the statistical profile of the nation's health developed by the National Center for Health Statistics, Health: United States, periodically should include a special supplement or profile on low birthweight and its prevention.

Because many of the risk factors for low birthweight are widely distributed throughout the population, and because a substantial amount of low birthweight occurs among women judged to be at low risk, the committee concluded that a public information program on low birthweight should embrace a broad audience. Within this program, however, a special subset of messages should be developed to reach several high-risk target groups: pregnant smokers, young teenagers, and socioeconomically disadvantaged women. In the full report, several specific messages are suggested.

This public information program needs an organizational home and strong leadership. The committee recommends that the responsibility be assumed by the Healthy Mothers, Healthy Babies Coalition, a 4-year-old consortium of voluntary, professional, and governmental groups. The coalition should establish a formal executive secretariat to provide stability and permanence. Both public and private funds should be provided to the coalition in amounts adequate to the task of leading a major public information campaign, which would include the production and distribution of high-quality, well-tested public information materials.

Cost Issues

The fiscal implications of the strategies recommended by the committee for reducing low birthweight are difficult to evaluate. In general, estimates of the costs of measures that should be implemented in the period before pregnancy to reduce the risks associated with low birthweight are not available. Lack of information also prevented the committee from attempting to estimate the additional public expenditures that would be required to finance the recommended public information campaign and research efforts.

With regard to extending the availability of prenatal care, however, the committee found that a straightforward, common sense analysis could be performed regarding some of the financial implications involved in the provision of prenatal services to pregnant women. The committee defined a target population of high-risk women (women with less than a high school education and on welfare) who often do not begin prenatal care in the first trimester of pregnancy. The current low birthweight rate in this group is about 11.5 percent. The committee estimated the increased expenditures that would be required to provide routine prenatal care to all members of the target population from the first trimester to the time of delivery. These expenditures were compared with savings that could be anticipated through a decreased incidence of low birthweight resulting from the improved utilization of prenatal care by the target population. These savings were estimated for a single year and consisted of initial hospitalization costs, rehospitalization costs, and ambulatory care costs associated with general illness. The many assumptions that shaped these calculations are detailed in the report.

The analysis showed that if the expanded use of prenatal care reduced the low birthweight rate in the target group from 11.5 percent to only 10.76 percent, the increased expenditures for prenatal services would be approximately equal to a single year of cost savings in direct medical care expenditures for the low birthweight infants born to the target population. If the rate were reduced to 9 percent (the 1990 goal set by the Surgeon General for a maximum low birthweight rate among high-risk groups), every additional dollar spent for prenatal care within the target group would save $3.38 in the total cost of caring for low birthweight infants, because there would be fewer low birthweight infants requiring expensive medical care.

With regard to extending the availability of prenatal care, however, the committee found that a straightforward, common-sense analysis could be performed comparing some of the financial implications involved in the provision of prenatal services to pregnant women. The committee selected a target population of high-risk women (women with less than a high school education) and [illegible] who often do not [illegible] [illegible] 11.5 percent. The committee estimated the [illegible] mothers of the target population [illegible] these expenditures compared [illegible] anticipated [illegible] lower incidence of low birthweight resulting from the [illegible] would [illegible] within the target population [illegible] savings [illegible] for [illegible] costs associated with [illegible] rehospitalizations [illegible] calculations [illegible] in the report.

The analysis showed that the expenditures of prenatal [illegible] target population [illegible] percent [illegible] would be approximately equal to a single year of [illegible] in direct medical care expenses for the low birthweight infants born to the target population. [illegible] set by the Surgeon General for a maximum low birthweight rate among high-risk groups, every additional dollar spent on prenatal care within the target group would save $3.38 in the total cost of the care of low birthweight infants, because there would be fewer low birthweight infants requiring expensive medical care.

PART I

Definitions, Risk Factors, and Trends

CHAPTER 1

The Significance of Low Birthweight

The observation that babies born too small are less likely to survive than other newborns dates back centuries,[1] but concern over the effects of low birthweight on a child's health and development is relatively recent. This chapter traces the changes in perspective that have occurred as infant mortality from other causes has declined, and as modern technologies have provided the capability to sustain even the tiniest neonate. It also examines the contribution of low birthweight to morbidity and mortality in general and the need for improved strategies to prevent low birthweight.

Although the earliest references to the practice of weighing infants at birth date from Talmudic times, the potential significance of birthweight does not appear to have been recognized until the end of the seventeenth century, when it was discussed by the French obstetrician Mauriceau. Unfortunately, Mauriceau's widely cited measurements were incorrect--his estimate of a normal birthweight was about 15 pounds. A more accurate assessment of normal birthweight did not enter the English literature until late in the eighteenth century. Almost another hundred years passed before systematic weighing of infants at birth revealed sufficient variability in birthweights to support the concept that weight could be used to assess nutritional status and physical growth.[2]

By the early 1900s, physicians had begun to assess the relationships among inadequate growth (low birthweight), shortened gestation (prematurity), and mortality. In 1930, the Finnish pediatrician, Yllpö, advocated 2,500 grams as the birthweight below which infants were at high risk of adverse neonatal outcome, presumably on the basis of inadequate fetal growth.[3] This recommendation was formally adopted by the World Health Organization (WHO) on two separate occasions. The first was at the First World Health Assembly in 1948: "For the purpose of this classification, an immature infant is a liveborn infant with a birthweight of 5-1/2 pounds (2,500 grams) or less, or specified as immature. In some countries, however, this criterion will not be applicable. If weight is not specified, a liveborn infant with a period of gestation of less than 37 weeks or specified as 'premature' may be considered as the equivalent of an immature infant for purposes of this classification."[4]

In 1950, the WHO Expert Group on Prematurity reinforced the use of the 2,500-gram limit: "The Expert Group on Prematurity recognizes the necessity for uniform terminology for international usage. Since the primary goal is to lower fetal and neonatal mortality, the aim can best be achieved by providing specialized care for infants of low birth-weight. The group suggests that a premature infant be defined as one whose birth-weight is 2,500 g. (5-1/2 pounds) or less. The limitations of this criterion are recognized, however, since data on birth-weight will not always be available and other criteria of prematurity must be used, for example, gestation."[5]

Both recommendations indicated that the use of a birthweight marker for risk served as a shorthand notation for a variety of interrelated physiologic processes affecting fetal growth and duration of gestation. The complexity of the issue was underscored by subsequent epidemiological studies, which confirmed that infants born weighing 2,500 grams or less were at increased risk of mortality,[6] but also showed that a birthweight of 2,500 grams was not synonymous with short gestation--some full-term infants weigh 2,500 grams or less.[7,8]

These observations led to further clarification of the definitions by the 1961 WHO Expert Committee on Maternal and Child Health.[9,10] This group recommended that the word "premature" be reserved for infants born before 37 weeks from the first day of the last menstrual period. Infants born weighing 2,500 grams or less were now to be considered "low birthweight." The classification was divided further to distinguish between the low birthweight infant (gestation of 37 weeks or longer, birthweight 2,500 grams or less) and the premature low birthweight infant (gestation less than 37 weeks, birthweight 2,500 grams or less). The former were considered to be "stunted" for duration of gestation and characterized by different risks of mortality and morbidity than infants who were premature and whose birthweights were, therefore, more consistent with gestational age.[10]

While these gestational age/birthweight classifications proved useful in delineating subpopulations of low birthweight infants with different etiologies and prognoses, they posed some of the same ambiguities as birthweight alone:

- Birthweight is a continuous variable and the limit at 2,500 grams does not represent a biologic category, but a single point on a continuous curve. The infant born at 2,499 grams does not differ significantly from one born at 2,501 grams on the basis of birthweight alone.
- Although 37 weeks of gestation may reflect biologic processes more directly, because certain biochemical changes indicative of increasing fetal maturity occur about this time, variation is such that not all 37-week infants are equally mature.
- The population of infants who weigh 2,500 grams or less and are less than 37 weeks gestation is not homogeneous with respect to outcome; further distinctions are required to classify those at increased risk.
- The risk of mortality as it applies to the birthweight/gestational age distribution varies for different populations.

With the emergence of modern approaches to the management of low birthweight infants, interest increased in the outcomes of subgroups of low birthweight infants. The fate of the smallest infants was of particular concern.[11] [12] Conventionally, very low birthweight infants were considered to be those born weighing 1,500 grams or less. Even with more specific birthweight categories, it was recognized that infants with similar birthweights could be of different gestational ages. Those whose birthweights were consistent with their gestational ages differed in outcome from those whose birthweights were not (especially when the birthweight was substantially lower than expected).[13] [14] As with the 2,500-gram limit, designation of very low birthweight infants as those weighing 1,500 grams or less reflected convention rather than biologic criteria.

Current Concepts of Fetal Growth

Current descriptions of fetal growth parallel the "growth curve" approach used to describe growth throughout childhood. At any given age (whether in utero or after birth), most individuals tend to be similar in size and weight, although variation exists. Since the advent of statistical concepts, particularly that of the "normal distribution," observations incorporating both similarity among the majority and wide variation are described in terms of "means" and "deviations from the mean." The term "average" growth refers to the value about which the majority cluster. Thus, the expected birthweight at any given gestational age would be the average or mean birthweight of infants at that gestational age.

The definition of abnormal growth requires identification of those whose growth deviates from what would be expected given normal or anticipated variation. Normally distributed data such as weight and other measures of physical growth form smooth curves, which theoretically extend to infinity without clear discontinuities, so "abnormality" is most practically defined in terms of the likelihood that an individual observation will fall within the normal variation expected for a given population. The lower this probability, the more likely the individual observation represents an abnormality. Commonly, an "abnormal" observation is considered to be one that falls outside the range described by two standard deviations on either side of the mean. This range includes 95 percent of a population, so an observation outside that range would have only a 5 percent chance of reflecting normal variation.[15]

Application of this approach to the distribution of birthweights in different populations indicates that two standard deviations below the mean does not always fall at 2,500 grams. In fact, one study of birthweights by country showed that two standard deviations below the mean ranged from 1,850 to 2,250 grams.[3] (The coding of birthweights, i.e., in exact grams, or by 250- or 500-gram intervals, also can affect mean values and standard deviations.[3]) These observations have been used to argue for different ways of defining high-risk groups to allow more accurate comparisons of birthweight-related infant mortality figures.[3] [16] [17]

The use of different birthweight limits to designate high-risk subgroups of a population has special relevance in the United States, where an effort has been made to identify racial differences in birthweight distributions.[18] Nonwhite low birthweight infants have lower neonatal mortality rates than white infants of the same birthweight.[8 19] It has been argued, therefore, that the lower birthweight of nonwhites may reflect prior genetic or nutritional factors but not contribute to current risk[18] and that the 2,500-gram birthweight limit may not have the same implications for nonwhite infants as for whites (i.e., that low birthweight should perhaps be defined differently for nonwhite infants). This line of reasoning is overshadowed by the more imposing fact that nonwhite infants are twice as likely to be born at low birthweight and twice as likely to die in the neonatal period. Chapter 2 discusses race as a risk factor for low birthweight in more detail.

Recent publications[20 21] on birthweight distributions at different gestational ages have improved the physician's ability to identify preterm infants who have experienced inadequate growth (Figure 1.1). Growth curves tied to gestational age also allow standardization of terms such as "small for gestational age" and "appropriate for gestational age"; precise definition of these terms is essential for future clinical and epidemiological studies.

In view of the more sophisticated data available, the continued reliance on a single standard, 2,500 grams, as a measure of risk for adverse perinatal outcome could be questioned. The rationale for retaining this standard rests on four arguments. First, although birthweight/gestational age combinations provide useful information, they require accurate assessments of gestational age, which is considerably more difficult to measure than birthweight.[21] Second, birthweight appears to be relatively more important in determining prognosis than gestational age.[21] Third, the use of standard birthweight limits allows comparisons across time and populations. Most important, as will be illustrated in the remainder of this chapter, a substantial literature exists to support the use of low birthweight as a marker or risk factor for mortality and morbidity.

Birthweight and Infant Mortality

The contribution of low birthweight to infant mortality in the United States is relatively greater now than it was in the past. Support for this assertion is indirect and is based on the fact that two-thirds of infant deaths early in the century occurred in the postneonatal period (between 28 days and 11 months of age).[22] Postneonatal deaths are considered a reflection of environmental factors, particularly infections resulting in diarrhea or respiratory illness.[22 23] In developing countries, where infant mortality rates remain high, low birthweight accounts for less than half (20 to 40 percent) of postneonatal deaths.[24]

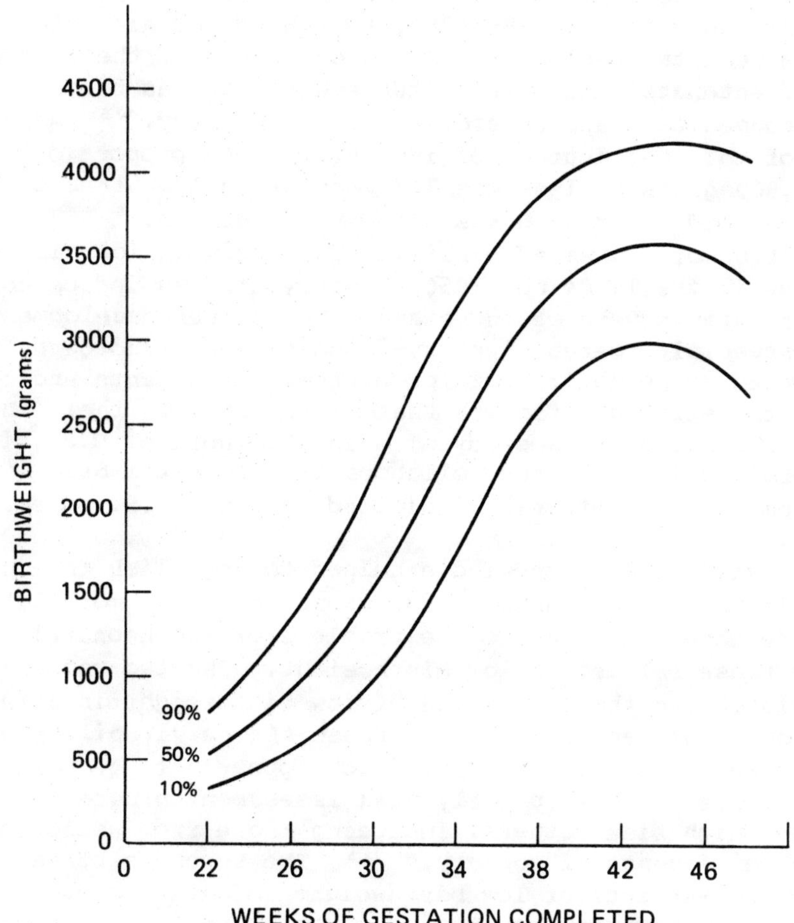

FIGURE 1.1 Birthweight percentiles for fixed gestations for single births, California, 1970 to 1976.

SOURCE: Williams RL, Creasy RK, Cunningham GC, Hawes WE, Norris FD, and Tashiro M: Fetal growth and perinatal viability in California. Obstet. Gynecol. 59:624-632, 1982.

Over the first half of the century, infant mortality rates in the United States declined from 100 per 1,000 live births to about 50 per 1,000.[25] Most of this decrease occurred among postneonatal deaths, so the majority of observers attribute this decline to changes in the environment, including a reduction in infectious diseases and improved nutrition.[22 23 25] The contribution of shifts in birthweight distribution is unknown, but probably was not significant. Data for the past 30 years reveal relatively slow changes in birthweight distribution,[26] suggesting that major shifts probably did not occur in the past.

With the reduction in postneonatal mortality, a shift in the timing of infant deaths occurred. By 1950, two-thirds of all infant deaths were in the neonatal period.[25] The major causes of these neonatal deaths were antenatal and intrapartum events such as birth injury, asphyxia, congenital malformations, and "immaturity."[25] As an indicator of the contribution of immaturity, the proportion of infants weighing 2,500 grams or less was 7.5 percent in 1950,[26] but these infants accounted for two-thirds of neonatal deaths.[25]

Recognition of increased morbidity in surviving low birthweight infants grew in the 1950s and 1960s. Early studies indicated that low birthweight infants were at increased risk of neurodevelopmental problems, especially cerebral palsy[27] and seizure disorders.[28] This increased vulnerability of low birthweight infants and the nature of some of the etiologic factors that contributed to their increased risk were established in a study of a large cohort of U.S. births followed prospectively in the Collaborative Perinatal Study.[29,30] Reports from other countries[31] indicated that the U.S. experience was not unique.

This growing body of knowledge helped to establish the context for modern perinatal care. Further reductions in infant mortality seemed likely to require solutions to the problems of the neonatal period, especially those related to low birthweight. The two major alternatives in this effort were the prevention of low birthweight in infants and the development of techniques to increase the survivability of low birthweight neonates. The former, which appeared to be more desirable, included efforts to develop early risk assessment programs[32,33] and services for high-risk mothers, including those from socioeconomically disadvantaged segments of society.[34,35] The second alternative, increasing the survival of low birthweight infants, induced clinicians to develop new management strategies, such as neonatal intensive care units. This approach was associated with the potential disadvantage of an increase in the number of children suffering from handicaps related to antenatal and intrapartum events, especially neurodevelopmental problems. This risk of increased morbidity has led clinicians to evaluate neonatal intensive care not only in terms of survival, but also in terms of developmental outcomes.

Since the early 1950s, the proportion of low birthweight infants has declined modestly.[26] Recent figures for the United States indicate that 6.8 percent of all neonates weigh 2,500 grams or less.[36] Almost no change in the proportion of infants born at very low birthweights (1,500 grams or less) has occurred, and these infants constitute just over 1 percent of all births. Thus, of the 3,494,398 live births in 1979, 252,511 weighed 2,500 grams or less, and 40,186 weighed 1,500 grams or less.

Assessing the contribution of low birthweight infants to mortality in the population requires birthweight-specific mortality rates derived from files containing infant death certificates matched to the corresponding birth certificates, as well as morbidity information on surviving children. Unfortunately, such data are not available for the United States as a whole. However, some indirect evidence of an association between low birthweight and mortality on a national level can be gleaned from racial differences in neonatal mortality figures.

Infants born to blacks are twice as likely to weigh 2,500 grams or less than those born to whites (12.7 percent versus 5.9 percent); this increased risk also pertains to the proportion in the lowest birthweight group of 1,500 grams or less (2.4 percent versus 0.9 percent).[36] Parallel to this difference in birthweight distribution is a difference in infant mortality. Between 1977 and 1979, the overall infant mortality rate was 13.6 per 1,000 live births, 11.9 for white births and 22.8 for black births.[36] Black births accounted for 16.5 percent of all live births in this period, but for 30 percent of all low birthweight births, 34 percent of very low birthweight births, and 28 percent of infant deaths.

More direct estimates of the effect of birthweight on mortality can be derived from several recent large-scale analyses relying on matched infant death and birth files. While these analyses do not deal with the nation as a whole, the results probably can be generalized.

The relationship between birthweight and infant mortality has been documented repeatedly in a variety of settings.[19-21 24 25 31 37-39] The lowest mortality rates are experienced by infants weighing 3,000 to 3,500 grams. For infants weighing 2,500 grams or less, the mortality rate increases rapidly with decreasing birthweight. Most of the infants weighing 1,000 grams or less die (Figure 1.2), although among those that live until admission to a neonatal intensive care unit, survival rates are believed to be improving considerably. Compared with normal birthweight infants, low birthweight infants are almost 40 times more likely to die in the neonatal period; for very low birthweight infants, the relative risk* of a neonatal death is almost 200 times greater.[19]

Not only are low birthweight infants at increased relative risk of neonatal mortality, but the attributable risk or proportion of all neonatal deaths occurring among low birthweight infants also is high

---

*In The Risk Approach in Health Care,[40] the World Health Organization defines and discusses both relative and attributable risk. Relative risk "expresses the ratio between the incidence of the illness or cause of death [or, in this case, low birthweight] in the population of those with the risk factor (or factors) and the corresponding incidence in the population of those without the risk factor (or factors). It is therefore a measure of the strength of the association between risk factor and outcome. . . . Attributable risk brings together three ideas: the frequency of the unwanted outcome [here, low birthweight] when the risk factor is present, the frequency of the outcome when the risk factor is absent, and the frequency of occurence of the risk factor in the community. It therefore indicates what might be expected to happen to the overall [incidence of the unwanted] outcome in the community if the risk factor were removed" (pp. 21-22). A more extensive discussion of the concepts of relative and attributable risk, along with methods for their calculation, appears in Foundations of Epidemiology, by Lilienfeld and Lilienfeld, 2nd Edition. New York: Oxford University Press, 1980.

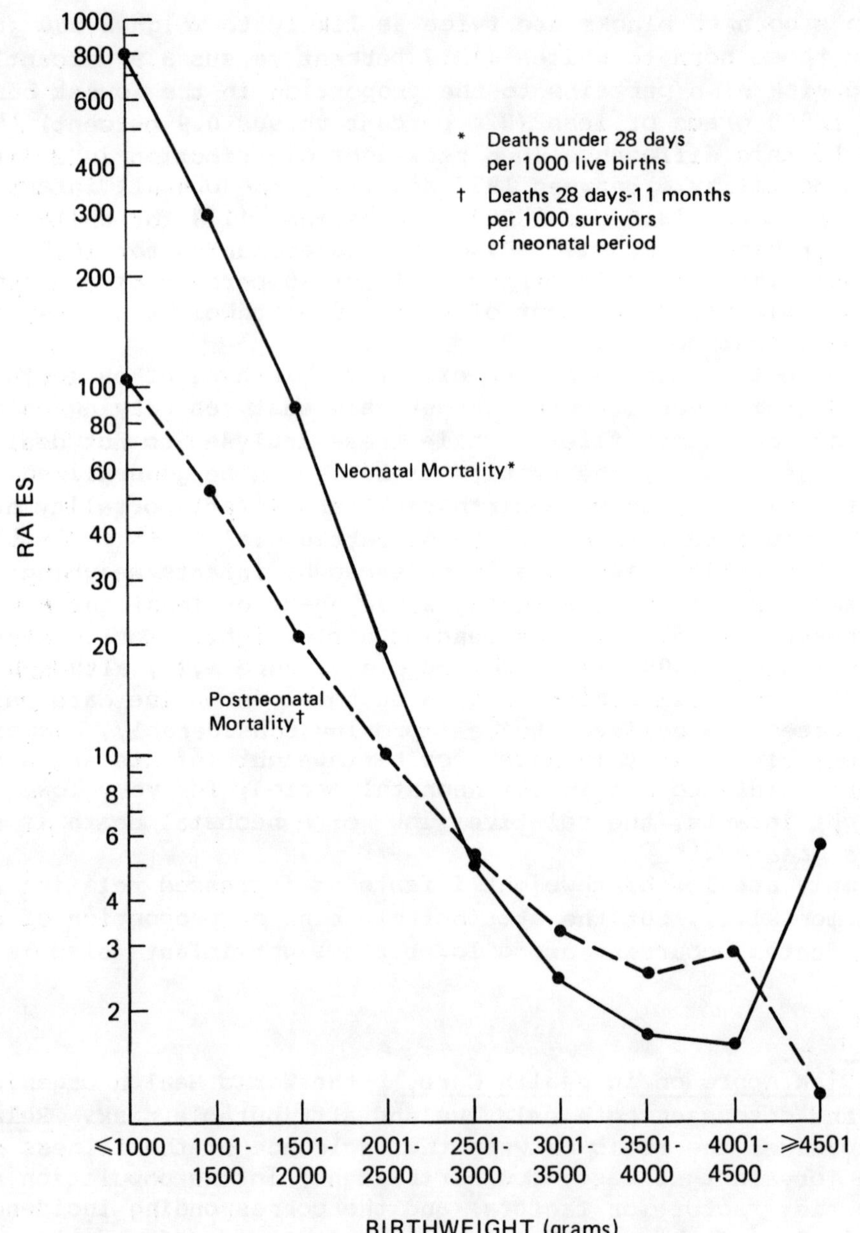

FIGURE 1.2 Neonatal and postneonatal deaths by birthweight, single live births, 1974 to 1975, based on data from eight areas of the United States.

SOURCE: Shapiro S, McCormick MC, Starfield BH, Krischer JP, and Bross D: Relevance of correlates of infant deaths for significant morbidity at 1 year of age. Am. J. Obstet. Gynecol. 136:363-373, 1980.

(see definition of attributable risk above). Infants born weighing 2,500 grams or less still account for two-thirds of neonatal deaths;[19] those 1,500 grams or less account for half of neonatal deaths.[41] As mortality among normal birthweight infants decreases, this attributable risk is likely to increase. Thus, in industrialized populations, the proportion of very low birthweight infants is a major predictor of neonatal mortality.[42] Even controlling for other factors known to affect the risk of neonatal mortality, low birthweight remains the major determinant of neonatal death.[43]

Postneonatal Mortality

The relationship between postneonatal mortality and birthweight is not as sharp as that for neonatal mortality; however, low birthweight infants are 5 times more likely than normal birthweight infants to die later in the first year and account for 20 percent of all postneonatal deaths.[19,44] For very low birthweight infants, the relative risk of postneonatal death is 20 times that of normal birthweight infants, and these infants account for between 25 and 30 percent of postneonatal deaths.[45] As suggested by previous reports,[23,25] the effect of birthweight on postneonatal mortality is modified by socioeconomic factors.[43]

Effect of Gestational Age and Other Risk Factors

Within birthweight groups, the risk of mortality is not uniform and varies with gestational age. For a given birthweight, the longer the duration of gestation up to 42 weeks, the lower the mortality.[20,21] Similarly, for a given gestational age, again up to 42 weeks, the heavier infants have lower mortality rates.[20,21]

In general, small for gestational age (SGA) infants have lower neonatal and postneonatal mortality rates than appropriate for gestational age (AGA) infants of comparable birthweights.[10,46] The exception is the full-term infant weighing 2,500 grams or less,[10] which has a higher mortality rate than term infants of normal birthweight.

The relative proportion of AGA and SGA infants among low birthweight infants varies with different low birthweight rates. For populations in which the proportion of low birthweight infants exceeds 10 percent, SGA infants represent the majority of low birthweight infants.[47,48] At lower rates, of 5 to 7 percent, premature AGA infants are in the majority.[47,48]

The relative contributions of AGA and SGA infants to neonatal mortality in the United States are not well established. Despite the difference in mortality rates between SGA and AGA infants at a given birthweight, the shift towards a higher proportion of AGA infants is unlikely to have much effect on the estimate of the proportion of perinatal deaths accounted for by low birthweight infants. When the relative effects of birthweight and gestational age on mortality have been examined, birthweight has been the dominant factor.[20 49] As noted below, however, the shift may have implications for morbidity among surviving infants.

Besides gestational age, other factors are associated with an increased risk of neonatal mortality. As noted earlier, race is one such factor; others include maternal age at the extremes of the childbearing age range, low maternal educational attainment, and a history of prior adverse obstetrical outcomes such as fetal death.* These risk factors also are associated with high rates of low birthweight. Controlling for birthweight distribution sharply reduces or eliminates the differentials in neonatal mortality associated with several of these factors, namely, nonwhite race (especially black and American Indian), adolescent motherhood, and low maternal educational attainment.[19 50] This finding indicates that the proportion of low birthweight infants largely accounts for the adverse neonatal mortality experiences of these subgroups.

Differences in birthweight do not eliminate the increased risk of neonatal death associated with advanced maternal age and prior history of fetal loss.[19] These factors are associated with a combination of increased risk of low birthweight and increased obstetrical vulnerability.

The situation is different for postneonatal mortality. Even after controlling for birthweight, postneonatal mortality rates remain higher for nonwhite infants, infants of adolescent mothers, and infants of mothers of low educational attainment.[19 50] Thus, factors indicative of socioeconomic disadvantage are linked to increased infant mortality through both higher low birthweight rates and an increased risk of postneonatal death, regardless of birthweight.

Current Decline in Neonatal Mortality

After a period of relative stagnation in the 1960s, the infant mortality rate began its current rapid decline. In 1980, the infant mortality rate was 13.1 per 1,000 live births, a 47 percent decrease from the rate in 1965.[36] In contrast to the first half of the century, this recent change is primarily the result of a decrease in neonatal mortality.

The accumulating evidence indicates that a major factor in this rapid decline has been the increased survival of low birthweight infants, in part as a result of more intensive, hospital-based management and of improvements in perinatal care, particularly for high-risk pregnancies. Several different factors support this conclusion:

---

*In Chapters 2 and 3, these risk factors are discussed in more detail and an effort is made to isolate their independent effects.

• The decrease in neonatal mortality has occurred in the context of only modest decreases in the proportion of low birthweight infants.[51-53]

• There has been a progressive decline in neonatal mortality among very low birthweight infants who receive intensive care.[11 12]

• Decreases in neonatal mortality for geographically defined areas have followed the introduction of perinatal intensive care units.[54-56]

• Low birthweight infants born in hospitals with intensive care facilities have a higher survival rate than infants born in hospitals without such units,[57-59] even after controlling for other risk factors known to affect survival.[59] This enhanced survival rate persists even in comparisons involving infants transported to regional perinatal care centers shortly after birth.[60 61]

• Decreases in neonatal mortality in geographically defined regions have been shown to accompany an increase in the proportion of low birthweight and very low birthweight births occurring in tertiary centers.[41]

Thus, the current decline in neonatal mortality can be attributed largely to increased survival of high-risk infants. In many areas of the country, birthweight-specific mortality rates are now similar for high- and low-risk groups. This means that efforts to sustain the decline in neonatal mortality will have to focus on the prevention of low birthweight in infants.

Low Birthweight and Morbidity

The contribution of low birthweight to morbidity in childhood is less well established than its contribution to infant mortality. In part, this results from the relative lack of population-based morbidity data involving sufficient numbers of low birthweight infants. In addition, the types of morbidity that occur in low birthweight survivors, especially those at very low birthweight, are still being identified. Finally, perinatal events are only one determinant of child health, and disentangling the effect of low birthweight from other factors and from the interactions among these factors has proved difficult. Still, the existing literature indicates that low birthweight infants appear to be at increased risk of a number of health problems and that this increased risk has implications for health services, and possibly for educational services and family function as well. Several health problems are discussed below; additional morbidity data are in Chapter 10.

Neurodevelopmental Handicaps

The prevalence of neurodevelopmental handicaps has been a primary focus in the follow-up of low birthweight infants because the increased risk of cerebral palsy, seizure disorders, and other neurodevelopmental problems in these infants was documented in the 1950s.[27-30] At that time, the risk of neurodevelopmental problems for all low birthweight infants was 3 times that of normal birthweight infants, and that for very low birthweight infants was 10 times that of normal birthweight infants.[30]

Much of the recent literature on neonatal birthweight has focused on the very low birthweight group.[13,62-64] Recent reviewers[11,12] of this literature have concluded that the prevalence of neurodevelopmental handicaps among very low birthweight survivors appears to be decreasing, although variations in data suggest cautious interpretation. Despite the evidence of a decrease, low birthweight infants remain 3 times as likely as normal birthweight infants to experience adverse neurologic sequelae,[65] and the risk increases with decreasing birthweight, so that 8 to 19 percent of very low birthweight infants may be severely affected.[13,66,67]

Variations in outcome among very low birthweight survivors may be related to several factors. One that has received significant attention is cerebral intraventricular hemorrhage, probably caused by asphyxia. Although very low birthweight infants without intraventricular hemorrhage remain at increased risk of adverse neurodevelopmental outcomes as compared with a normal population, those with large hemorrhages (Grades 3 and 4) are at substantially increased risk of severe handicap.[66]

The risk of other developmental problems, especially those related to success in school, is less well established. It does appear, however, that low birthweight may be a significant predictor of school failure,[67] and this may be particularly characteristic of those who are small for gestational age.[14,68] Even in the SGA groups, however, the proportion of handicapped may be dependent on the presence of birth asphyxia, rather than on birthweight per se.[69]

The risk of developmental delay is not independent of factors that act to increase the risk of low birthweight. Thus, the low birthweight infants of disadvantaged mothers are more likely to experience school failure,[68] or to have lower intelligence quotients (IQs), than infants of similar birthweight in more advantaged families.[30,70]

The Risk of Congenital Anomalies

Although less intensively studied, the increased relative risk of congenital anomalies among low birthweight survivors is well documented. As compared with normal birthweight infants, low birthweight infants are twice as likely to have a nontrivial anomaly, and very low birthweight infants are 3 times as likely to have one.[71] Among the low birthweight infants, the risk of an anomaly is higher for those who are small for gestational age than for those whose birthweight is more consistent with the duration of gestation.[10,46]

Congenital anomalies and neurodevelopmental handicaps are not mutually exclusive occurrences. The percentage of infants affected with one or both ranges from 19 percent of normal birthweight infants to 42 percent of very low birthweight infants (anomalies include the presence of extra digits and strabismus, as well as more serious problems); those severely affected range from 2 percent of normal birthweight infants to 14 percent of very low birthweight infants.[19]

Respiratory Tract Conditions

Low birthweight also is a risk factor for the development of lower respiratory tract conditions.[72] Abnormal chest x-rays and pulmonary function and repeated lower respiratory tract infections often have been reported in low birthweight infants who had hyaline membrane disease or respiratory distress syndrome as newborns.[73-78] They also may occur in low birthweight infants who were asymptomatic in the neonatal period.[77] The persistence of abnormal cardiopulmonary function into early childhood is particularly characteristic of those infants who required prolonged ventilatory support.[79,80]

Overall, 8 percent of very low birthweight infants have evidence of chronic pulmonary disease at 40 weeks of age (corrected for duration of gestation), but this proportion decreases to 3 percent by 20 months of age.[81] The implications of these abnormalities for acute respiratory illness among surviving infants, especially illnesses that do not require hospitalization, have been only partially delineated.

Complications of Neonatal Care

Intensive care technology required for the survival of these infants is not without hazard, and may result in complications. The most well known is that seen with oxygen administration to immature infants, who may develop retrolental fibroplasia.[82,83] Other diagnostic and therapeutic techniques also have been shown to be hazardous.[1] Today's special care units expose infants to many substances, machines, and environmental conditions.[84-86] The potential side effects are still being defined.

Nonspecific Morbidity

Early studies suggested that low birthweight infants might be at greater risk of illness in general.[87] Relatively few investigators have examined this issue, however, and their findings have varied.[88,89] Recent data suggest that very low birthweight infants may be at increased risk of relatively serious or protracted illness. At one year, about one-third of these infants have had an illness requiring hospitalization and/or requiring prolonged care, as compared with 20 percent of all low birthweight infants and 17 percent of normal birthweight infants.[19] This may vary with age, because the proportion of very low birthweight infants with selected chronic conditions varies from 23 percent at 40 weeks of age (corrected for duration of gestation) to 3 percent at 20 months.[81] The susceptibility of high-risk survivors to acute or less serious illness remains to be established.

Injury

The risk of accidental injury for low birthweight infants remains relatively unexplored. Up to 1 year of age, little difference in the risk of injury by birthweight occurs.[89] Few studies have examined this association in older children. The relatively extensive literature identifying low birthweight as a risk factor for intentional injury (abuse) has been reviewed recently; the conclusion was that the evidence for such an association is not strong.[90]

Use of Health Services

Morbidity among low birthweight infants has significant implications for health services. Most of the interest in medical care use by low birthweight infants has focused on the intensive care services required to increase the survival of very low birthweight infants. The length of hospital stay in the neonatal period for infants who survive to the first year of life averages 3.5 days for normal birthweight infants, but is much longer for smaller infants: 7 days for those between 2,001 and 2,500 grams at birth; 24 days for those between 1,501 grams and 2,000 grams; 57 days for those less than 1,500 grams;[45] and 89 days for those less than 1,000 grams.[91] The length of stay for nonsurviving infants tends to be much less, although not proportionally less expensive.[91] [92] Wide variations both in length of stay and direct medical costs per day occur within birthweight groups, depending on the need for ventilation, the presence of congenital anomalies, the need for surgery, and other factors.[93]

The cost-effectiveness of neonatal intensive care has been questioned. A recent review has concluded that it is generally cost-effective.[11] Some individuals have expressed doubts, however, as to whether this conclusion will hold for the very smallest infants (1,000 grams or less). The results depend on the adjustments made for future costs incurred by handicapped survivors.[94]

In addition to undergoing prolonged hospitalization at birth, a substantial proportion of very low birthweight infants are rehospitalized during the first year.[95] [96] Up to 40 percent of these infants will have almost two hospitalizations, for an average of 16 days. This compares with 19 percent of all low birthweight infants for an average of 12.5 days, and 8.7 percent of normal birthweight infants for an average of 8 days.[95] A major determinant of rehospitalization for all birthweight groups is the presence of a chronic condition, congenital anomaly, or poor developmental outcome.[95] [96] After infancy, hospital use diminishes sharply.[96]

The average number of physician visits also is higher for low birthweight infants than for normal birthweight infants, but the relationship to birthweight is not as sharp as that for hospitalization. In one study, average visits in the first year ranged from 14 to 16 for those less than 1,500 grams at birth, to 10 for normal birthweight infants. As with hospitalization, a major determinant of physician utilization is the presence of a congenital anomaly and/or developmental delay.[97]

It is perhaps worth emphasizing that, on a population basis, the conditions for which medical services are used by low birthweight infants, even very low birthweight infants, are similar to those occasioning the use of services by normal birthweight infants.[95 97] These include congenital anomalies; respiratory infections such as pneumonia, bronchiolitis, and otitis media; and gastrointestinal problems. The increased use of services by low birthweight infants reflects the increased prevalence of these conditions. The etiologic basis for this increased morbidity and increased use of services has been only partially defined. Contributing factors may include biologic vulnerability due to immaturity, residual effects from the therapeutic maneuvers required to support the infants, socioeconomic disadvantages characteristic of many low birthweight infants, and increased surveillance by health care providers and parents.

Family Function

Finally, the birth of a high-risk infant may have major implications for family function. Early attempts to manage low birthweight infants produced an incidental observation of an apparent decrease in attachment between the mother and the surviving low birthweight infant.[98] Much recent work suggests that the bonds between mothers and critically ill infants may be disrupted so extensively that inappropriate parenting behaviors emerge.[99 100] In the extreme, this is seen as overprotectiveness[101 102] or physical abuse,[103 104] although the data on the latter may be questioned on methodological grounds.[90] More subtle indications of this disruption include altered perceptions and attitudes toward the low birthweight infant, which could have adverse consequences for the child's future development.[105 106]

The etiology of this maladaptive parenting remains unclear. Early investigators linked these changes to separation of the mother and infant required for intensive management.[99 100] Other work has suggested that the physical appearance of the child,[107] parental anxiety generated by the critical status of the infant at birth,[105] continued illness after discharge from the nursery,[104] and temperamental differences in the infant[108] also may contribute to altered parent-child interactions. Most likely, many of these factors operate together.[106]

Little information is available on other effects of high-risk infants on family function. Numerous studies of children with different chronic or catastrophic illnesses suggest, however, that the usual patterns of family function may be disrupted substantially. Serious and/or chronic illness in children has been associated with marital instability,[109] altered parental employment opportunities and family income,[110] decreased social contacts and vacations as a result of the burden of care for the child and the lack of alternate care-givers,[111] problems in other children in the family,[112] and increased workload for the mothers.[113]

Long-term assessments of family function following the birth of a low birthweight infant are just beginning to be reported. At least one study supports concerns in this regard. In this study,[70] high levels of behavior problems were found among preschoolers who were born at very low birthweight, and these problems were associated with decreased performance on standardized IQ tests.

Financial Stress

The degree of financial stress experienced by the families of high-risk infants may be another relevant factor. In the neonatal period, a substantial proportion of direct medical charges may be borne by the parents, up to 5 percent of the total for those with insurance and up to a third for those without insurance.[92] The amount of postdischarge care, both inpatient and ambulatory, absorbed by the family is not known, but likely to be high. In general, 15 to 20 percent of the costs of hospital care and 70 percent of the costs of outpatient care and medical supplies[114-117] for children are paid out of pocket by the family. It has been shown that insurance coverage affects the use of inpatient services regardless of health problems for low birthweight infants[95] and that family income, as well as insurance, affects the use of ambulatory services.[97] Almost no information is available on indirect costs, such as alterations in opportunities for maternal participation in the work force and time lost from work to obtain medical care, although the costs of visiting the child in the neonatal period have been estimated recently.[118] Whatever the expenditures, stress levels in some of these families are likely to be high, because these are young parents just beginning their working lives.

Overall Contribution of Low Birthweight to Morbidity

Despite the many conditions to which low birthweight infants may be vulnerable, the overall contribution (attributable risk) of birthweight-related conditions to morbidity is quite small. Low birthweight infants are only 1.6 times more likely to have a congenital anomaly, with or without developmental delay, than a normal birthweight infant; they account for 6 percent of infants with these conditions--about their representation in the population.[19] For very low birthweight infants, the relative risk is only 3.3 times that of normal birthweight infants.[19] For more severe conditions, the relative and attributable risks are smaller.[19] In particular, the proportion of very low birthweight survivors with serious illnesses diminishes rapidly after the first year,[81] so the effect of low birthweight infants on morbidity later in the preschool period is likely to be small. The contribution of low birthweight infants to the population of children with school and behavioral problems cannot be estimated, but again the effect is unlikely to be as overwhelming as that of low birthweight on mortality.

These conclusions may seem inconsistent with data on increased risk of morbidity, but the risk of morbidity from low birthweight is much smaller than the risk of mortality. In addition, because of their higher mortality rates, low birthweight infants constitute a smaller proportion of all infants who survive their first year of life than of live births. Thus, the effect of low birthweight in infants on childhood morbidity is substantially less than its effect on mortality.

This optimistic assessment must be tempered, however, by the realization that the full range of morbidity experienced by these infants is still being defined. Outcomes among the newest group of surviving babies, those weighing less than 1,000 grams, are generally unknown. Although they represent a relatively small proportion of surviving children, these high-risk infants often have health problems that require special services. This suggests that more research is required to evaluate the morbidity experienced by these infants and to determine the appropriate structure and target population for effective management strategies.

Decreasing Mortality: The Effect on Morbidity

Reviews of the outcomes among survivors of intensive care have documented decreases in the proportion of infants with adverse outcomes over time.[11 12] Interpretation of these reviews must be cautious, however, because the proportion of children with adverse outcomes has varied significantly among the studies and because selection factors affecting referral to intensive care units might alter the results.

More recent data based on clinical series [65 81] and population-based morbidity surveys[119] indicate that the increased survival of low birthweight infants has not been associated with an increase in the number with handicaps. The proportion with severe congenital anomalies and/or developmental delay has remained the same[64 119] whereas the proportion with less severe morbidity associated with antenatal and intrapartum events has declined.[119] As noted earlier, however, concerns remain about the effect of increased survival of the very smallest infants, those less than 1,000 grams.[96]

Summary

Low birthweight is a major determinant of infant mortality. Most infant deaths occur in the first month of life, or neonatal period. The majority of these deaths are a consequence of inadequate fetal growth as indicated by low birthweight (birthweight of 2,500 grams or less). Inadequate fetal growth may result from shortened duration of gestation or prematurity (duration of pregnancy less than 37 weeks from the last menstrual period), poor weight gain for a given duration of pregnancy (intrauterine growth retardation), or a combination of the two. The risk of mortality increases with decreasing birthweight so the smallest infants (very low birthweight or infants born weighing 1,500 grams or less) are at greatest risk.

The proportion of low birthweight infants is not only a major determinant of the overall neonatal mortality rate for a given population, but also is an important factor in the differences in neonatal mortality rates among different subgroups in the population. Thus, the higher neonatal mortality rates seen for nonwhite mothers, teenage mothers, and mothers of low educational attainment are explained by higher proportions of low birthweight infants among these groups.

In addition to increasing the risk of mortality, low birthweight increases the risk of morbidity. Although low birthweight is not a major determinant of the total burden of morbidity among infants and children, the relative risk of morbidity among low birthweight infants is high. The association of neurodevelopmental handicaps and congenital anomalies with low birthweight has been well established; low birthweight infants also may be susceptible to a wide range of other conditions, such as lower respiratory tract infections, learning disorders, behavior problems, and complications of neonatal intensive care interventions. Moreover, the birth of a low birthweight infant and its subsequent problems may place substantial emotional and financial stress on a young family; the consequences of this stress are still being studied.

Although the neonatal mortality rate in the United States has dropped significantly over the past 15 years, this change has not been associated with a comparable decrease in the incidence of low-weight births. Instead, the decline has resulted from the increased survival of low birthweight infants, due largely to more specialized, hospital-based management through neonatal intensive care. The proportion of infants born at low birthweight has changed only modestly since the late 1960s, and little change has been seen in the proportion of infants born at very low birthweight. The current statistics suggest that further reductions in neonatal mortality and decreases in the differentials between high- and low-mortality subgroups will require the prevention of low birthweight in infants.

References and Notes

1. Silverman WA: Retrolental Fibroplasia: A Modern Parable. New York: Grune and Stratton, 1980.
2. Cone TE Jr: De pondere infantum recens natorum: The history of weighing the newborn infant. Pediatrics 28:490-498, 1961.
3. Rooth G: Low birthweight revised. Lancet I:639-641, 1980.
4. World Health Organization: Manual of the International Statistical Classification of Diseases, Injuries and Causes of Death, Sixth Revision, Adopted 1948. Geneva: World Health Organization, 1948.
5. World Health Organization: Report on the Second Session of the Expert Committee on Health Statistics. Technical Report Series, No. 25. Geneva: World Health Organization, 1950.
6. Shapiro S: Influence of birthweight, sex and plurality on neonatal loss in the United States. Am. J. Public Health 44:1142-1153, 1954.

7. McKeown T and Gibson JR: Observations on all births (23,970) in Birmingham, 1947. II. Birthweight. Br. J. Soc. Med. 5:98-112, 1951.
8. Taback M: Birthweight and length of gestation with relation to prematurity. JAMA 146:897-901, 1951.
9. World Health Organization Expert Committee on Maternal and Child Health: Public Health Aspects of Low Birthweight. Third Report of the Expert Committee on Maternal and Child Health. Technical Report Series, No. 217. Geneva: World Health Organization, 1961.
10. Van den Berg BJ and Yerushalmy J: The relationship of intrauterine growth of infants of low birthweight to mortality, morbidity, and congenital anomalies. J. Pediatr. 69:531-545, 1966.
11. Office of Technology Assessment, U.S. Congress: The Implications of Cost-Effectiveness Analysis of Medical Technology. Background Paper No. 2: Case studies of medical technologies. Case Study No. 10: The costs and effectiveness of neonatal intensive care. Prepared by P Budetti, MA McManus, N Barrand, and LA Heinen. GPO Stock No. 052-003-00845-9. Washington, D.C.: U.S. Government Printing Office, 1981.
12. Stewart AL, Reynolds EO, and Lipscomb AP: Outcomes for infants of very low birthweight: Survey of world literature. Lancet I:1038-1040, 1981.
13. Fitzhardinge PM: Follow-up studies of the low birthweight infant. Clin. Perinatal. 3:503-516, 1976.
14. Fitzhardinge PM and Steven EM: The small-for-date infant. II. Neurologic and intellectual sequelae. Pediatrics 50:50-57, 1972.
15. Blalock NM: Social Statistics. New York: McGraw-Hill, 1960.
16. Wilcox AJ and Russell IT: Birthweight distribution and perinatal mortality. I. On the frequency distribution of birthweight. Int. J. Epidemiol. 12:314-318, 1983.
17. Wilcox AJ and Russell IT: Perinatal mortality: Standardizing for birthweight is biased. Am. J. Epidemiol. 118:857-864, 1983.
18. Weaver JL: Policy responses to complex issues: The case of black infant mortality. J. Health Politics Policy Law 1:433-443, 1977.
19. Shapiro S, McCormick MC, Starfield BH, Krischer JP, and Bross D: Relevance of correlates of infant deaths for significant morbidity at 1 year of age. Am. J. Obstet. Gynecol. 136:363-373, 1980.
20. Williams RL, Creasy RK, Cunningham GC, Hawes WE, Norris FD, and Tashiro M: Fetal growth and perinatal viability in California. Obstet. Gynecol. 59:624-632, 1982.
21. Koops BL, Morgan LJ, and Battaglia FC: Neonatal mortality risk in relation to birth weight and gestational age: Update. J. Pediatr. 101:969-977, 1982.
22. Morris JN and Heady JA: Social and biological factors in infant mortality. Lancet I:343-349, 1955.
23. Pharoah POD and Morris JN: Post-neonatal mortality. Epidemiol. Rev. 1:170-183, 1979.
24. Puffer RR and Serrano CV: Patterns of Mortality in Childhood. Washington, D.C.: Pan American Health Organization, 1973.

25. Shapiro S, Schlesinger ER, and Nesbitt REL: Infant, Perinatal, Maternal and Childhood Mortality in the United States. Cambridge, Mass.: Harvard University Press, 1968.
26. National Center for Health Statistics: Factors Associated with Low Birthweight: United States, 1976. Prepared by S Taffel. Vital and Health Statistics, Series 21, No. 37. DHEW No. (PHS) 80-1915. Public Health Service. Washington, D.C.: U.S. Government Printing Office, April 1980.
27. Lilienfeld AM and Parkhurst E: A study of the association of factors of pregnancy and parturition with the development of cerebral palsy: A preliminary report. Am. J. Hyg. 53:262-282, 1951.
28. Lilienfeld AM and Pasamanick E: Association of maternal and fetal factors with the development of epilepsy: Abnormalities in the prenatal and perinatal periods. JAMA 155:719-724, 1954.
29. Niswander KR and Gordon M: The Women and Their Pregnancies: The Collaborative Perinatal Study of the National Institute of Neurologic Diseases and Stroke. Philadelphia: W.B. Saunders, 1972.
30. Hardy JB, Drage JS, and Jackson EC: The First Year of Life: The Collaborative Perinatal Study of the National Institute of Neurological and Communicative Disorders and Stroke. Baltimore: Johns Hopkins University Press, 1979.
31. Abramowicz M and Kass EH: Pathogenesis and prognosis of prematurity. N. Engl. J. Med. 275:878-885, 938-943, 1001-1007, 1053-1059, 1966.
32. Aubrey RH and Pennington JC: Identification and evaluation of high-risk pregnancy: The perinatal concept. Clin. Obstet. Gynecol. 16:3-27, 1973.
33. Hobel CJ, Youkeles L, and Forsythe A: Prenatal and intrapartum high-risk screening. II. Risk factors reassessed. Am. J. Obstet. Gynecol. 135:1051-1056, 1978.
34. Davis K and Schoen C: Health and the War on Poverty: A Ten Year Appraisal. Washington, D.C.: The Brookings Institute, 1978.
35. Select Panel for the Promotion of Child Health: Analysis and Recommendations for Selected Federal Programs. Better Health for Our Children: A National Strategy. Vol. II. DHHS No. (PHS) 79-55071. Public Health Service. Washington, D.C.: U.S. Government Printing Office, 1981.
36. National Center for Health Statistics: Health, United States, 1982. DHHS No. (PHS) 83-1232. Public Health Service. Washington, D.C.: U.S. Government Printing Office, December 1982.
37. Susser M, Marolla FA, and Fleiss J: Birthweight, fetal age and perinatal mortality. Am. J. Epidemiol. 96:197-204, 1972.
38. Rooth G: Better perinatal health: Sweden. Lancet II:1170-1172, 1979.
39. Lumley J: Better perinatal health: Australia. Lancet I:79-81, 1980.
40. Backet EM, Davies AM, and Petros-Barvazian A: The Risk Approach in Health Care: With Special Reference to Maternal and Child Health, Including Family Planning. Public Health Papers, No. 76. Geneva: World Health Organization, 1984.

41. McCormick MC, Shapiro S, and Starfield BH: The regionalization of perinatal services: Summary of the evaluation of a national demonstration program. JAMA, in press.
42. Lee KS, Paneth N, Gartner LM, and Pearlman M: The very low-birthweight rate: Principal predictor of neonatal mortality in industrialized populations. J. Pediatr. 97:759-764, 1980.
43. Shah FK and Abbey H: Effects of some factors on neonatal and postneonatal mortality: Analysis by a binary variable multiple regression model. Milbank Mem. Fund Q. 49:33-57, 1971.
44. Hack M, Merkatz IR, Jones PK, and Fanaroff AA: Changing trends of neonatal and postneonatal deaths in very-low-birth-weight infants. Am. J. Obstet. Gynecol. 137:797-800, 1980.
45. Unpublished data from the Evaluation Project of the Robert Wood Johnson Foundation National Perinatal Regionalization Program, Health Services Research and Development Center, Johns Hopkins School of Hygiene and Public Health, Baltimore, Md.
46. Starfield BH, Shapiro S, McCormick MC, and Bross D: Mortality and morbidity in infants with intrauterine growth retardation. J. Pediatr. 101:978-983, 1982.
47. Villar J and Belizan JM: The relative contribution of prematurity and fetal growth retardation to low birthweight in developing and developed countries. Am. J. Obstet. Gynecol. 143:793-798, 1982.
48. Kessel SS, Villar J, Berendes HW, and Nugent RP: The changing pattern of low birthweight in the United States: 1970-1980. JAMA 251:1978-1982, 1984.
49. Hoffman HJ, Stark CR, Lundin FE Jr, and Ashbrook JD: Analysis of birthweight, gestational age, and fetal viability, U.S. births, 1968. Obstet. Gynecol. Surv. 29:651-681, 1974.
50. McCormick MC, Shapiro S, and Starfield BH: High-risk young mothers: Infant mortality and morbidity in four areas in the United States, 1973-78. Am. J. Public Health 74:18-23, 1984.
51. Kleinman JC, Kovar MG, Feldman JJ, and Young CA: A comparison of 1960 and 1973-74 early neonatal mortality in selected states. Am. J. Epidemiol. 108:454-469, 1978.
52. Lee KS, Paneth N, Gartner LM, Pearlman MA, and Gruss L: Neonatal mortality: An analysis of the recent improvements in the United States. Am. J. Public Health 70:15-21, 1980.
53. Williams RL and Chen PM: Identifying the sources of the recent decline in perinatal mortality rates in California. N. Engl. J. Med. 306:207-214, 1982.
54. Usher RH: Clinical implications of perinatal mortality statistics. Clin. Obstet. Gynecol. 14:885-925, 1971.
55. Schlesinger ER: Neonatal intensive care: Planning for services and outcome following care. J. Pediatr. 82:916-920, 1973.
56. Horwood SP, Boyle MH, Torrance GW, and Sinclair JC: Mortality and morbidity of 500- to 1499-gram birthweight infants live-born to residents of a defined geographic region before and after neonatal intensive care. Pediatrics 69:613-620, 1982.

57. Williams RL and Hawes WE: Cesarean section, fetal monitoring and perinatal mortality in California. Am. J. Public Health 69:864-870, 1979.
58. Hein HA and Brown CJ: Neonatal mortality review: A basis for improving care. Pediatrics 68:504-509, 1981.
59. Paneth N, Kiely JL, Wallenstein S, Marcus M, Pakter J, and Susser M: Newborn intensive care and neonatal mortality in low-birthweight infants. N. Engl. J. Med. 307:149-155, 1982.
60. Haines TR, Isaman J, and Giles HR: Improved neonatal survival through maternal transport. Obstet. Gynecol. 52:294-300, 1978.
61. Modanlou HD, Dorchester W, Freeman RK, and Rommal C: Perinatal transport to a regional perinatal center in a metropolitan area: Maternal versus neonatal transport. Am. J. Obstet. Gynecol. 138:1157-1164, 1980.
62. Sabel KG, Olegard R, and Victoria L: Remaining sequelae with modern perinatal care. Pediatrics 57:652-658, 1976.
63. Stewart A, Turcaro D, Rawlings S, Hart S, and Gregory S: Outcome for infants at high risk of major handicap. In Major Mental Handicap: Methods and Costs of Prevention. CIBA Foundation Symposium 59, pp. 151-171. Amsterdam: Elsevier-Excerpta Medica, 1978.
64. Hack M, Fanaroff AA, and Merkatz IR: The low-birthweight infant: Evolution of a changing outlook. N. Engl. J. Med. 301:1162-1165, 1979.
65. McCormick MC, Wessel KW, Krischer JP, Welcher DW, and Handy JB: Preliminary analysis of developmental observations in a survey of morbidity in infants. Early Hum. Devel. 5:377-393, 1981.
66. Papile L, Munsick-Bruno G, and Schaefer A: Relationship of cerebral intraventricular hemorrhage and early neurologic handicaps. J. Pediatr. 103:273-277, 1983.
67. Ramey CT, Stedman DJ, Borders-Patterson A, and Mengel W: Predicting school-failure from information available at birth. Am. J. Ment. Defic. 82:525-534, 1978.
68. Harvey D, Prince J, Bunton J, Parkinson C, and Campbell S: Abilities of children who were small-for-gestational-age babies. Pediatrics 69:296-300, 1982.
69. Westwood M, Kramer MS, Munz D, Lovett JM, and Watters GV: Growth and development of full-term nonasphyxiated small-for-gestational-age newborns: Follow-up through adolescence. Pediatrics 71:376-382, 1983.
70. Escalona SK: Babies at double hazard: Early development of infants at biologic and social risk. Pediatrics 70:670-676, 1982.
71. Christianson RE, Van den Berg BJ, Milkovich L, and Oechsli FW: Incidence of congenital anomalies among white and black live births with long-term follow-up. Am. J. Public Health 71:1333-1341, 1981.
72. McCall MG and Acheson HG: Respiratory disease in infancy. J. Chronic Dis. 21:349-359, 1968.
73. Outerbridge EW, Nogrady MB, Beaudry PH, and Stern L: Idiopathic respiratory distress syndrome. Am. J. Dis. Child. 123:99-104, 1972.

74. Shephard FM, Johnston RB Jr, Klatte EC, Burko H, and Stahlman M: Residual pulmonary findings in clinical hyaline-membrane disease. N. Engl. J. Med. 279:1063-1071, 1968.

75. Westgate HD, Fisch RO, Langer LO Jr, and Staub HP: Pulmonary and respiratory function changes in survivors of hyaline membrane disease. Dis. Chest 55:465-470, 1969.

76. Bryan MH, Hardie MJ, Reilly BJ, and Swyer PR: Pulmonary function studies during the first year of life in infants recovering from the respiratory distress syndrome. Pediatrics 52:169-178, 1973.

77. Coates AL, Bergsteinsson M, Desmond K, Outerbridge EW, and Beaudry PH: Long-term sequelae of premature birth with and without idiopathic respiratory distress syndrome. J. Pediatr. 90:611-616, 1977.

78. Lamarre A, Linao L, Reilly BJ, Swyer PR, and Levison H: Residual pulmonary abnormalities in survivors of idiopathic respiratory distress syndrome. Am. Rev. Respir. Dis. 108:56-61, 1973.

79. Harrod JR, L'Heureux P, Wangenstren OD, and Hunt CE: Long-term follow-up of severe respiratory distress syndrome treated with IPPB. J. Pediatr. 84:277-286, 1974.

80. Smyth JA, Tabachnik E, Duncan WJ, Reilly BJ, and Levison H: Pulmonary function and bronchial hyperreactivity in long-term survivors of bronchopulmonary dysplasia. Pediatrics 68:336-340, 1981.

81. Hack M, Caron B, Rivers A, and Fanaroff AA: The very low birthweight infant: The broader spectrum of morbidity during infancy and early childhood. J. Behav. Devel. Pediatr. 4:243-249, 1983.

82. James LS and Lanman JT, eds.: History of oxygen therapy and retrolental fibroplasia. Pediatrics 57(supplement):591-642, 1976.

83. Lucey JF and Dangman B: A reexamination of the role of oxygen in retrolental fibroplasia. Pediatrics 73:82-96, 1984.

84. Speidel BD: Adverse effects of routine procedures on preterm infants. Lancet I:864-866, 1978.

85. Aranda JV, Cohen S, and Neims AH: Drug utilization in a newborn intensive care unit. J. Pediatr. 89:315-317, 1976.

86. Gottfried AW, Wallace-Lande P, Sterman-Brown S, King J, Coen C, and Hodgman J: Physical and social environment of newborn infants in special care units. Science 214:673-675, 1981.

87. Perkins GB: A year's follow-up study of illness in a sample of premature infants. Am. J. Public Health 45:774-783, 1955.

88. Van den Berg BJ: Morbidity of low birthweight and/or pre-term children compared to that of the "mature." 1. Methodologic considerations and findings for the first 2 years of life. Pediatrics 42:590-597, 1968.

89. McCormick MC, Shapiro S, and Starfield BH: Injury and its correlates among 1-year-old children: Study of children with both normal and low birth weights. Am. J. Dis. Child. 135:159-163, 1981.

90. Leventhal JM: Risk factors for child abuse: Methodologic standards in case-control studies. Pediatrics 68:684-690, 1981.

91. Pomerance JJ, Ukrainski CT, Ukra T, Henderson DH, Nash AH, and Meredith JL: Cost of living for infants weighing 1,000 g or less at birth. Pediatrics 61:908-910, 1978.

92. McCarthy JT, Koops BL, Honeyfield PR, and Butterfield LJ: Who pays the bill for neonatal intensive care? J. Pediatr. 95:755-761, 1979.

93. Phibbs CFS, Williams RL, and Phibbs RH: Newborn risk factors and the costs of neonatal intensive care. Pediatrics 68:313-321, 1981.

94. Boyle MH, Torrance GW, Sinclair JC, and Horwood SP: Economic evaluation of neonatal intensive care of very-low-birthweight infants. N. Engl. J. Med. 308:1330-1337, 1983.

95. McCormick MC, Shapiro S, and Starfield BH: Rehospitalization in the first year of life for high-risk survivors. Pediatrics 66:991-999, 1980.

96. Hack M, DeMonterice D, Merkatz IR, Jones P, and Fanaroff AA: Rehospitalization of the very low birthweight infant--a continuum of perinatal and environmental morbidity. Am. J. Dis. Child. 135:263-266, 1981.

97. McCormick MC, Shapiro S, and Starfield BH: Factors associated with the use of hospital, ambulatory and preventive services among infants using different sources of ambulatory care. Paper presented at the Annual Meeting of the Ambulatory Pediatric Society, San Francisco, California, April 1981.

98. Silverman WA: Incubator-baby side shows. Pediatrics 64:127-141, 1979.

99. Kennell JH and Klaus MH: Care of the mother of the high-risk infant. Clin. Obstet. Gynecol. 14:926-954, 1971.

100. Lozoff B, Brittenham GM, Trause MA, Kennell JH, and Klaus MH: The mother-newborn relationship: Limits of adaptability. J. Pediatr. 91:1-12, 1977.

101. Green M and Solnit AJ: Reactions to the threatened loss of a child: A vulnerable child syndrome. Pediatrics 34:58-66, 1964.

102. Levy, JC: Vulnerable children: Parents perspectives and the use of medical care. Pediatrics 65:956-963, 1980.

103. Klein M and Stern L: Low birthweight and the battered child. Am. J. Dis. Child. 122:15-18, 1971.

104. Lynch MA: Ill health and child abuse. Lancet II:317-318, 1975.

105. Bidder RT, Crowe EA, and Gray DP: Mothers' attitudes to infants. Arch. Disease Child. 49:766-770, 1974.

106. McCormick MC, Shapiro S, and Starfield BH: Factors associated with maternal opinion of infant development--clues to the vulnerable child? Pediatrics 69:537-543, 1982.

107. LaVeck B, Hammond MA, and LaVeck GS: Minor congenital anomalies and behavior in different home environments. J. Pediatr. 96:940-943, 1980.

108. Stone NW and Chesney BIT: Attachment behaviors in handicapped infants. Ment. Retard. 16:8-12, 1978.

109. Pless IB and Pinkerton R: Chronic Childhood Disorder: Promoting Patterns of Adjustment. London: Henry Kimpton, 1975.

110. Salkever D: Children's health problems: Implications for parental labor supply and earnings. In Economic Aspects of Health, edited by VR Fuchs, pp. 221-251. Chicago: University of Chicago Press, 1980.

111. Stein RK and Riessman CK: The development of an impact-on-family scale: Preliminary findings. Med. Care 18:465-472, 1980.

112. Breslau N, Weitzman W, and Messenger K: Psychological functioning of siblings of disabled children. Pediatrics 67:344-353, 1981.

113. Breslau N: Care of disabled children and women's time use. Med. Care 21:620-629, 1983.

114. Blendon RJ: Paying for medical care for children: A continuing financial dilemma. Adv. Pediatr. 29:229-246, 1982.

115. National Center for Health Services Research: Charges and Sources of Payment for Visits to Physician Offices. Data Preview 5. DHHS No. (PHS) 81-3291. Public Health Service. Washington, D.C.: U.S. Government Printing Office, 1981.

116. National Center for Health Services Research: Dental Services: Use, Expenditures, and Sources of Payment. Data Preview 8. DHHS No. (PHS) 82-3319. Public Health Service. Washington, D.C.: U.S. Government Printing Office, 1982.

117. National Center for Health Services Research: Medical Equipment and Supplies: Purchases, Rentals, Expenditures and Sources of Payment. Data Preview 10. DHHS No. (PHS) 82-3321. Public Health Service. Washington, D.C.: U.S. Government Printing Office, 1982.

118. Smith MA and Baum JD: Cost of visiting babies in special care units. Arch. Dis. Child. 58:56-59, 1983.

119. Shapiro S, McCormick MC, Starfield BH, and Crawley B: Changes in morbidity associated with decreases in neonatal mortality. Pediatrics 72:408-415, 1983.

CHAPTER 2

Etiology and Risk Factors

Despite important new research findings and improvements in the science of obstetrics, our understanding of the basic causes of preterm labor and intrauterine growth retardation is limited. In the absence of adequate knowledge about etiology, a large body of information has developed about factors associated with low birthweight, often termed "risk factors," because their presence in an individual woman indicates an increased chance, or risk, of bearing a low birthweight infant. This chapter outlines data both on the etiology of prematurity and IUGR and on the risk factors associated with these outcomes of pregnancy. It also describes the process of risk assessment and analyzes several risk assessment systems.

Etiology

As described in the previous chapter, the term low birthweight can refer to three often intertwined outcomes of pregnancy: preterm delivery, intrauterine fetal growth retardation (IUGR), and a combination of both. Although little is known about the various mechanisms that produce these conditions, several theoretical models have been developed as a basis for further research and are outlined in this section.

Prematurity

The mechanism for the initiation and maintenance of normal human labor is not known, but substantial progress has been made in understanding some of the important associated physiologic and biochemical events.[1] Information about the onset of preterm labor is more fragmentary and speculative.[2]

Endocrine changes in the uteroplacental environment appear to be the principal factors leading to the development of uterine contractions.[3] These endocrine changes involve hormones from both the mother and the fetus; cortisol, estrogen, and progesterone appear to play major roles. Much of this information is based on studies of sheep in which the process starts about 10 days before labor.

The first event in sheep is an elevation in fetal cortisol, probably in response to fetal ACTH. This cortisol rise generates a decline in maternal progesterone due to the induction of 17 a-hydroxylase enzyme activity in the placenta, which increases the conversion of progesterone to dehydroxyprogesterone.[4] Progesterone withdrawal is associated with increased uterine muscle excitability, or responsiveness to electrical and hormonal stimuli. Dehydroxyprogesterone also is a precursor of the rise in maternal estrogen, which occurs a few days before the onset of labor. Estrogens increase rhythmic uterine contractions and also the responsiveness of the uterus to oxytocin. In sheep, estrogen elevation also causes a rise in prostaglandin (PGF_{2a}) production hours before the onset of uterine activity. The combined changes in maternal hormones are thought to affect uterine muscle by enhancing myometrial excitability and the conduction of action potential.

In contrast to sheep, the human hormonal changes appear to occur during the last 5 weeks of pregnancy, and evidence for fetal cortisol initiating the onset of labor is lacking. Amniotic fluid cortisol and maternal blood estrogen increase at 34 to 36 weeks of gestation. The former correlates with fetal pulmonary maturity and the latter may play a role by increasing prostaglandin production. Unlike in sheep, the role of progesterone in human labor is unclear.[3] A decline in peripheral blood levels before labor has been suggested in at least one study,[5] although others have failed to confirm this finding. The presence of a fetal membrane progesterone binding protein, possibly facilitated by estrogen, indicates that a local withdrawal effect may occur. Several reports indicate that prostaglandins do play a role in human labor; they are synthesized from a fatty acid precursor in the chorioamnion and/or decidua at a time when estrogen levels are increasing.[6,7] Last, increased levels of maternal oxytocin are not thought to contribute to initiating labor (although a threshold level may be important as a permissive factor), but may be necessary for the development of more intense contractions during the second stage of labor. Fetal oxytocin may play a role, however, as indicated by high concentrations of this hormone in umbilical cord blood.

The way in which hormonal changes act to induce labor is not clear.[2,3] Animal studies demonstrate that low resistance myometrial pathways (gap junctions) form during labor and suggest that the structural and biochemical organization of myometrial muscle may be important in the development of contractions. The development of gap junctions under the influence of steroids and prostaglandins and in relation to the estrogen/progesterone ratio is probably of major importance to the organization of the myometrium.[8] The contraction of uterine muscle is significantly influenced by an increase in the concentration of free calcium on the myofibrils resulting from the action of prostaglandins, which counteracts progesterone-induced calcium binding in the sarcoplasmic reticulum.

Knowledge about the etiology, initiation, and maintenance of preterm labor is limited.[1,2,9,10] The underlying pathophysiology is postulated on the basis of variations from the normal patterns of hormonal effects detected in animals and man or on the basis of inferences made about the possible untoward effects of certain clinical conditions on uteroplacental physiology. Observations suggest that infection, stress, hypertension, and other conditions may be associated with variations in the endocrine environment and metabolic state of the uterus and the cervix. These variations probably result from complex interactions involving progesterone, estrogen, oxytocin, and other hormones; prostaglandins; calcium ions; adrenergic agents and receptors; catecholamines; and uteroplacental blood flow.

From the foregoing, it is clear that at this time it is not possible to identify a single etiology for premature birth.[2] It is possible, however, to enumerate a variety of factors and clinical conditions that have been associated with the preterm onset of labor. This list includes, but is not limited to, abruptio placentae, amnionitis, congenital malformations, erythroblastosis fetalis, incompetent cervix, placenta previa, polyhydramnios, preeclampsia, premature rupture of membranes, severe maternal illness, multiple pregnancies, and urinary tract infections. In general, these are conditions in which there is an inability of the uterus to retain the fetus, interference with the course of the pregnancy, premature separation of the placenta, or a stimulus to effective uterine contractions before term. Several of these conditions are discussed later in the chapter as risk factors for preterm birth, although it is apparent that the distinction between a risk factor and a causal mechanism is not always clear. Finally, in many cases of premature birth, no association with a pathologic factor can be identified.

Intrauterine Growth Retardation (IUGR)

Delay in the growth and development of the fetus has been associated with a variety of factors that can be grouped in terms of the locus of their impact: the placenta, the pregnant woman herself, the fetus, or some combination of these. In general, IUGR is associated with conditions that interfere with the circulation to and efficiency of the placenta, with the development or growth of the fetus, or with the general health and nutrition of the pregnant woman; however, for many growth-retarded infants no relevant pathogenic factors can be identified.

Vascular and inflammatory lesions of the placenta; placental separation and infarction; and decreases in placental weight, cellularity, and surface area may act alone or in combination to produce IUGR.[11] It is postulated that such conditions result directly or indirectly in a reduction in the supply of nutrients to the fetus.[12] Multiple pregnancies (for example, twins or triplets) also may be associated with IUGR because the placenta may be unable to supply sufficient nutrients to multiple fetuses. Other placental conditions associated with IUGR include hemangioma of the placenta or umbilical cord and the parabiotic transfusion syndrome. Insufficient placental transfer of nutrients may be primarily related to abnormal transport across the placenta, to alterations in placental metabolism, or to changes in the uteroplacental circulation.[13]

Certain conditions or diseases of pregnant women also are associated with IUGR.[14, 15] They are thought to directly or indirectly hamper delivery of nutrients or oxygen to the uteroplacental circulation, which results in an inability to maintain normal fetal growth and development.[16] The most frequent, recognized problem is the presence of a maternal vascular disease, such as chronic hypertension or chronic renal disease. The duration and severity of the disorder are roughly related to the severity of the IUGR. Pregnancy-induced hypertension also can cause IUGR, but commonly the fetus is delivered before severe growth retardation develops. This condition, superimposed on chronic hypertension, often is associated either with IUGR or premature delivery of a fetus that has grown and developed normally up to the time of delivery. Severe forms of diabetes mellitus also are frequently associated with vascular disease and IUGR. Sickle-cell disease may be associated with IUGR and placental lesions.

Several conditions that lead to hypoxia in pregnant women have been associated with IUGR, including cyanotic heart or pulmonary disease and residence at high altitudes.[16, 17] A variety of mechanisms have been postulated for the development of IUGR associated with cigarette smoking, alcohol and narcotic ingestion, and the administration of antimetabolites, but no definitive statement can be made concerning these etiologies. Similarly, the precise pathogenic mechanisms linking maternal malnutrition and chronic illness during pregnancy to low birthweight (IUGR or prematurity) are unknown.

Fetal factors implicated by association in the etiology of IUGR include chromosomal disorders, such as certain autosomal trisomies; chronic fetal infections, such as congenital rubella, syphilis, and cytomegalovirus inclusion disease; certain congenital malformations and diseases; and radiation injury.[15, 18] Although a variety of pathogenic mechanisms have been suggested by these associations, the specific etiologies have not been established conclusively.[15]

Finally, IUGR and prematurity occur together in about 30 percent of low birthweight cases. In some instances, both the prematurity and the IUGR occur without a demonstrable association with a suspected pathogenic factor. In other cases, various combinations of the factors discussed above can be identified.

Risk Factors: An Overview

Recent research on the risk factors associated both with preterm delivery and IUGR has helped to identify possible causes of low birthweight. Risk factor analysis also helps guide clinical practice and suggests possible prevention strategies at both the individual and population level.

Unfortunately, the risk factor literature has many methodological and conceptual problems that make its interpretation difficult. For example, many studies analyze the relationship of a given risk factor to "low birthweight" rather than to the more specific outcomes of preterm delivery and intrauterine growth retardation; also, these studies commonly rely on estimates of gestational age, which often are approximate. Risk factors often are defined differently in different studies, and studies of small groups often do not produce information that can be applied to other populations, thereby hampering comparisons and pooling of data. More importantly, many studies examine risk factors as independent entities, although several factors may cluster in an individual and may be causally related. Finally, known confounding variables may not be controlled, and the cross-sectional design of many risk factor studies makes it difficult to separate cause and effect. Such problems make it hard to reach conclusions about the magnitude of risk posed by single factors.

Some of these limitations can be overcome by more careful statistical design and definition. Others are more difficult to correct. For example, many population-based studies must rely on data derived from birth certificates; in most states, these forms include only a limited number of risk factor variables relevant to low birthweight. Birth certificates in most states do not provide information on such factors as maternal height, weight, weight gain during pregnancy, or smoking practices.

A chart listing the principal risk factors for low birthweight is shown in Appendix A. Based on the studies noted in the appendix, in this chapter, and in Chapter 3, the chart records whether a given factor has been reported to increase the risk of preterm delivery or IUGR, or whether it has simply been linked to low birthweight. For some factors, the chart also records attributable and relative risk values (defined in Chapter 1). Appendix A includes a mixture of factors for which the evidence of risk is strong and those for which the association with prematurity and/or IUGR is less clear.

Because some studies have calculated relative or attributable risk values for certain factors, the committee explored the possibility of ranking the risks in order of magnitude to help set priorities for interventions and for further research. Unfortunately, the data do not permit such ordering. For some factors (including many of the infections), the committee was able to locate no risk values at all. For many others, only a single value was located, and the committee judged this to be an inadequate data base from which to construct a ranking of magnitude of risk. Another problem is that risks important at an individual level are not always so for populations. It is also apparent that the estimates of risk vary significantly, probably due to definitional variations and to differences in populations studied. The committee also concluded that, because of the numerous interrelationships among factors, it would be unwise to address them in a way that suggests each always has an independent influence on preterm delivery or IUGR.

Even without an orderly ranking of risk, the committee found that the factors could be grouped in a way that helps to structure preventive interventions, which is the principal focus of the report. In Table 2.1, which summarizes Appendix A, the risk factors are separated into demographic characteristics, medical risks that can be detected before conception, risks that can be detected during pregnancy, behavioral and environmental risks, health care risks, and a final category of factors whose role in low birthweight is still being defined.

TABLE 2.1 Principal Risk Factors for Low Birthweight

I. Demographic Risks
- A. Age (less than 17; over 34)
- B. Race (black)
- C. Low socioeconomic status
- D. Unmarried
- E. Low level of education

II. Medical Risks Predating Pregnancy
- A. Parity (0 or more than 4)
- B. Low weight for height
- C. Genitourinary anomalies/surgery
- D. Selected diseases such as diabetes, chronic hypertension
- E. Nonimmune status for selected infections such as rubella
- F. Poor obstetric history, including previous low birthweight infant, multiple spontaneous abortions
- G. Maternal genetic factors (such as low maternal weight at own birth)

III. Medical Risks in Current Pregnancy
- A. Multiple pregnancy
- B. Poor weight gain
- C. Short interpregnancy interval
- D. Hypotension
- E. Hypertension/preeclampsia/toxemia
- F. Selected infections such as symptomatic bacteriuria, rubella, and cytomegalovirus
- G. First or second trimester bleeding
- H. Placental problems such as placenta previa, abruptio placentae
- I. Hyperemesis
- J. Oligohydramnios/polyhydramnios
- K. Anemia/abnormal hemoglobin
- L. Isoimmunization
- M. Fetal anomalies
- N. Incompetent cervix
- O. Spontaneous premature rupture of membranes

IV. Behavioral and Environmental Risks
- A. Smoking
- B. Poor nutritional status
- C. Alcohol and other substance abuse
- D. DES exposure and other toxic exposures, including occupational hazards
- E. High altitude

V. Health Care Risks
- A. Absent or inadequate prenatal care
- B. Iatrogenic prematurity

VI. Evolving Concepts of Risk
- A. Stress, physical and psychosocial
- B. Uterine irritability
- C. Events triggering uterine contractions
- D. Cervical changes detected before onset of labor
- E. Selected infections such as mycoplasma and Chlamydia trachomatis
- F. Inadequate plasma volume expansion
- G. Progesterone deficiency

This grouping leads to the observation that many of the risk factors for low birthweight (categories I, II, and IV of the table) can be identified before pregnancy occurs; detection and possible intervention need not always wait until the prenatal period. Chapter 5 develops this theme more fully. The grouping also helps to highlight the importance of behavioral and environmental risks and the need for interventions that go beyond medical care. The demographic measures can help to define target populations. The cluster of health care issues highlights the fact that not all risks for low birthweight derive from characteristics of women themselves. And finally, the category of evolving concepts of risk suggests some important research areas for improved understanding of low birthweight. These themes appear throughout Part II of this report.

In the following detailed discussion of risk factors, the committee chose to focus on those that are widely distributed throughout the population, amenable to prevention or treatment, or especially controversial. These include the demographic risk factors of race, age, and socioeconomic status; the medical and obstetric risks of hypertension/preeclampsia, diabetes, obstetric history (including previous induced abortion), multiple pregnancy, and infection; nutrition; the behavioral and environmental risks of smoking and alcohol use; and iatrogenic prematurity. The committee also examines certain risk factors that are more speculative in nature, including stress, uterine irritability, cervical changes, inadequate plasma volume expansion, and progesterone deficiency.

Chapter 3, a review of state and national vital statistics data, provides additional information on some of the demographic factors and on the issues of pregnancy interval, obstetric history, and parity in relation to age. Chapter 6 explores another risk factor for low birthweight, absent or inadequate prenatal care.

Demographic Risks

The interrelationships among the major demographic risk factors are numerous and it is often difficult to determine the precise association between any single factor and low birthweight. Nonetheless, through careful statistical design, the independent effect of each is gradually being defined.

Race

Table 2.2 shows the frequency of low birthweight for different racial and ethnic groups. The approximate 2:1 low birthweight ratio between black and nonblack ethnic groups has remained fairly constant for the past 20 years. When low birthweight infants are subdivided into those born at term and those born prematurely, blacks remain approximately twice as likely as whites to be in either category.[19] In one large but now dated study of approximately 50,000 pregnancies, black newborns were on average 233 grams lighter than their white counterparts.[20]

That black neonates are at high risk of low birthweight is unquestioned. The reason or reasons for this risk are uncertain, however. Maternal age may account for part of the increased risk. Teenage mothers are at high risk of low birthweight, and black mothers are more likely to be teenagers than are mothers of other ethnic groups. In 1980, 26.5 percent of all black births were to teenagers. In contrast, 12.1 percent of white births and 15.3 percent of Hispanic births were to teenagers.[21] When black and white mothers of the same

TABLE 2.2 Percentage of Live Births Less Than 2,500 Grams

	Percent Less Than 2,500 Grams	Percent Less Than 1,500 Grams
White	5.7[a]	0.9[a]
Black	12.5[a]	2.4[a]
Chinese	4.9[a]	0.6[a]
Mexican-American	5.3[b]	0.9[b]
American Indian	6.9[c]	--

SOURCES:
[a]National Center for Health Statistics: Characteristics of Asian Births: United States, 1980. Prepared by S Taffel. Monthly Vital Statistics Report, Vol. 32, No. 10 (supplement). Public Health Service. Washington, D.C.: U.S. Government Printing Office, February 1984.
[b]National Center for Health Statistics: Births of Hispanic Parentage, 1979. Prepared by SJ Ventura. Monthly Vital Statistics Report, Vol. 31, No. 2 (supplement). Public Health Service. Washington, D.C.: U.S. Government Printing Office, May 1982.
[c]National Center for Health Statistics: Factors Associated with Low Birthweight, 1976. Prepared by S Taffel. Vital and Health Statistics, Series 21, No. 37. DHEW No. (PHS) 80-1915. Public Health Service. Washington, D.C.: U.S. Government Printing Office, April 1980.

age are compared, however, blacks are at higher risk of low birthweight in every age group.[22] The relationship of low birthweight to maternal age using 1976 data is shown in Table 2.3; Appendix Table B.7 displays more recent and more detailed data on the same subject.

Low level of maternal education is another risk factor for low birthweight and is often used as a proxy for socioeconomic status. Table 2.4 shows the relationship between race, education, and low birthweight. In general, black mothers are less educated than white mothers. In 1980, 35 percent of black women who delivered live-born babies had completed less than 12 years of school, versus 20 percent of whites. At the other end of the educational spectrum, 16 percent of white mothers and 6 percent of black mothers were college graduates.[21] Educational differences do not account for the racial differences in low birthweight, however. When matched for both age and education, blacks are still at higher risk of low birthweight.[22] See also Appendix Table B.9.

Black women are more likely than white women to delay initiation of prenatal care.[21] However, when receipt of prenatal care is held constant, black women are still at increased risk of delivering a low birthweight baby.[23] A limitation of most studies in this area is the

TABLE 2.3 Maternal Age and Percentage of Infants Less Than 2,500 Grams, 1976

Maternal Age (years)	White (percent)	Black (percent)
Less than 15	11.8	17.1
15-19	8.1	14.7
20-24	6.0	12.6
25-29	5.3	11.3
30-34	5.8	11.6
35-39	7.0	13.1
40-44	8.3	12.8
45-49	9.4	16.3

SOURCE: National Center for Health Statistics: Factors Associated with Low Birthweight, 1976. Prepared by S Taffel. Vital and Health Statistics, Series 21, No. 37. DHEW No. (PHS) 80-1915. Public Health Service. Washington, D.C.: U.S. Government Printing Office, April 1980.

inability to adjust for the quality or content of prenatal care received. Chapter 6 takes up this issue in detail.

To control for the effects of other variables that may be related to race, such as maternal stature, smoking, and others that are not included on birth certificates, one can look at special studies, such as the Collaborative Perinatal Study, which, though dated, remains an important and detailed survey of a number of important issues and processes in pregnancy. At the time of that project, fewer black than white women smoked, and among the smokers, white women smoked more than black women. When smoking status was controlled, blacks were still twice as likely as whites to have low birthweight infants. The height distributions of blacks and whites were almost identical, while blacks tended toward slightly higher prepregnant weights. At almost every combination of height and weight, and for almost every combination of weight and weight gain, black women were at higher risk of low birthweight than white women. Furthermore, black women were at higher risk of low birthweight at all combinations of age and parity.[20] Finally, it has been shown that women whose last infant was of low birthweight are at increased risk of low birthweight in the current pregnancy.[24] Yet in the Collaborative Study, when women were stratified by whether or not their last child was low birthweight, blacks were still at increased risk of low birthweight during the

TABLE 2.4 Percentage of Single Live Births Less Than 2,500 Grams by Race and Educational Attainment of Mother

Maternal Educational Attainment (years)	White		Black	
	1972 (percent)	1977 (percent)	1972 (percent)	1977 (percent)
Less than 12	7.29	6.99	13.59	13.04
12	5.16	4.74	10.85	10.31
13-15	4.43	4.09	9.76	9.41
16 or more	3.97	3.63	8.92	8.15

NOTE: Adjusted for maternal age and total birth order. Women under age 20 excluded.

SOURCE: National Center for Health Statistics: Trends and variations in birth weight. Prepared by JC Kleinman. In Health, United States, 1981, pp. 7-13. DHHS No. (PHS) 82-1232. Public Health Service. Washington, D.C.: U.S. Government Printing Office, 1981.

current pregnancy.[20] In summary, anthropometric and obstetric differences do not appear to account for the increased risk of low birthweight seen in blacks.

In trying to understand the nature of this risk factor, it is worthwhile to examine the low birthweight incidence among Mexican-Americans, who are economically and sociodemographically similar in some respects to black Americans, yet have been reported to have a very low incidence of low birthweight. In 1979, 5.3 percent of Mexican-American newborns weighed less than 2,500 grams, compared with 5.7 percent of white babies and 12.8 percent of black babies.[21] This low incidence among Mexican-Americans is not readily explained. It may be due in part to problems in data reporting. Selby et al. recently showed, for example, that the Spanish surname infant mortality rate may appear lower than it actually is because of uneven reporting of infant mortality in this population and that it is therefore an inaccurate indicator of Mexican-American health status.[25] Similar data problems may skew reporting of low birthweight. The large difference between black and Mexican-American low birthweight rates also raises the possibility that cultural differences may play a role in pregnancy outcome. The very low incidence of childbearing among unmarried Mexican-American women, unlike that among black women, and their different dietary practices and family structures support this notion. The forthcoming Hispanic HANES survey should provide information on the physical stature and health-related behavior of Mexican-Americans and perhaps help to clarify the reasons for the low rate of low birthweight observed in Mexican-Americans.

The issue of race and low birthweight is further complicated by the different birthweight-specific neonatal mortality rates of white and black infants that have been noted in a variety of populations. Black infants born at less than 2,500 grams have long been recognized to have better rates of survival in the neonatal period than low birthweight white infants of similar birthweights.[26 27]

The conclusion to be drawn from the complicated data on race, low birthweight, and race- and birthweight-specific mortality is that the reasons for the risk differential between white and black neonates are not well understood. The cumulative effects over time of poverty and social neglect, and the interaction of such factors with biological parameters, undoubtedly have played a role in these racial differences; other factors remain to be defined. Research should be pursued to obtain a better understanding of these issues.

Age

U.S. vital statistics data show that in 1978, 17 percent of all births were to teenagers, yet 24 percent of all low birthweight infants had a teenage mother.[28] The relationship of low birthweight to age was shown in Table 2.3 The rate for both whites and blacks is highest at very young ages. It falls throughout the teenage years and reaches its lowest point between 25 and 29 years. Thereafter, the low birthweight rate rises slowly with increasing maternal age.

Teenage mothers, particularly the youngest (under age 15), have many other risk factors that could be responsible for an adverse pregnancy outcome. First births are more likely than later births to be low-weight, and young mothers are more likely to be having their first birth. However, when only first births are examined, teenagers are still at higher risk than older mothers.[22] Very young teenagers having higher-order births are a particularly high-risk group, probably in part because such births imply a short interval between pregnancies, which itself is a risk factor for low birthweight. Thirty percent of second- and higher-order births to women less than 15 in 1978 were low birthweight. Fortunately, there were fewer than 350 such births in the United States in 1978.

Young mothers are more likely to be black and of low socioeconomic status, to report late for prenatal care, and to be unmarried.[28] They tend to be shorter and lighter than their older counterparts.[29] Young teenagers, not being old enough to have completed their schooling, are less educated than older women. These factors in combination appear to account for the higher rate of low birthweight in teenage mothers. For example, in one study, 422 consecutive primigravidas less than 16 years old delivering at a hospital were matched by race to 422 primigravidas aged 20 to 24 delivering at the same hospital. The adolescent mothers delivered infants that were 40 grams lighter on average than the young adult mothers, but the difference was not statistically significant. It was noted that the adolescents were more likely to be clinic patients, unmarried, and live in a census tract with low buying power. They were shorter and lighter as well. When these factors were controlled, newborns of the adolescent mothers were actually slightly heavier than newborns of the older mothers, but again the difference was not significant.[30]

Such studies point to the conclusion that being young biologically is not an independent risk factor for low birthweight and that the increased risk probably comes from other attributes of teenage mothers--such as low socioeconomic status, poor nutritional status, and late receipt of prenatal care. They also illustrate the point made at the beginning of the section on risk factors--that many of the individual risk measures are heavily intertwined and that only a few exert an independent effect.

Socioeconomic Status

Low socioeconomic status (SES) measured in several different ways (social class, income, education, or census tract) is clearly associated with an increased risk of low birthweight and preterm delivery. The literature suggests that at least some of the excess risk is due to other variables that are also associated with both low social class and low birthweight. These include low maternal weight gain and short stature; certain obstetric complications such as hypertension and preeclampsia; possible infection; smoking; and access, source, and utilization of prenatal care. The effect of socioeconomic status is probably the sum of multiple factors, many of which may be affected by specific interventions.

Population-based studies of the role of SES in the pathogenesis of low birthweight are severely limited. Income and occupation data are not generally available, and maternal and paternal education are the only markers of SES present on most birth certificates. For young teenagers and often for other groups as well, SES of the mother's parents probably would be more relevant than the mother's education. Some studies[30] have used the mother's census tract of residence, which is available on birth certificates, to define SES. Most of the studies specifically addressing the role of SES have come from the United Kingdom, particularly the Perinatal Mortality Surveys of 1958 and 1970, in which social class is defined using the Registrar General's system of five social classes represented by Roman numerals I (most privileged) to V (least privileged). British studies may not be directly applicable to the United States. Social class in the United Kingdom is more rigidly defined than it is in the United States, and at the time some of these studies were carried out, the racial/ethnic mixture of the British population was significantly different from that of the United States. More important, the absence of a U.S. analogue of the National Health Service in Britain, which is intended to ensure relatively equal access to and quality of health care regardless of social class, limits the direct application of British data in this area to the United States.

Poverty has been cited by many as a major risk factor for low birthweight. This is supported by reports of a risk of preterm delivery 50 percent higher and a risk of term low birthweight delivery

95 percent higher among women in social classes IV and V as compared with social classes I and II in data derived from the First British Perinatal Mortality Survey.[31] [32] Similarly, a case control study conducted in New Haven, Connecticut, reported a higher rate of preterm delivery among women who were of lower socioeconomic status.[33] The risk diminished, but did not disappear, after adjusting for prepregnant weight, weight gain, alcohol and tobacco consumption, race, parity, and source of prenatal care.

Marital status is a measure related to socioeconomic status and also is important in measuring risk of low birthweight. Of babies born in the United States in 1980, the low birthweight ratio for those whose mothers were unmarried was 11.6 percent, exactly twice as high as the ratio (5.8 percent) for babies with married mothers.[34] Although an increased risk of low birthweight associated with being unmarried apparently exists in all subgroups of the population, the degree of that risk varies with age, race, and other factors. Chapter 3 explores such variations. The significance of marital status as a risk factor is underscored by the dual facts that the proportion of births occurring to unmarried women has been increasing for both white and black women for several decades and that the proportion of out-of-wedlock births to teenagers is also increasing.

Investigators recently have engaged in studies attempting to understand how socioeconomic status, as determined by various measures, affects the risk of low birthweight, i.e., is the relationship a direct one or mediated by other variables known to be associated with both low socioeconomic class and low birthweight? For example, the 1970 British Mortality Survey found that mothers of Social Class I had babies that were on average 161 grams heavier than did mothers of Social Class V. Smoking was inversely correlated with class--upper-class women were less likely to smoke. Among nonsmokers, the weight difference between Social Class I and V was only 90 grams. Thirty-seven percent of the social class difference in birthweight was attributed to smoking.[35] Women of low SES also were shorter than those of high SES in this study. Lower-SES mothers also were more likely to be relatively young or old, and they registered for prenatal care later than did higher-SES women.

Another aspect of low socioeconomic status that may help to explain its relationship to low birthweight is derived from two separate bodies of data: the information that various classes of genital tract infections are associated with low birthweight and the possibility that these organisms may be more prevalent in low SES women. The subject of genital tract infection is discussed in more detail later in this chapter.

Medical and Obstetric Risks

A large number of medical and obstetric factors have been linked to low birthweight, as noted on Table 2.1. Some can be detected before pregnancy, including chronic illness in the mother and a history of obstetric problems; others, such as preeclampsia, arise only during pregnancy. This section focuses on a subset of these major medical and obstetric risks: hypertension/preeclampsia; diabetes; obstetric history, including the role of previous induced abortion; multiple pregnancy; and infection.

Hypertension/Preeclampsia

Hypertension is the disease most often associated with fetal growth retardation and also can be associated with preterm delivery. In a study by Low and Galbraith, 27 percent of IUGR with an identifiable cause could be attributed to severe preeclampsia, chronic hypertensive vascular disease, or chronic renal disease. Infants with IUGR were born to 30 percent of patients with a diagnosis of chronic hypertension and 46 percent of patients with severe preeclampsia.[36]

Low birthweight is strongly linked to maternal blood pressure elevation. Growth retardation of the fetus occurs with hypertension, and preterm delivery may occur (because of abruptio placentae, for example) or be undertaken to terminate the pregnancy when maternal preeclampsia or chronic hypertension are present. In a study of 2,997 normal patients registering early (before the sixteenth week) for prenatal care, Breart et al. examined the relationship between IUGR (defined as a birthweight less than fifth percentile for a given gestational age) and a variety of maternal factors. They reported risk factors for IUGR as mother's age, number of previous pregnancies, birth of a previous low birthweight infant, smoking, and elevation in diastolic blood pressure. IUGR occurred in only 3 percent of births when the diastolic blood pressure was less than 90-mm Hg, 6 percent when it reached 90-mm Hg during pregnancy, and 16 percent when it was 110-mm Hg or more. In their determination of the number of infants with IUGR attributable to hypertension, Breart et al. used the hypothesis that, in the absence of hypertension, the observed rate would be 3.2 percent. According to this hypothesis, 44 of 141 growth-retarded infants, 31 percent, were attributable to hypertension.[37]

Using data from the Collaborative Perinatal Study, Friedman reported on perinatal mortality rates for various levels of systolic and diastolic blood pressure, with and without proteinuria. Mortality rates were higher with elevations in blood pressure and further increased when both elevated blood pressure and proteinuria were present.[38]

Lin et al. reported on fetal outcome among 157 hypertensive patients whose underlying disease had been established by renal biopsy. The perinatal mortality rate was very high, 134 per 1,000. Three-quarters of the deaths were stillbirths; 22 percent of the infants were small for gestational age; and 40 percent were born before term. The highest perinatal mortality was among women with preeclampsia.[39] The fetal growth retardation associated with maternal hypertension is currently attributed to uterine ischemia.[40]

Diabetes

Maternal diabetes mellitus, most often thought of in relation to babies that are large for gestational age, is also associated with an increased risk of both preterm delivery and intrauterine growth retardation. Although these risks have decreased in recent years due to improved management of diabetes, clinicians caring for diabetic women still consider the illness a serious threat to fetal well-being.

In the past, diabetes-related premature births often resulted from physician interventions to avoid unexpected intrauterine deaths. In some cases, the early delivery was appropriate; in others, errors were made in judging fetal maturity. With improved techniques to assess fetal well-being, gestational age, and pulmonary maturity, the number of unnecessary early deliveries associated with maternal diabetes has decreased.[41]

Also in the past, women with insulin-dependent diabetes often suffered from polyhydramnios, probably related to poor control of maternal diabetes. Polyhydramnios contributed to premature labor, which also resulted in the delivery of low birthweight infants. Such polyhydramnios is unusual today; however, Roversi recently observed an increased risk of spontaneous preterm delivery in pregnant patients with diabetes and associated this with poor diabetic control even in the absence of hydramnios.[42] Roversi's findings have not been confirmed by other authors. Premature delivery may be necessary for pregnant women with insulin-dependent diabetes complicated by diabetic vasculopathy. In such cases, preterm delivery may be indicated because of worsening maternal retinopathy, nephropathy, or hypertension. These infants are often both premature and growth retarded.

IUGR has been observed in pregnancies complicated by insulin-dependent diabetes mellitus. As noted above, hypertension and maternal vasculopathy, particularly nephropathy, increase the risks of growth retardation and premature delivery. In a recent series by Kitzmiller, 8.8 percent of women with nephropathy were delivered before 34 weeks as compared to 4.3 percent of other women with diabetes mellitus. The incidence of growth retardation in women with diabetic nephropathy was almost 21 percent, a figure 10 times higher than that for other patients with diabetes mellitus.[43]

Increasing evidence indicates that poor control of maternal diabetes during the early weeks of pregnancy may contribute to both poor fetal growth and congenital anomalies. Molsted-Pedersen, studying women with insulin-dependent diabetes, demonstrated the phenomenon of early growth delay, in which the crown-rump length of the fetus measured in the first trimester by ultrasound lags behind normal development.[44] Such cases are typically found in mothers with poor diabetic control. The fetuses remain small throughout pregnancy, never achieving the weight seen in infants without early growth delay. Furthermore, these fetuses more often have congenital malformations.[45] Fuhrmann has shown that excellent control of maternal diabetes before and during the early weeks of pregnancy will prevent the development of malformations.[46] The effects of such control on the phenomenon of early growth delay have not been explored.

At present, gestational diabetes or carbohydrate intolerance of pregnancy has not been associated with an increased risk of preterm labor in the absence of other contributing factors. Several investigators have observed that hypoglycemia measured by means of glucose tolerance testing may be related to intrauterine growth retardation.[47] Whether this hypoglycemia signals a decrease in the nutrients available to the fetus requires further research.

Obstetric History

The history of a woman's previous pregnancies is of prime importance in the prediction of a subsequent low birthweight infant. Based on a detailed study of the weights and gestational ages of all births in Norway from 1967 through 1973, Bakketeig concluded that a premature first birth is the best predictor of a preterm second birth, and that growth retardation of a first birth is the most powerful predictor of growth retardation during a second pregnancy. The risk of the birth of a subsequent low birthweight infant is 2 to 5 times higher than average for mothers who have had a previous low birthweight delivery and increases with the number of prior low-weight births.[24]

Previous fetal and neonatal deaths also are strongly associated with preterm low birthweight; again, the risk increases as the number of previous poor fetal outcomes goes up. A history of abruptio placentae or isoimmunization is associated with increased risk of premature delivery; the large number of preterm births among previously isoimmunized women may be due in part to medically necessary early cesarean sections or inductions of labor.[48 49]

Although previous pregnancy history is the most reliable predictor of low birthweight in a current pregnancy, this information obviously is not available for women who are having their first baby. Almost 43 percent of all U.S. births in 1980 were to primiparous women, and 87 percent of births to girls under 18 years of age were first births.[50]

Previous Induced Abortion The large number of legal induced abortions--about 1,500,000 occur annually in the United States--makes it important to assess the potential effect of induced abortion on preterm delivery and IUGR in subsequent pregnancies. Hogue et al. have completed two major reviews of studies regarding the effects of induced abortion on subsequent reproduction and the impact of particular abortion techniques on subsequent pregnancy outcomes.[51 52] Most of the studies reviewed by Hogue and her colleagues had important methodological problems, including poor control of confounding variables and conceptual difficulties in defining appropriate comparison groups. Conclusions from these review articles include the following:

- The risk of midtrimester spontaneous abortion, low birthweight, or preterm delivery in a pregnancy following one that is terminated by vacuum aspiration abortion in the first trimester (the most frequently performed abortion procedure in the United States) is no greater than the risk of adverse outcome expected for a first pregnancy.

• Increased risk of both low birthweight and preterm delivery following a first trimester abortion by dilatation and curettage (D and C) under general anesthesia, as distinct from vacuum aspiration, has been reported in some countries, but not in others. Failure to adjust for confounding factors may be responsible for these discrepancies; also, abortion is illegal yet frequently performed in some of these countries, which may affect the data.

• Thirteen epidemiologic studies of pregnancy outcome following more than one induced abortion have failed to disclose a clear pattern. Studies that showed multiple abortions to have adverse effects on rates of ectopic pregnancy, spontaneous abortion, preterm delivery, and low birthweight are offset by investigations that found no increase in the incidence of ectopic pregnancy, spontaneous abortion, preterm delivery, or low birthweight. The studies that demonstrated positive, significant associations between multiple induced abortions and these reproductive problems have generally focused on D and C procedures, especially those requiring relatively wide dilatation of the cervix. Studies of vacuum aspiration have involved too few women to allow for a definitive conclusion about whether that procedure also may have adverse effects when performed more than once. The world literature is too scanty to allow assessment of the effects of the D and E (dilatation and evacuation) procedure (a midtrimester abortion technique), although some concern exists that cervical dilatation of more than 12 mm (required in most D and E procedures) may lead to problems of cervical incompetence.

An additional conclusion that is reasonable to draw from the two review articles of Hogue et al. is that research is needed to investigate further the relationship of induced abortion to subsequent pregnancy outcome. The fact that some studies have suggested an increased risk of preterm delivery associated with induced abortion in some circumstances, coupled with the large number of such procedures in the United States annually, underscore the importance of this research topic.

Multiple Pregnancy

Multiple pregnancies (such as twins or triplets) are associated both with shorter gestation and low birthweight infants. The National Center for Health Statistics reports that, in 1976, plural births were about 9 times as likely to be of low birthweight as single births.[22] The overall incidence of low birthweight in 1976 was 54.3 percent for infants in plural deliveries, compared with 6.3 percent for infants in single deliveries. At full term, infants in plural deliveries were 11 times more likely to be of low birthweight than singleton deliveries. Additionally, plural deliveries are associated with more frequent low Apgar scores, breech position, and maternal complications of labor. Perinatal and neonatal mortality is greatly increased in twin pregnancies and morbidity is high among survivors.

Infections

A variety of infections have been associated with both preterm delivery and intrauterine growth retardation. For some infectious agents, a causal role in low birthweight can be asserted; for others, the situation is less clear. This section highlights selected infections in both categories. Interest in the consequences of infections for both mother and fetus is heightened by the fact that many are amenable to therapy or prevention.

Intrauterine Infection of the Fetus Congenital rubella syndrome in the newborn, resulting from maternal rubella virus infection, is most often thought of in terms of the congenital anomalies that typify the condition. Growth retardation is another cardinal sign of the syndrome. Before introduction of the rubella vaccine, the incidence of fetal infection in the United States was 4 to 30 cases per 1,000 live births.[53] Today, the major reservoir of infection has been decreased significantly by compulsory vaccination of infants and young children, and the number of congenitally infected neonates has been reduced dramatically. Nevertheless, fetal infection with rubella will continue to be seen in the United States until the cohort of women immunized in childhood predominates among women in the childbearing years.

Cytomegalovirus infection, like rubella, also causes fetal growth retardation. Infection with cytomegalovirus is very common in women in the childbearing years: the incidence is 40 to 150 infected mothers per 1,000 pregnancies and 5 to 25 infected fetuses per 1,000 live births.[53] A prototype vaccine for cytomegalovirus has been developed and has resulted in slight protection in susceptible, nonpregnant volunteers.

Genitourinary Infection of the Mother Infections of the genitourinary tract also are relevant to low birthweight. Bacteriuria is present in 3 to 8 percent of pregnant women and varies with parity; the incidence is higher in women of parity greater than three.[54] Untreated or inadequately treated symptomatic urinary tract infections, which may include pyelonephritis, are known to have adverse effects on both mother and fetus, including low birthweight. Among the 55,697 pregnancies followed in the Collaborative Perinatal Study, 1,906 (3.4 percent) had symptomatic urinary tract infections.[55]

The effect on the fetus of untreated asymptomatic genitourinary tract infections during pregnancy is controversial. Studies by Kass and Elder et al. in the 1960s identified a relationship between asymptomatic maternal bacteriuria and low birthweight.[56] [57] The results of other investigations have not consistently demonstrated this relationship. The importance of asymptomatic urinary tract infection may be the subsequent increased incidence of acute pyelonephritis, which, as noted above, is closely associated with low birthweight. In a series reviewed by Kunin, 13 to 40 percent of pregnant women with asymptomatic bacteriuria who were left untreated developed overt signs of urinary tract infection. Most of these symptomatic episodes were acute pyelonephritis.[58] For women with asymptomatic bacteriuria who do not go on to develop acute pyelonephritis, data are not consistent as to whether treatment has a significant positive effect on birthweight or gestational age at birth.[54]

Asymptomatic pregnant women should be screened routinely for bacteriuria, because symptomatic urinary tract infections can be prevented in most patients by treatment of asymptomatic infections. Many tests for bacteriuria have been developed, including various chemical tests and direct cultures. Direct culture is most reliable and is available in an inexpensive and easy-to-use form, the dip slide. This technique utilizes a glass slide coated on both sides with an agar medium. The slide is dipped into the specimen of urine and incubated at room temperature, which is adequate for gram-negative bacteria, the most common cause of bacteriuria. Patients with known infections can be given dip slides and taught to culture their urine at home.[59]

Mycoplasma infection is another possible cause of low birthweight. Braun et al. found that women who were colonized in the genital tract by mycoplasma had more low birthweight infants than women who were not colonized. Multivariate analysis of the data indicated that the relationship of genital mycoplasmas to birthweight was independent of other variables, such as age, race, parity, and maternal weight.[60] Kass et al. reported that mycoplasma-infected pregnant women treated with a 6-week course of erythromycin in the third trimester showed a markedly reduced incidence of low birthweight.[61] These findings are consistent with results from other studies suggesting that infection due to mycoplasma or other organisms susceptible to erthromycin may play a role in fetal development and birthweight. Additional research is needed to confirm such findings and explore their significance.

Chlamydia trachomatis is present in the genital tracts of between 2 and 30 percent of pregnant women. In one recent study, isolation of C. trachomatis from the cervix did not predict low birthweight, prematurity, or premature rupture of the membranes. Increased risk of low birthweight and premature rupture of the membranes did occur, however, among women with immunoglobulin antibody to C. trachomatis.[62] Ascending primary infection due to chlamydia or mycoplasma may cause inflammation of the placenta resulting in poor diffusion of nutrients to the fetus or premature rupture of the membranes.

Interest in the association between certain pathogens and low birthweight also centers on their possible role in triggering preterm labor. Bejar et al. recently postulated that many genital bacteria, including gram-negative enteric organisms and anaerobic bacteria, may provide a stimulus capable of prematurely initiating the biochemical sequence that leads to labor.[63] To determine the importance of such genital infections in the outcome of pregnancy, future studies must comprehensively define the cervical and vaginal flora, and identify local and systemic immune responses.

These research findings, suggesting the important though complicated role of selected infections in low birthweight, led the National Institutes of Health to sponsor a research planning workshop in 1981 on maternal genitourinary infections and the outcome of pregnancy.[54] This workshop was the stimulus for the initiation of a multicenter study of the role of genitourinary infections in the etiology of low birthweight. Women colonized with specific organisms will be invited to participate in a randomized, double-blind trial of one or more antimicrobial agents or placebos from 24-26 weeks until 38 weeks of pregnancy. All women screened will be followed to determine pregnancy outcome. This study, now under way, will help to determine which organisms are associated with prematurity and IUGR, among other outcome measures, and whether antimicrobial treatment could reduce the associated incidence of low birthweight.

Nutrition

This section focuses on a series of nutrition-related factors that have been associated with low birthweight. Some material pertains to the interval before pregnancy, some to the prenatal period.

Four types of research have been used to examine the effect of nutrition during pregnancy on birth outcomes: animal studies; human war famine studies; nutritional intake/fetal outcome correlational studies; and experimental nutrition intervention studies. They all point to a common conclusion: good nutrition has a positive influence on birthweight, but the magnitude of the effect is unclear.

Controlled studies of extreme nutritional deprivation of research animals has shown that consistent restriction of diet during pregnancy (such as reducing dietary intake by 50 percent) results in a marked (25 to 30 percent) decrease in litter birthweight;[64] [65] however, the birthweight reduction is always less than the magnitude of the dietary reduction. Metabolic, tissue, and cellular deficits also have been found with dietary restrictions.[66] [67] Restrictions of diet during the final stage of pregnancy are associated with the largest birthweight deficits.[68] Findings from these animal models cannot, however, be translated directly into human terms. Fetal development consumes a much larger proportion of material resources for small primates than for humans;[69] hence, small primate vulnerability to nutritional restrictions is greater.

Human famines caused by war are an unfortunate analogue of the animal laboratory nutrition reduction studies and have been examined to shed light on the impact of dietary restrictions on human birth outcomes. Studies of the effects of famine on pregnancy outcome during World War II in Leningrad[70] and Holland[71] indicate that extreme, sustained nutritional deprivation can compromise pregnancy outcome and increase the incidence of low birthweight. For example, studies from Leningrad--which experienced extreme food restrictions from September 1941 to February 1942--show marked fetal impact, including a 500-gram reduction in average birthweight, a 50 percent low birthweight rate, a 41.2 percent prematurity rate, and a 32.3 percent overall infant mortality rate. It should be noted, however, that the famine model of absolute deprivation may have only limited applicability to the problem of low birthweight in other settings characterized more by dietary imbalances and/or chronic caloric deprivation.

Studies of nutritional intake/fetal outcome examine the correlation between maternal nutritional intake during pregnancy (using either a direct estimate or an indirect estimate based on maternal weight gain) and the birthweight of the offspring. Nutritional intake, estimated directly from dietary surveys, has proved to be inconsistently related to birth outcomes.[72-75] The methodological limitations of dietary recall studies have hindered this line of research. Many cross-cultural studies show that women from poorer social classes have infants of smaller birthweight than more affluent women. While socioeconomic status factors other than poor nutrition may play a role in this relationship, restricted diets may be a key component.

Poor weight gain during gestation has been widely correlated with decreased fetal weight. Data from the Collaborative Perinatal Study clearly document that increased maternal weight gain is related to larger birthweight, decreased low birthweight rates, and decreased neonatal mortality.[20 76] Low birthweight occurred 4 times more frequently among women who gained less than 14 pounds than among those who gained 30 to 35 pounds.

Consistent with such data are those of Taffel and Keppel, who recently explored the relationship between a mother's weight gain during pregnancy and the occurrence of low birthweight by analyzing data from the 1980 National Natality and Fetal Mortality Surveys.[77] They found that many groups of women known to have an increased risk of delivering a low birthweight infant also were more likely to have inadequate weight gains. For example, they found that black mothers were twice as likely as white mothers to gain less than 16 pounds during pregnancy. Mothers 35 years of age or older and teenage girls were less likely to gain at least 16 pounds, as were unmarried women, poorly educated women, and women of lower socioeconomic status. For married women only, the investigators also examined the relationship between smoking and weight gain, and found that the weight gain of nonsmokers averaged 1.3 pounds more than that of mothers smoking at least 11 cigarettes daily. With regard to pregnancy outcome and weight gain, the authors concluded in their analysis of births to white mothers only that, "after controlling for mother's prepregnant weight, age, education, period of gestation, live birth order, and infant's sex, mothers who gained less than 21 pounds were still 2.3 times as likely to bear low birthweight infants as mothers who gained at least 21 pounds. Except for period of gestation, no other factor has this strong an impact on birthweight. Thus, it is apparent that weight gain is one of the most important correlates of birthweight" (pp. 3-4).

Experimental nutrition supplementation studies, another source of data on nutrition and low birthweight, developed from efforts to test or clinically apply the hypothesis that increased nutritional intake during pregnancy improves birth outcome. These studies are operationally and methodologically problematic and vary widely in quality; none is without critics. Considered together, however, they indicate that supplementation can have small but positive benefits. For example, Stein et al. conclude that prenatal dietary supplements can lead to a modest (40 to 60 grams) rise in birthweight; that a balanced calorie/protein intervention produces more positive benefits than protein-only interventions (which may be harmful, depending on the precise nature of the supplement); and that the optimal time for nutritional intervention remains to be clarified. Several of the supplementation studies specifically showed reductions in the incidence of low birthweight.[78] While the results are generally positive, these studies are sobering because they indicate that extensive nutritional interventions may have only a marginal impact on pregnancy outcome. This conclusion may reflect more on difficulties in assessing supplementation than on the relationship between nutrition and pregnancy.

Complicating the study of the impact of maternal nutrition on low birthweight risk is the fact that, while both nutritional status before pregnancy and nutritional intake during pregnancy influence birthweight, they are not independent. Prepregnancy weight and weight gain during pregnancy are negatively correlated.[79 80] Substantial prepregnancy weight can compensate for low pregnancy weight gain, and vice versa.[81 82] A combined deficit appears to be the most detrimental.[83] The existence of these two compensating maternal nutrition systems--prior nutritional storage and nutritional intake--is clearly protective for the developing fetus; it helps guarantee that adequate nutrition will be available. However, it makes analysis of the impact of nutrition on pregnancy outcome difficult. Maternal dietary inputs or absences during pregnancy do not translate directly into fetal growth or its retardation. The relationship and trade-offs between these two maternal nutrition systems remain to be fully explored.

In sum, the magnitude of nutritional effects on low birthweight is not easily assessed because nutritional status is difficult to isolate from other socioeconomic characteristics and because of the complicated relationship between prepregnant weight and weight gain during pregnancy. While researchers have found positive correlations between birthweight and nutritional status, there is wide variability in the degree of these associations. A reasonable conclusion is that poor nutritional status before pregnancy and inadequate nutritional consumption during pregnancy appear to have a negative impact on fetal weight gain, thereby increasing the risk of low birthweight.

Behavioral and Environmental Risks

This section describes two factors that can contribute to low birthweight, smoking tobacco and drinking alcohol.

Smoking

Smoking is one of the most important preventable determinants of low birthweight in the United States.[84] In 1979, the Surgeon General of the United States warned clearly of the risks to infants of mothers who smoke cigarettes: "Smoking slows fetal growth, doubles the chance of low birthweight and increases the risk of stillbirth. Recent studies suggest that smoking may be a significant contributing factor in 20 to 40 percent of low weight infants born in the United States and Canada."[85]

In so stating, the Surgeon General was summarizing a body of literature on smoking and pregnancy that is by now extensive. In 1957, Simpson first reported that infants of women who smoked during gestation were of significantly lower weight than the infants of comparable nonsmokers.[86] Since that time, more than 50 studies have been published, involving more than half a million births from a broad spectrum of ethnic groups and nationalities, documenting the adverse effect of maternal smoking on birthweight.[87]

After surveying many of these studies, Stein et al. concluded ". . . Smoking during pregnancy is associated with a reduction in birthweight of offspring in the range of 150-250 grams. The relation of number of cigarettes smoked to varying decrements in birthweight is less well defined. Yet smoking, defined grossly by presence or absence, or somewhat more finely in terms of half-packs, has maintained a relatively constant relationship to birthweight over a period of at least 20 years. This constancy has persisted in spite of the reported reduction in the average tar and nicotine yields of the cigarettes marketed. Thus, for reasons that are not yet fully understood, cigarette smoking retards intrauterine growth and it decreases mean gestation by about 1 to 2 days. . . . The association between cigarette smoking and intrauterine growth, over time, through the social classes, over age groups, ethnic groups, and geographic locations remains firm and stable. This consistency brings a weight and certainty to the public health message for reproduction as it does for cancer of the lung. For epidemiologists, consistency is one of the most powerful criteria for judging cause. In cancer of the lung, the processes are also poorly understood, but the label on the cigarette pack is correct. The label should also read that cigarette smoking could be harmful to the fetus" (p. 1154).[88]

The risk of smoking for low birthweight is of heightened concern because of the prevalence of smoking among pregnant women. Although exact rates of smoking during pregnancy are not known, a 1980 Surgeon General's report estimated that 20 to 30 percent of pregnant women in the United States smoke.[89] Such estimates are consistent with figures on smoking rates for U.S. women of childbearing age. In 1980, about a third of women of childbearing age (17 to 39 years of age) smoked.[90] Although smoking is less prevalent among teenagers than among older individuals, it is troublesome to note that teenage girls are more likely to smoke than teenage boys; in 1979, 26 percent of girls 17 to 18 years old smoked, compared to 19 percent of boys in the same age group.[89]

Alcohol

The data on maternal alcohol consumption and its association with low birthweight are not as uniform as for smoking. It is reasonably certain that pregnant women who drink heavily are at risk of delivering a baby with fetal alcohol syndrome--characterized by IUGR and a variety of congenital abnormalities.[91] With regard to moderate or even light alcohol use, however, the data are less clear. Stein et al. recently reviewed a large body of studies on the role of alcohol use in IUGR and concluded that it is "unlikely that regular drinking of fewer than 2 drinks daily either before or during pregnancy is an important determinant of intrauterine growth retardation" (p. 1156).[88]

In contrast, two other recent studies suggest that moderate use of alcohol during pregnancy can compromise birthweight. Mills et al. reported on a prospective study of more than 30,000 pregnancies in women who were part of a health maintenance organization; the study demonstrated a significant increase in the risk of IUGR associated with drinking one to two drinks per day even after adjusting for other important risk factors, such as maternal age, race, education, marital status, maternal weight for height, smoking, parity, prior reproductive history, hypertension, and preeclampsia.[92]

An unpublished report by Graves et al., based on an analysis of the data from the 1980 National Natality and Fetal Mortality Surveys, also demonstrated a significant increase in the rate of low birthweight in married women drinking one or more drinks per day during pregnancy. Again, the researchers controlled for many other variables known to be associated with the rate of low birthweight, including maternal age and race, family income, maternal prepregnant weight and weight gain, maternal and paternal weight-to-height ratios, and maternal smoking.[93]

Because moderate alcohol use during pregnancy may pose added risks to fetal development, common sense suggests avoiding both heavy and moderate alcohol use in pregnancy. Consistent with this cautionary stance, in 1981 the Surgeon General advised pregnant women not to drink alcoholic beverages.

Iatrogenic Risks

Iatrogenic prematurity refers to the birth of a physiologically immature and/or low-weight infant who is delivered prematurely as a result of medical intervention. Justifiable iatrogenic prematurity may result from cesarean sections performed before term to avoid even more serious consequences for the mother or the infant. Some cases of iatrogenic prematurity are accidental, however, resulting either from mistiming of induced labor or nonemergency cesarean section, or from unintentional induction of labor during an oxytocin challenge test or some other procedure. Accidental iatrogenic prematurity is probably most frequently associated with an overestimation of gestational age by physicians responsible for scheduling repeat cesarean sections.

Three studies conducted in the early and mid-1970s found that from 4 to 8 percent of infants admitted to neonatal intensive care units in three different cities had been born prematurely as a result of labor inductions and electively timed cesarean sections.[94-96] In one of these studies, 12 percent of infants admitted to a neonatal intensive care unit over a 6-month period with respiratory distress syndrome (RDS), which is often associated with premature birth, were born after elective intervention.[94] In another study, a full third of cases of RDS in infants seen in a neonatal intensive care nursery, also over a 6-month period, were judged to be the result of inappropriate obstetric intervention.[97] It is difficult to estimate the extent of the problem in more recent years, however.

In 1981, Bowers et al. described 71 cases of newborn RDS following repeat cesarean sections. Although 29 (41 percent) were judged to be at term on the basis of both physical examination and birthweight, at least one critical element of prenatal gestational-age documentation (the date at which unamplified fetal heart tones were first heard) was missing in all 71 cases. Other important pieces of data that were often missing included documentation of the date of quickening, evidence of a positive pregnancy test, and a record of uterine size at the first prenatal visit. In 37 percent of the cases, the recorded uterine fundal height measurement was inconsistent with the date of the last menstrual period, but the inconsistency was ignored. Although ultrasound was used to measure the fetal head in 32 cases, the resulting information was not used correctly in 20 cases.[98]

Such findings are unfortunate, given that it is increasingly possible to prevent a large portion of iatrogenic prematurity by combining accurate prenatal assessment of gestational age with prenatal fetal maturity testing. Taffle et al. describe a study of 252 consecutive, elective, repeat cesarean sections performed at a Naval medical center, in which no cases of iatrogenic prematurity occurred. The authors attribute these results to an obstetric care setting in which the scheduling of repeat sections was controlled by rigid adherence to a clearly defined process of assessing fetal age and maturity.[99] Iatrogenic prematurity also could be reduced by decreasing the persistently high rate of both repeat and primary cesarean sections. Quilligan estimates that the total number of such operations could be reduced by more than half.[100]

Evolving Concepts of Risk

This section explores several risk factors more speculative in nature than those described earlier. They are currently being studied in a variety of settings and may over time evolve into important predictors of low birthweight. These factors are stress; uterine irritability and the notion of "triggering factors"; certain cervical changes; inadequate plasma volume expansion; and progesterone deficiency.

Stress

The relationship between socioeconomic status and low birthweight suggests that a woman's response to and interaction with her environment may have an impact on pregnancy outcome. This concept has led to a variety of studies on the potential effects of certain environmental characteristics. It may be, for example, that poverty is a risk factor for low birthweight partially because of the high levels of stress associated with being poor; the same might be true for the risk factor of being unmarried. Currently, two types of factors are receiving considerable attention: physical stress and fatigue, particularly as related to work during pregnancy; and psychological distress resulting from maternal attitudes toward the pregnancy or from external stressors in the environment.

Physical Stress Numerous studies have examined the risks for both preterm delivery and IUGR posed by physical stress, especially in the work place. The literature in this area is hard to interpret for many reasons. Problems of definition are common, issues of physical and psychosocial stress are often intertwined, and the quality of the study methods varies. Moreover, the studies imply that employment may be more physically stressful than being unemployed--a questionable perspective for some employed pregnant women with young children at home. Studies on employment and pregnancy outcome are further limited by the many differences between working women as a group and unemployed women. The Cardiff Birth Survey clearly documents that women who decide to keep working during pregnancy differ in age and health status from those who do not.[101]

Naeye et al. analyzed data on 7,722 births from the Collaborative Perinatal Study (the data for which were collected between 1959 and 1966) to determine effects of maternal work status during pregnancy. They found that although gestations were not shortened, the newborns of women who worked in the third trimester weighed an average of 150 to 400 grams less than the newborns of nonemployed mothers. The growth retardation was greatest among infants whose mothers' jobs required standing much of the time and increased as the mothers worked further into the third trimester. Low prepregnancy weight, poor weight gain during pregnancy, and hypertension were also associated with lower birthweights.[102] A similar association between prematurity and some occupational categories was noted by Mamelle et al.[103] In contrast, the Cardiff Birth Survey found virtually no ill-effects associated with employment. In fact, a significantly higher proportion of births were growth retarded in the unemployed groups than in the employed groups, even after controlling for adverse medical and obstetric history.[101]

In general, the work-related studies and a major study of overall physical stress by Papiernik et al.[104] indicate that there is probably some association between low birthweight, manifested as both IUGR and prematurity, and activities that require long periods of standing or other substantial amounts of physical stress. It cannot be concluded, however, that maternal employment as such increases the risk of low birthweight.

Psychological Stress Historically, concern about the effect of psychological stress emerged in the context of studies exploring the normal emotional changes that occur as a woman faces the many changes occasioned by pregnancy and motherhood.[105] More recently, researchers have addressed the effect of maternal stress on pregnancy outcome. The results have been mixed. In some studies, the proportion of women with evidence of adverse psychological states has been found to be higher among women who had deliveries considered "abnormal" by their obstetricians[106-113]; this effect appeared to depend partly on the timing of the stress in relation to delivery[112] and on the presence of psychosocial supports.[113] In other studies, however, no association has been found between increased stress and adverse pregnancy outcome; for example, no differences in outcome were noted between women refused abortions and comparison groups.[114-116]

Many studies have noted a relationship between stress and conditions that increase the risk of IUGR and preterm labor, such as toxemia, but data supporting a specific relationship between maternal psychological distress and low birthweight are not strong. Other adverse outcomes have been associated with maternal psychosocial distress, including perinatal death and congenital anomalies,[118] fetal distress,[108] neonatal motor immaturity,[107] and depressed Apgar scores[118] (this particular association was not found by another group[119]). However, only one study has linked psychosocial stress with premature labor; researchers found higher stressful event scores among women in preterm labor as compared to those in labor at term.[117]

In summary, numerous studies suggest a link between maternal psychological stress and adverse pregnancy outcome generally, but the impact of stress on low birthweight specifically needs further investigation. Many studies suffer from a serious methodological flaw--the stress is ascertained after the event (the study by Nuckolls et al.[113] is an important exception). Such retrospective studies introduce the potential of recall bias, which could increase the reporting of stress and stressful events among mothers with adverse outcomes. The studies are also difficult to interpret in the aggregate because concepts and definitions of stress vary significantly. Sample sizes, too, are often very small, which makes it difficult to isolate the specific outcome of low birthweight; all poor outcomes are usually combined into a single measure. Also, the studies usually fail to control for smoking behavior, a major correlate of low birthweight.

Uterine Irritability

The precise role that uterine irritability plays in the pathophysiology of preterm labor is not well understood. The contractile state of the uterus is modified by various physiologic and endocrine states. This subject was recently reviewed by Hobel.[14] The natural history or the evolution of uterine activity and its sensitivity to oxytocin has been studied by Calderyo-Barcia.[120] Before 30 weeks, the uterus shows minimal spontaneous uterine activity. Between 30 weeks and term, however, the uterus exhibits more spontaneous activity and is more sensitive to oxytocin.

The notion that uterine activity might be a risk factor for preterm labor was first suggested by Wood et al. in 1965.[121] In 1981, Suranyi and Szomolya published evidence suggesting that contractility in the subclinical phase of preterm labor could be a reliable method for predicting the onset of preterm labor.[122] Recently Tamby Raja et al. studied the diurnal rhythm of uterine activity in normal, low-risk pregnancies and found, as noted above, minimal activity before 30 weeks.[123] Between 30 and 36 weeks, however, women had mild spontaneous uterine contractions, primarily in the morning and afternoon from 7 A.M. until 5 P.M. During the remainder of the 24-hour cycle, the uterus was quiet at this gestational stage. Between 36 weeks and term, mild uterine contractions began to be detected from 6 P.M. to midnight as well, although from midnight until 6 A.M. the uterus remained quiet as it was at earlier gestational stages. By contrast, patients at high risk for preterm labor were found to have uterine activity throughout the 24-hour cycle in this latter part of pregnancy.

Such studies suggest that excessive uterine activity may be a component of the events leading up to true preterm labor. Assessing the extent of uterine activity could be a part of the surveillance of patients at risk for preterm labor.

Closely related to assessing uterine activity is the possibility that certain events can "trigger" uterine contractions, which in turn can lead to preterm labor. For example, all of the prematurity prevention programs described in Appendix C include patient education for high-risk women concerning the concept of triggering factors, self-detection of uterine contractions, and the advisability of avoiding events or situations that appear to stimulate such contractions. Program personnel describe wide variation in the types of events that women report as stimulating uterine contractions--sexual activity, climbing several flights of stairs, lifting heavy loads, and others.

Sexual intercourse also has been discussed as a risk factor for preterm labor because of the possibility that coitus can be a means of transferring pathogenic bacteria to the urinary tract or to the cervical opening and thus to the amniotic membranes. Also, it has been suggested that absorbed seminal prostaglandins may initiate uterine contractions. Research in all these areas is inconclusive, however.[124]

Cervical Changes

Several studies have suggested that cervical assessment may be another means to detect heightened risk for preterm labor. For example, part of Papiernik's and Creasy's approach to identifying women at risk of preterm delivery, described in Appendix C, involves serial pelvic exams to evaluate the cervix--primarily its shortness and state of dilatation.[104, 158] The station of the presenting part and thinness of the lower uterine segment also may be important.

The value of cervical assessment in later pregnancy may lie in its ability to identify changes that occur several days, and sometimes even weeks before preterm labor. These changes may be early signs of risk and, if identified, could lead to interventions designed to prevent further changes within the cervix. A second reason for identifying early changes is that once the cervix opens, the uterine environment is exposed to ascending pathogenic bacteria and the risk of infection increases. There may, however, be a potential risk in the repeated pelvic exams required to monitor cervical changes. A recent prospective study by Lenihan of patients at term showed a significant relationship between weekly pelvic exams and premature rupture of the membranes.[125] At present, no data exist on the risks of frequent pelvic exams in patients prior to term. The technique of the pelvic exam may be important, an issue not described in the Lenihan study.

Another potential problem associated with cervical assessment is that the identification of a short cervix, either by ultrasound or by pelvic exam, increases the likelihood of the physician initiating some form of intervention, including cervical cerclage, which itself carries risks. Recently, concern has been expressed about the marked increase in the use of cervical cerclage in some developed countries. This concern has led to the initiation of prospective randomized trials in both France and Great Britain.[126] These studies, when complete, should identify the types of patients, other than those with classical incompetent cervix, who might benefit from this more aggressive form of therapy.

Inadequate Plasma Volume Expansion

Plasma volume increases at least 30 percent during pregnancy.[127] Most of this increase occurs before 24 weeks gestation. Because plasma volume increases more than red blood cell volume between the twenty-fourth and thirty-fourth weeks, normal pregnant women generally have lowered hematocrits. Failure to expand blood volume has been associated with an increased risk of pregnancy-induced hypertension, IUGR, and preterm labor.

Goodlin et al. found significantly lower maternal plasma volumes in all three of the above disorders.[128] They also showed that therapy for preterm labor--betamimetics, bedrest, hydration, and plasma volume expansion with 5 percent albumin--increased plasma volume at least 15 percent. Prospective randomized trials are needed to determine whether plasma volume expansion prevents preterm labor in women with low plasma volumes.

Progesterone Deficiency

Progesterone, a key hormone for the maintenance of pregnancy, preserves uterine quiescence. It helps to stabilize the physiologic properties of both the muscle cell wall[129] and fetal membranes, and prevents the release of arachidonic acid, a precursor of prostaglandins.[130] A few studies have suggested that progesterone deficiency and decreasing progesterone levels are associated with preterm[131-133] and term labor,[5] respectively; this possible association remains controversial, however.

In 1977, Cousins et al. reported significantly lower maternal serum progesterone levels in patients in preterm labor when compared to normal controls.[133] At about the same time, Csapo and Herezeg also reported significantly lower progesterone concentrations in patients with preterm labor.[131] These investigators reported that maternal progesterone concentrations increased in patients successfully treated with isoxsuprine hydrochloride, a labor-suppressing agent. Neither group, however, measured progesterone before preterm labor to determine whether the low progesterone levels were a consequence of preterm labor or a factor predictive of preterm labor. There are limited data to suggest that low progesterone levels precede preterm labor.[132 134]

Studies to show the efficacy of progestational agents in the prevention of preterm labor are limited.[132 135-137] Potential risks to the fetus associated with the use of progestational agents have led the FDA to recommend that there is no justification for using progestogens in threatened abortion or as a pregnancy test in the first 4 months of pregnancy.[138] The risks of these agents after 20 weeks is unknown.

Risk Assessment

In an effort to use risk factor data to help structure prenatal care for pregnant women, researchers have developed a variety of techniques to measure risk status--that is, to distinguish women at high risk of preterm labor or IUGR from women at low risk. The following section discusses the evolving science of risk assessment and includes a critical review of several risk assessment instruments.

Risk management techniques originated in 1962 with the development of "risk registers" in England; however, until 1969, little appeared in the obstetric literature. A detailed review of the literature since that time indicates that much of the work to date has been directed toward predicting perinatal and neonatal mortality.[139-141] Relatively less work has been devoted to predicting low birthweight.

Papiernik was the first to report on a method developed solely for identifying the patient at risk for preterm labor.[142 143] Other European work has focused on the development of a screening system and program to prevent low birthweight related to both prematurity and IUGR.[144]

In the United States, these approaches have been modified and augmented in an effort to improve their predictive power. Several researchers have attempted to incorporate biochemical, ultrasound, and other diagnostic information into more sophisticated mathematical models.[145-148] Others have tried to simplify the content of the risk instruments while retaining their predictive value.[149 150] However, both the difficulty of such an undertaking, especially for distinguishing women at risk for intrauterine growth retardation, and the need for further improvement continue to receive attention.[151-153]

Screening for Obstetric Risk

The design of a risk assessment instrument begins with decisions about what outcome is to be predicted and which factors are to be reviewed to predict risk. In obstetrics, the factors generally constitute a subset of the risk factors listed in Table 2.1, selected on the basis of the literature or the experience of the designer. The factors are given numerical weights and grouped in some fashion to provide a score. This score is used to assess the probability that an individual woman is at risk of, for example, a preterm delivery.

The basis of selection of the risk factors, the determination of a numerical weight for each factor, and the cut-off point indicating "high risk" are relatively controversial.[154-157] Moreover, the scores are statements of probability and cannot be viewed as definitive predictors for a specific woman. Also, the instruments achieve standardization in the characterization of risk at the expense of an appreciation of the dynamic nature of the individual course. Nonetheless, these instruments have been shown to be useful clinical tools.

Understanding the use of risk assessment instruments requires an appreciation of certain screening principles. First, accuracy in the prediction of risk is defined in terms of sensitivity (the ability of the instrument to identify those with adverse outcomes such as low birthweight) and specificity (the ability to detect those without adverse outcomes) (Table 2.5). These are called true positives (a) and true negatives (d), respectively. Those who score in the high-risk range but do not have an adverse outcome are labelled false positives (b); those scoring in the low-risk range but experiencing adverse outcomes are called false negatives (c). For any instrument, the sensitivity and specificity can be changed by selecting a different cut-off point to designate "high-risk," but this always involves a trade-off. Selecting a lower score (i.e., fewer risk factors) will increase the sensitivity, but more false positives also will be identified (i.e., fewer will be identified as true negatives). The converse occurs when a higher cut-off point is selected, i.e., an increase in specificity (true negatives) but a decrease in sensitivity (true positives).

A high sensitivity (i.e., a high rate of detecting those with adverse outcomes) appears desirable until the implications of large numbers of false positives are appreciated. These implications are best conveyed by an examination of the proportion of those predicted at high risk who eventually experience the adverse outcome, the predictive value positive (PV+). A low PV+ indicates that many more women are predicted to be at high risk than actually have adverse outcomes. This overdiagnosis will affect the cost of services, because women classified as high risk will receive special (and often more expensive) care, but do not develop the problem(s) being predicted by the risk assessment. In addition, women misclassified as high risk may experience complications of unnecessary diagnostic and therapeutic procedures. The risk of overdiagnosis is dependent on the prevalence of the adverse outcome in the population. For a risk assessment

TABLE 2.5 Validity Measures of Screening Tests

Risk Status	Adverse Outcome[a] Present	Absent	Total
High Risk	(a)	(b)	(a+b)
Low Risk	(c)	(d)	(c+d)
Total	(a+c)	(b+d)	(a+b+c+d)

Sensitivity = a/a+c
Specificity = d/b+d[b]

Predictive Value + (of high risk) = a/a+b[c]
Predictive Value - (of low risk) = d/c+d[c]

[a]Preterm labor or intrauterine growth.
[b]Properties of instrument, not dependent on nature of population.
[c]Depends on prevalence of outcome in population.

instrument of a given sensitivity and specificity, the lower the prevalence of the adverse outcome in the population, the more likely it is that a woman classified as high risk will be a false positive.

Instruments designed to predict low birthweight and preterm birth are summarized in Table 2.6. To illustrate the points above, the sensitivity and specificity of these instruments and their PV+ in different populations are summarized in Table 2.7. The sensitivity values extend over a wide range, but the majority correctly identify as high risk approximately 65 percent or more of those with eventual adverse outcomes. The sensitivity is higher for multiparous women than for primiparous women, probably because prior obstetric experience is such a strong predictor of subsequent obstetric risk. In general, more than half of women with low birthweight infants will be identified by these instruments. This also means, however, clinicians must continue to expect the occurrence of low-weight births among women determined to be at low risk of such an outcome.

Even using some of the better risk-assessment systems, several women who are judged to be high risk but eventually turn out not to be so will receive special care for every truly high-risk woman identified with a risk assessment instrument. Although this may seen undesirable, the alternative must be considered. As shown in the Table 2.7, the proportion with low birthweight or preterm labor in the populations studied ranges from 2 to 8 percent. To reduce the risk of adverse outcome without some form of risk assessment would require special services for all.

TABLE 2.6 Scoring Methods for Low Birthweight and Preterm Birth Risk Classification

		Risk Assessment Method												
				Scoring Method										
		Factors[a]		Manner of Weighting[b]			Outcome Used For Calculating Weights[c]				Score For Risk Group			Problems System Used to Predict (Definition if Given)
Authors	Date	No.	Sys.	Arbit. & Lit	Mvar.	R.R.	All LBW	All PTB	P-LBW	T-LBW	High Risk	Medium Risk	Low Risk	
Papiernik-Berkhauer	1969	30	RPD[d]	X			?	X			≥10	9-5	<5	P-LBW, T-LBW
Kaminski et al.	1973	13			X		X				>8.5	8.5-5.6	≤5.5	LBW (≤2,500 grams)
					X			X			>13	13.0-9.1	≤9.0	PTB (≤36 weeks)
Kaminski & Papiernik	1974	35	RPD		X		X				≥7	6-4	≤3	LBW (≤2,500 grams)
Creasy et al.	1980	35	RPD	X			?	X			≥10	9-5	<5	PTB (≤37 weeks)
Giffei & Saling	1974	36	PDP[e] list II	X ?			X		X	X	≥6		0-5	LBW, T-LBW (≤2,500 grams)
Fedrick	1976	10				X			X		≥1		<1	P-LBW (≤37wk & <2,500 grams)
Adelstein & Fedrick	1978	(Same as Fedrick)				X				X	≥1		<1	T-LBW (>38 weeks and ≤2,500 grams)
Wennergren & Karlsson	1982	8	gravido-gram		X		X				≥4		<4	LBW (≤-2 SD)[f]
Ross et al.	1984	24	POPRAS[g]		X			X			>-2.8		≤-2.7	PTB (≤36 weeks but >20 weeks)
Sokol et al.	1983	8-9	POPRAS			X				X ?		???		T-LBW

Belizan et al.	1978	2	X	X	X	<10th percentile	10-90th percentile	P-LBW and T-LBW weight <10th percentile for gestational age
Quaranta et al.	1981	2	X	X	X	<10th percentile	10-90th percentile	P-LBW and T-LBW weight ≤10th percentile for gestational age
Nielson et al.	1980	3	X	X	X	<10th percentile	10-90th percentile	P-LBW and T-LBW weight <5th percentile for gestational age

NOTE: Horizontal lines group instruments that assess sets of factors derived from similar risk assessment systems.

[a]No. = number; Sys. = system
[b]Arbit. & Lit. = arbitrary decision and from literature; Mvar. = multivariate analysis technique; R.R. = relative risk
[c]Outcome served as the denominator in analysis to assign points (weights) to each factor in system.
"All LBW" means authors used, all low-weight births without regard for gestational age. "All PTB" means authors used all preterm births without regard for birthweight. P-LBW = preterm and low birthweight; T-LBW = term and low birthweight.
[d]RPD = Risk of preterm delivery.
[e]PDP = Prematurity & dysmaturity prevention.
[f]SD = Standard deviation.
[g]POPRAS = Problem oriented perinatal risk assessment system.

TABLE 2.7 Sensitivity, Specificity and Predictive Value of Risk Classification System for Predicting Low Birthweight and Preterm Birth

				Percentage in Each Risk Group			System Accuracy[c]						
Author	Date	Outcome Predicted[a]	System Used[b]	High Risk	Medium Risk	Low Risk	Percentage in Pop.	Sens. (percent)	Spec. (percent)	FP (percent)	FN (percent)	PV+ (percent)	R.R.
Kaminski et al.	1973	LBW ≤2,500 grams	16	22	62	4	39	63	15	36	10	4	
Kaminski & Papiernik	1974	LBW ≤2,500 grams	RPD	?[e]	?	?	--	54	64	17	27	NC[f]	
			DFA	?	?	?	--	66	67	14	26	NC	
Giffei & Saling	1974	LBW ≤2,500 grams	PDP	42	-- (includes those not treated)	58	6	84	60	40	16	11	7
Wennergren & Karlsson	1982	LBW <-2 SD[g]	historical and gravidogram	7	--	93	2	100	95	5	0	34	Inf.[h]
Kaminski et al.	1973	PTB ≤36 weeks		16	22	62	8	30	68	13	42	17	3
Creasy et al.	1980	PTB ≤37 weeks	RPD	68 ALL DELIVERIES	19	13	6	64	12	68	20	6	0.6
				9 PRIMIGRAVIDAS	25	66	6	31	68	7	44	21	5
				15 MULTIGRAVIDAS	16	69	6	77	72	10	12	33	31
Ross et al.	1984	PTB ≤36 weeks	POPRAS	35 ALL DELIVERIES	--	65	6	59	64	36	41	9.8	2
				? PRIMIGRAVIDAS	--	?	?	46	71	29	54	?	?
				? MULTIGRAVIDAS	--	?	?	64	61	39	36	?	?

Fedrick	1976	P-LBW ≤37 weeks and <2,500 grams		40 PRIMIPARAS	--	60	2	70	60	40	30	3	4
				26 MULTIPARAS	--	74	2	74	75	25	26	5	8
Adelstein & Fedrick	1978	T-LBW >38 weeks and ≤ 2,500 grams	Fed[i]	19 PRIMIPARAS	--	81	3	46	82	18	55	5	4
				12 MULTIPARAS	--	88	2	58	89	11	42	12	10
Sokol et al.	1983	T-LBW ?	POPRAS	?	--	?	?	50	?	?	?	34	?
			plus oligo-hydramnios	?	--	?	?	76	?	?	?	47	?
Belizan et al.	1978	P&T-LBW	uterine height	34	--	66	32	86	90	10	14	79	12
Quaranta et al.	1981	P&T-LBW	uterine height	39	--	61	32	73	77	23	24	60	4
Nielson et al.	1980	P&T-LBW	ultra-sound	18	--	82	8	94	88	12	6	39	76

NOTE: Horizontal lines group risk classification systems predicting the same outcome, listed under the column, "Outcome Predicted."

[a]LBW = low birthweight; PTB = preterm birth; T-LBW = term and low birthweight; P-LBW = preterm and low birthweight.
[b]RPD = Risk of preterm delivery; DFA = discriminant function analysis; PDP = prematurity and dysmaturity prevention; POPRAS = Problem oriented perinatal risk assessment system
[c]Only highest risk group included in sensitivity and false negative results; only lowest risk group included in specificity and false positive results. Sens. = sensitivity; Spec. = specificity; FP = false positive; FN = false negative; PV+ = predictive value of high risk; RR = relative risk.
[d]Percentage of the population with the condition.
[e]? = not stated.
[f]NC = not calculated.
[g]SD = standard deviation
[h]Inf. = infinity
[i]Fed. = Fedrick

Strengths and Limitations

Well-constructed risk assessment instruments have the potential to reduce the misdiagnosis of both IUGR and preterm labor and are useful adjuncts to clinical judgment in evaluating the risk of low birthweight.[145] In addition, they offer the possibility of grouping risk factors by their modifiability or preventability, thereby suggesting potential interventions. The effects of such an approach have been explored by at least two investigators.[140 144] Finally, risk assessment systems encourage more appropriate referrals for care and more reasonable expenditures of resources for the management of preterm birth.[134 158 159]

The limitations also must be recognized. First, because the performance of a risk assessment instrument is to some extent dependent on the prevalence of adverse outcome in a population, it is unlikely to produce the same results in every setting. Second, the instrument cannot be used in a rote manner as a substitute for high-quality professional care. Errors in classification occur, so some degree of continued monitoring of low-risk women is required, as well as attention to the more generic needs of all pregnant women for support and education to make pregnancy a positive experience and to enhance their ability to care for a new child.

Improving Risk Assessment

Further refinement of our knowledge about the etiology, natural history, and epidemiology of low birthweight, and about associated risk factors, will contribute to improvements in the science of risk assessment. Information is needed to permit a clearer delineation of which outcomes to predict, which factors to monitor, and which weights to assign to individual factors. Other ways to strengthen the impact of risk assessment include establishing more uniform outcome definitions to allow comparisons among risk assessment instruments; testing various risk assessment methods in the same population; testing risk assessment instruments on populations other than those contributing to their development (Papiernik has shown a clear drop in the correlation of risk value and outcome between the group from which a risk assessment instrument was developed and a test group[160]); and designing systems to permit some degree of individualization of the risk score, if such systems are not too complicated to use. Finally, users of risk assessment instruments should receive more explanation of the utility and expectations of risk scores and of the probabilities they represent.

Conclusions

The risk factor literature suggests several conclusions. A variety of factors are clearly and consistently linked to low birthweight and can be used to help define high-risk groups and to target resources for intervention. Important ones listed at the beginning of the chapter include several sociodemographic factors; various medical and obstetric risks; certain behavioral, environmental, and occupational factors; and selected risks based in health care practices. It is also apparent that risks for low birthweight are widely distributed throughout the population and that a substantial amount of low birthweight will continue to occur outside of groups defined as high risk. This fact highlights the need for greater understanding of risk and etiology; it should not be used to minimize the value of using existing risk information for targeting interventions.

Risk factor data also suggest another conclusion. Many of the established risk factors are amenable to prevention or therapy, and of these, many can be recognized before pregnancy occurs. Smoking is perhaps the best example. Other examples include poor nutritional status, certain chronic illnesses, and susceptibility to infections such as rubella. Even demographic risk factors such as age can be managed before conception, for instance, by avoiding pregnancy at extremes of the reproductive age span; and the risks posed by high parity and brief interval between pregnancies can be decreased through family planning.

Another major conclusion that emerges from the literature on the etiology of low birthweight is that more research is needed to answer a very long list of questions. Our understanding of the basic causes of preterm labor and IUGR is seriously inadequate. A 1983 workshop sponsored by the National Institute of Child Health and Human Development[161] outlined promising research areas pertinent to IUGR, and a recent review article by Huszar and Naftolin[1] touches on a number of topics that should be studied to provide a better understanding of the normal onset of labor and of the pathogenesis and process of preterm labor. In the absence of more complete information about basic causal mechanisms, efforts to prevent low birthweight will remain limited.

Factors whose role in low birthweight are uncertain need additional analysis. Stress, for example, may be a significant risk factor for both IUGR and preterm labor, but more research is needed to understand the nature and magnitude of this risk. Other possibilities that merit study include, for example, the role of selected genitourinary infections in low birthweight, the natural history of uterine activity throughout pregnancy (to determine the value of uterine activity assessment as an index in evaluating the risk of preterm labor), and related topics mentioned in the section on evolving concepts of risk.

Well-established risk factors also require more attention. For some factors, such as race, research is needed to understand why the risk exerts its effect. For others, such as alcohol, the magnitude of risk at various levels of consumption needs to be better defined.

For both known and less-certain risk factors, efforts should be made to distinguish risks for very low birthweight (1,500 grams or less) from risks for moderately low birthweight (1,500 to 2,500 grams) at various gestational ages. As Chapter 3 suggests, the incidence trends and sequelae of these two classes of low birthweight differ. Relating individual risk factors to more refined measures of low birthweight should provide clues to both cause and prevention.

The committee's review of risk assessment systems and instruments suggests that they are helpful in distinguishing between high- and low-risk women. The significant incidence of low birthweight deliveries in low-risk individuals and groups suggests, however, that additional research is needed to improve the predictive capability of these systems. It also indicates that clinicians must be alert to the possibility of low birthweight even in pregnant women judged to be at low risk of such an outcome.

References

1. Huszar G and Naftolin F: The myometrium and uterine cervix in normal and preterm labor. N. Engl. J. Med. 311:571-581, 1984.
2. Barden TP: Premature labor. In Neonatal-Perinatal Medicine, edited by AA Fanaroff and RJ Martins, pp. 139-144. St. Louis: The C.V. Mosby Co., 1983.
3. Speroff L, Glass RH, and Kase NG, eds.: Clinical Gynecologic Endocrinology and Infertility, 3rd Edition, pp. 316-322. Baltimore/London: Williams and Wilkins, 1983.
4. Liggins GC: Premature delivery of foetal lambs infused with ghicocorticoids. J. Endocrinol. 45:515-523, 1969.
5. Turnbull AC, Flint APF, Jeremy JY, Patten PT, Keirse MJNC, and Anderson ABM: Significant fall in progesterone and rise in estradiol levels in human peripheral plasma before onset of labour. Lancet I:101-104, 1974.
6. Novy MJ and Liggins GC: Role of prostaglandins, prostacyclin and thromboxanes in the physiologic control of the uterus and in parturition. Seminar Perinatol. 4:45-66, 1980.
7. Challis JRG and Mitchell F: Hormonal control of preterm and term parturition. Seminar Perinatol. 5:192-202, 1981.
8. Carsten MF: Calcium accumulation by human uterine microsomal preparations: Effects of progesterone and ocytocin. Am. J. Obstet. Gynecol. 133:598-601, 1979.
9. Tamby Raja RL, Anderson ABM, and Turnbull AC: Endocrine changes in premature labor. Br. Med. J. 4:67-71, 1974.
10. Creasy RK and Liggins GC: Actiology and management of preterm labour. In Recent Advances in Obstetrics and Gynecology edited by J Stallworthy and GG Bourne, pp. 21-45. Edinburg: Churchill Livingstone, 1979.
11. Shanklin DR: Influence of placental lesions on newborn infants. Pediatr. Clin. North Am. 17:25-42, 1970.
12. Gruenwald P: Chronic fetal distress and placental insufficiency. Biol. Neonat. 5:215-265, 1963.
13. Scott KE and Usher R: Fetal malnutrition: Its incidence, causes and effects. Am. J. Obstet. Gynecol. 94:951-963, 1966.
14. Hobel CJ: Prevention of preterm delivery. In Fetal Physiology and Medicine, edited by RW Beard and PW Nathaniels, pp. 757-779. New York: Marcel Dekker, 1984.
15. Kliegman R and Kins K: Intrauterine growth retardation: Determinants of aberrant fetal growth. In Neonatal-Perinatal

Medicine, edited by AA Fanaroff and RJ Martins, pp. 49-80. St. Louis: C.V. Mosby, 1983.

16. Behrman RE and Kliegman R: The fetus and the neonatal infant. In Nelson Textbook of Pediatrics, edited by RE Behrman and VC Vaughan III. 12th Edition, pp. 322-416. Philadelphia: W.B. Saunders, 1983.

17. Siegel LS: Reproductive, perinatal, and environmental variables as predictors of development of preterm (less than 1501 grams) and fullterm children at 5 years. Semin. Perinatol. 6:274-279, 1982.

18. Davies DD: Growth of "small for dates" babies. Early Hum. Devel. 5:95-104, 1981.

19. Kessel SS, Villar J, Berendes HW, and Nugent RP: The changing pattern of low birth weight in the United States: 1970-1980. JAMA, 251:1978-1982, 1984.

20. Niswander KR and Gordon M: The Women and Their Pregnancies: The Collaborative Perinatal Study of the National Institute of Neurologic Diseases and Stroke. Philadelphia: W.B. Saunders Company, 1972.

21. National Center for Health Statistics: Births of Hispanic Parentage, 1979. Prepared by SJ Ventura. Monthly Vital Statistics Report, Vol. 31, No. 2 (supplement). Public Health Service. Washington, D.C.: U.S. Government Printing Office, May 1982.

22. National Center for Health Statistics: Factors Associated with Low Birth Weight: United States, 1976. Prepared by S Taffel. Vital and Health Statistics, Series 21, No. 37. DHEW No. (PHS) 80-1915. Public Health Service. Washington, D.C.: U.S. Government Printing Office, April 1980.

23. Mark Klebanoff, Epidemiology and Biometry Research Program, National Institute of Child Health and Human Development, Bethesda, Md. Personal communication, 1984, based on an analysis of 1977-1981 birth certificate data from Baltimore, Maryland, and on the 1974-1977 Northern California Kaiser-Permanente Birth Defects Study.

24. Bakketeig LS, Hoffman HJ, and Harley EE: The tendency to repeat gestational age and birth weight in successive births. Am. J. Obstet. Gynecol. 135:1086-1103, 1979.

25. Selby ML, Lee ES, Tuttle DM, and Loe HD Jr: Validity of the Spanish surname infant mortality rate as a health status indicator for the Mexican American population. Am. J. Public Health 74:988-1002, 1984.

26. Williams RL: Measuring the effectiveness of perinatal medical care. Med. Care 17:95-110, 1979.

27. North AF and MacDonald HM: Why are neonatal mortality rates lower in small black infants than in white infants of similar birthweight? J. Pediatr. 90:809-810, 1977.

28. National Center for Health Statistics: Vital Statistics of the United States, 1978. Vol. I. DHHS No. (PHS) 82-1100. Public Health Service. Washington, D.C.: U.S. Government Printing Office, 1982.

29. Garn SM, and Petzold SB: Characteristics of mother and child in teenage pregnancies. Am. J. Dis. Child. 137:365-368, 1983.

30. Horon IL, Strobino DM, and MacDonald HM: Birth weights among infants born to adolescent and young adult women. Am. J. Obstet. Gynecol. 146:444-449, 1983.

31. Fedrick J and Anderson ABM: Factors associated with spontaneous preterm birth. Br. J. Obstet. Gynaecol. 83:342-350, 1976.

32. Fedrick J and Adelstein P: Factors associated with low birth weight of infants delivered at term. Br. J. Obstet. Gynaecol. 85:1-11, 1978.

33. Berkowitz GS: An epidemiological study of preterm delivery. Am. J. Epidemiol. 113:81-92, 1981.

34. National Center for Health Statistics: Vital Statistics of the United States, 1980. Vol. 1: Natality. Public Health Service. Washington, D.C.: U.S. Government Printing Office, in press.

35. Rush D and Cassano P: Relationship of cigarette smoking and social class to birthweight and perinatal mortality among all births in Britain, 5-11 April, 1970. J. Epidemiol. Commun. Health 37:249-255, 1983.

36. Low JA and Galbraith RS: Pregnancy characteristics of intrauterine growth retardation. Obstet. Gynecol. 44:122-126, 1974.

37. Breart G, Rabarison Y, Plouin PF, Sureau C, and Rumeau-Roquette C: Risk of fetal growth retardation as a result of maternal hypertension: Preparation for a trial on antihypertensive drugs. Dev. Pharmacol. Ther. 4(supplement): 116-123, 1982.

38. Friedman EA and Neff RK: Pregnancy outcome as related to hypertension, edema, and proteinuria. In Hypertension in Pregnancy, edited by MD Lindheimer, AI Katz, and FP Zuspan, pp. 13-22. New York: John Wiley & Sons, 1976.

39. Lin CC, Lindheimer MD, River P, and Moawad AH: Fetal outcome in hypertensive disorders of pregnancy. Am. J. Obstet. Gynecol. 142:255-260, 1982.

40. Lunell NO, Sarby B, Lewander R, and Nylund L: Comparison of uteroplacental bloodflow in normal and in intrauterine growth-retarded pregnancy: Measurements with indium-113m and a computer-linked gamma camera. Gynecol. Obstet. Invest. 10:106-118, 1979.

41. Gabbe SG: Management of diabetes in pregnancy: Six decades of experience. In 1980 Yearbook of Obstetrics and Gynecology, edited by RM Pitkin, pp. 37-49. Chicago: Yearbook Medical, 1980.

42. Roversi GD, Pedretti E, Gargiulo M, and Tronconi G: Spontaneous preterm delivery in pregnant diabetics: A high risk hitherto "unrecognized." J. Perinat. Med. 10:249-253, 1982.

43. Kitzmiller JL, Brown ER, Phillippe M, Stark AR, Acker D, Kaldany A, Singh S, and Hare JW: Diabetic nephropathy and perinatal outcome. Am. J. Obstet. Gynecol. 141:741-751, 1981.

44. Pedersen JF and Molsted-Pedersen L: Early growth retardation in diabetic pregnancy. Br. Med. J. 1:18-19, 1979.

45. Pedersen JF and Molsted-Pedersen L: Early growth delay predisposes the fetus in diabetic pregnancy to congenital malformation. Lancet I:737, 1982.
46. Fuhrmann K, Reiher H, Semmler K, Fischer F, Fischer M, and Glockner E: Prevention of congenital malformations in infants of insulin-dependent diabetic mothers. Diabetes Care 6:219-223, 1983.
47. Khouzami VA, Ginsburg DS, Daikoku NH, and Johnson JW: The glucose tolerance test as a means of identifying intrauterine growth retardation. Am. J. Obstet. Gynecol. 139:423-426, 1981.
48. Johnson JWC and Dubin NH: Prevention of preterm labor. Clin. Obstet. Gynecol. 23:51-73, 1980.
49. Kaltreider DF and Kohl S: Epidemiology of preterm delivery. Clin. Obstet. Gynecol. 23:17-31, 1980.
50. National Center for Health Statistics: Advance Report of Final Natality Statistics, 1980. Monthly Vital Statistics Report, Vol. 31, No. 8 (supplement). DHHS No. (PHS) 83-1120. Public Health Service. Washington, D.C.: U.S. Government Printing Office, November 1982.
51. Hogue CJR, Cates W Jr, and Tietze C: Impact of vacuum aspiration abortion on future childbearing: A review. Family Plan. Perspect. 15:119-126, 1983.
52. Hogue CJR, Cates W Jr, and Tietze C: The effects of induced abortion on subsequent reproduction. Epidemiol. Rev. 4:66-94, 1982.
53. Alford CA and Pass RF: Epidemiology of chronic congenital and perinatal infections of man. Clin. Perinatol. 8:397-414, 1981.
54. MacDonald P, Alexander D, Catz C, and Edelman R: Summary of a workshop on maternal genitourinary infections and the outcome of pregnancy. J. Infect. Dis. 147:596-605, 1983.
55. Sever JL, Ellenberg JH, and Edmonds D: Maternal urinary tract infections and prematurity. In The Epidemiology of Prematurity, edited by DM Reed and FJ Stanley, pp. 193-196. Baltimore, Md.: Urban and Schwarzenberg, Inc., 1977.
56. Kass EH: The role of asymptomatic bacteriuria in the pathogenesis of pyelonephritis. In Biology of Pyelonephritis, edited by EL Quinn and EH Kass, pp. 399-412. Boston: Little, Brown, 1960.
57. Elder HA, Santamarina BAG, Smith S, and Kass EH: The natural history of asymptomatic bacteriuria during pregnancy: The effect of tetracycline on the clinical cause and the outcome of pregnancy. Am. J. Obstet. Gynecol. 111:441-462, 1971.
58. Kunin CM: Asymptomatic bacteriuria. Annu. Rev. Med. 17:383-406, 1966.
59. Kunin CM: Detection, Prevention and Management of Urinary Tract Infections, 3rd Edition. Philadelphia: Lea and Febiger, 1979.
60. Braun P, Lee Y-H, Klein JO, Marcy SM, Klein TA, Charles D, Levy P, and Kass EH: Birthweight and genital mycoplasmas in pregnancy. N. Engl. J. Med. 284:167-171, 1971.

61. Kass EH, McCormack WM, Lin JS, Rosner B, and Munoz A: Genital mycoplasmas as a cause of excess premature delivery. Trans. Assoc. Am. Phys. 94:261-266, 1981.

62. Harrison HR, Alexander ER, Weinstein L, Lewis M, Nash M, and Sim DA: Cervical chlamydia trachomatis and mycoplasmal infection in pregnancy: Epidemiology and outcomes. JAMA 250:1721-1727, 1983.

63. Bejar R, Curbelo V, Davis C, and Gluck L: Premature labor. II. Bacterial sources of phospholipase. Obstet. Gynecol. 57:479-482, 1981.

64. Chow BF and Lee CJ: Effect of dietary restriction of pregnant rats on body weight gain of the offspring. J. Nutr. 82:10-18, 1964.

65. Berg BN: Dietary restriction and reproduction in the rat. J. Nutr. 87:344-348, 1965.

66. Winick M and Noble A: Quantitative changes in DNA, RNA and protein during prenatal and postnatal growth in the rat. Dev. Biol. 12:451-466, 1965.

67. Winick M and Noble A: Cellular response in rats during malnutrition at various ages. J. Nutr. 89:300-306, 1966.

68. Wallace LR: Effects of diet on foetal development. J. Phys. (Lond.) 104:34, 1945.

69. Widdowson EM: Effects of prematurity and dysmaturity in animals. In Nutricia Symposium: Aspects of Praematurity and Dysmaturity, edited by JHP Jonxis, HKA Visser, and JA Troelstra, pp. 127-137. Leiden, Holland: HE Stenfert-Kroese, 1968.

70. Antonov AN: Children born during siege of Leningrad in 1942. J. Pediatr. 30:250-259, 1947.

71. Stein A, Susser M, Saenger G, and Marolla F: Famine and Human Development: The Dutch Hunger Winter of 1944/45. New York: Oxford University Press, 1975.

72. Deckmann WJ, Turner DF, Meiller EJ, Savage LJ, Hill AJ, Straube MF, Pottinger RE, and Rynkiewicz LM: Observations on protein intake and the health of the mother and baby. 1. Clinical and laboratory findings. 2. Food intake. J. Am. Diet. Assoc. 27:1046-1052, 1951.

73. Woodhill MM, van den Berg AS, Burke BS, and Stare FJ: Nutrition studies of pregnant Australian women. Am. J. Obstet. Gynecol. 70:987-1003, 1955.

74. Kasius RV, Randall A, Tompkins WT, and Wiehl DG: Maternal and newborn nutrition studies at Philadelphia Lying-in Hospital: Newborn studies no. VI. Infant size at birth and parity, length of gestation, maternal age, height, and weight status. Milbank Mem. Fund Q. 36:335-362, 1958.

75. McGarity WJ, Cannon RO, Bridgforth EB, Martin MP, Densen PM, Newbill JA, McClellan GS, Christie A, Peterson JC, and Darby WJ: The Vanderbilt Co-operative study of maternal and infant nutrition. 6. Relationship of obstetric performance to nutrition. Am. J. Obstet. Gynecol. 67:501-527, 1954.

76. Singer JE, Westphal M, and Niswander K: Relationship of weight gain during pregnancy to birthweight and infant growth and development in the first year of life: A report from the

collaborative study of cerebral palsy. Obstet. Gynecol. 31:417-423, 1968.

77. Taffel SM and Keppel KG: Implications of mother's weight gain on the outcome of pregnancy. Paper presented at the American Statistical Association meeting, Philadelphia, Pennsylvania. August 13-16, 1984. Forthcoming in Proceedings of the American Statistical Association, Winter 1984-1985.
78. Stein Z, Susser M, and Rush D: Prenatal nutrition and birth weight: Experiments and quasi-experiments in the past decade. J. Reprod. Med. 21:287-297, 1978.
79. Love EJ and Kinch RAH. Factors influencing the birth weight in normal pregnancy. Am. J. Obstet. Gynecol. 91:342-349, 1965.
80. Committee on Maternal Nutrition: Maternal Nutrition and the Course of Pregnancy. National Research Council. National Academy of Sciences, Washington, D.C., 1970.
81. Weiss W and Jackson EC: Maternal factors affecting birth weight. In Perinatal Factors Affecting Human Development, pp. 54-59. Washington, D.C.: Pan American Health Organization, 1969.
82. Eastman NJ and Jackson E: Weight relationships in pregnancy. Obstet. Gynecol. Surv. 23:1003-1025, 1968.
83. Luke B: Maternal Nutrition, pp. 24-27. Boston: Little Brown and Co., 1979.
84. Committee on Nutrition of the Mother and Preschool Child: Alternative Dietary Practices and Nutritional Abuse in Pregnancy: Summary Report. National Research Council. Washington, D.C.: National Academy Press, 1982.
85. U.S. Department of Health, Education, and Welfare: Healthy People: The Surgeon General's Report on Health Promotion and Disease Prevention, pp. 24-25. DHEW No. (PHS) 79-55071. Public Health Service. Washington, D.C.: U.S. Government Printing Office, 1979.
86. Simpson WJ: A preliminary report on cigarette smoking and the incidence of prematurity. Am. J. Obstet. Gynecol. 73:808-815, 1957.
87. Committee to Study the Prevention of Low Birthweight: Efforts to change smoking and drinking behavior in pregnant women. Unpublished paper prepared by S Wilner. Washington, D.C.: Institute of Medicine, 1984.
88. Stein Z and Kline J: Smoking, alcohol and reproduction. Am. J. Public Health 73:1154-1156, 1983.
89. Office on Smoking and Health: The Health Consequences of Smoking for Women: A Report of the Surgeon General. Public Health Service. Washington, D.C.: U.S. Government Printing Office, 1980.
90. Marcus AC, Crane L, and Gritz E: Smoking behavior among pregnant women. Prev. Med., in press.
91. Ouellette EM, Rosett HL, Rosman NP, and Weiner L: Adverse effects on offspring of maternal alcohol abuse during pregnancy. N. Engl. J. Med. 297:528-530, 1977.
92. Mills JL, Graubard BI, Harley EE, Rhoads GG, and Berendes HW: Maternal alcohol consumption and birthweight: How much drinking during pregnancy is safe? JAMA 252:1875-1879, 1984.

93. Graves C, Malen H, and Placek P: The effect of maternal alcohol and cigarette use on infant birthweight. April 1983. Unpublished report, cited with permission of the authors. Contact Placek at National Center for Health Statistics, Hyattsville, Md.

94. Hack M, Fanaroff AA, Klaus MH, Mendalawitz BD, and Merkatz IR: Neonatal respiratory distress following elective delivery: A preventable disease? Am. J. Obstet. Gynecol. 126:43-47, 1976.

95. Maisels MJ, Rees R, Marks K, and Friedman Z: Elective delivery of the term fetus: An obstetrical hazard. JAMA 238:2036-2039, 1977.

96. Flaksman RJ, Vollman JH, and Benfield DG: Iatrogenic prematurity due to elective termination of the uncomplicated pregnancy: A major perinatal health problem. Am. J. Obstet. Gynecol. 132:885-888, 1978.

97. Goldenberg RL and Nelson K: Iatrogenic respiratory distress syndrome: An analysis of obstetric events preceding delivery of infants who develop respiratory distress syndrome. Am. J. Obstet. Gynecol. 123:617-620, 1975.

98. Bowers SK, MacDonald HM, and Shapiro ED: Prevention of iatrogenic neonatal respiratory distress syndrome: Elective repeat cesarian section and spontaneous labor. Am. J. Obstet. Gynecol. 143:186-189, 1981.

99. Taffle RC, Macfee MS, and Porreco RP: The management of elective repeat cesarian section. J. Reprod. Med. 21:377-380, 1978.

100. Quilligan EJ: Making inroads against the C-section rate. Contemp. Obstet. Gynecol. 21:221-225, 1983.

101. Murray JF, Dauncey M, Newcombe R, Garcia J, and Elbourne D: Employment in pregnancy: Prevalence, maternal characteristics, perinatal outcome. Lancet I:1163-1166, 1984.

102. Naeye RL and Peters EC: Working during pregnancy: Effects on the fetus. Pediatrics 69:724-727, 1982.

103. Mamelle N, Laumon B, and Lazar P: Prematurity and occupational activity during pregnancy. Am. J. Epidemiol. 119:309-322, 1984.

104. Papiernik E and Kaminski MH: Multifactorial study of the risk of prematurity at 32 weeks gestation. I. A study of the frequency of 30 predictive characteristics. J. Perinat. Med. 2:30-36, 1974.

105. Ferreira AJ: Emotional factors in prenatal environment. J. Nerv. Ment. Dis. 141:108-118, 1965.

106. Jones AC: Life change and psychological distress as predictors of pregnancy outcome. Psychosom. Med. 40:402-412, 1978.

107. Standley K, Soulle B, and Copons SA: Dimensions of prenatal anxiety and their influence on pregnancy outcome. Am. J. Obstet. Gynecol. 135:22-26, 1979.

108. Crandon AJ: Maternal anxiety and obstetric complications. J. Psychosom. Res. 23:109-111, 1979.

109. Davids A and DeVault S: Maternal anxiety during pregnancy and child birth abnormalities. Psychosom. Med. 24:464-470, 1962.

110. McDonald RL and Parham KJ: Relation of emotional changes during pregnancy to obstetric complications in unmarried primigravidas. Am. J. Obstet. Gynecol. 90:195-201, 1964.

111. McDonald RL and Christakos AC: Relationship of emotional adjustment during pregnancy to obstetric complications. Am. J. Obstet. Gynecol. 86:341-348, 1963.
112. Gorsuch RL and Key MK: Abnormalities of pregnancy as a function of anxiety and stress. Psychosom. Med. 36:352-362, 1974.
113. Nuckolls KB, Cassel J, and Kaplan BH: Psychosocial assets, life crisis and the prognosis of pregnancy. Am. J. Epidemiol. 95:431-441, 1972.
114. Hultin M and Ottosson J-O: Perinatal conditions of unwanted children. Acta Psychiatr. Scand. 221(supplement):59-76, 1971.
115. Arfwidsson L and Ottosson J-O: Pregnancy and delivery of unwanted children. Acta Psychiatr. Scand. 221(supplement):77-83, 1971.
116. Binkin N, Mhango C, Cates W Jr., Slovis B, and Freeman M: Women refused second-trimester abortion: Correlates of pregnancy outcome. Am. J. Obstet. Gynecol. 145:279-284, 1983.
117. Newton RW, Webster PA, Binu PS, Maskery N, and Phillips AB: Psychological stress in pregnancy and its relation to the onset of premature labor. Br. Med. J. 2:411-413, 1979.
118. Crandon AJ: Maternal anxiety and neonatal well being. J. Psychosom. Res. 23:113-115, 1979.
119. Beck NC, Siegel LJ, Davidson NP, Kormeier S, Breitenstein A, and Hall DG: The prediction of pregnancy outcome: Maternal preparation, anxiety and attitudinal sets. J. Psychosom. Res. 24:343-351, 1980.
120. Calderyo-Barcia R and Poseiro JJ: Oxytocin and contractility of the pregnant human uterus. Ann. N.Y. Acad. Sci. 75:813-830, 1959.
121. Wood C, Bannerman RHO, Booth RT, and Pinkerton JHM: The prediction of premature labor by observation of the cervix and external tocography. Am. J. Obstet. Gynecol. 91:396-402, 1965.
122. Suranyi S and Szomolya M: The clinical prediction of premature labor by self-observation of uterine contractility and external tocography. J. Perinat. Med. 9(supplement no. 1):140-141, 1981.
123. Tamby Raja R and Hobel CJ: Characterization of 24 hour uterine activity (UA) in the second half of pregnancy. Abstract No. 516, p. 280. Society for Gynecological Investigation Fifteenth Annual Meeting, Washington, D.C., March 17, 1983.
124. Bragonier JR, Cushner IM, and Hobel CJ: Social and personal factors in the etiology of preterm birth. In Preterm Birth: Causes, Prevention and Management, edited by F Fuchs and PG Stubblefield, pp. 64-85. New York: Macmillan, 1984.
125. Lenihan JP: Relationship of antepartum pelvic examinations to premature rupture of the membranes. Obstet. Gynecol. 63:33-37, 1984.
126. Chalmers I and Grant A: Cervical cerclage. Br. J. Obstet. Gynaecol. 89:497-498, 1982.
127. Hytlen FE and Paintin DB: Increase in plasma volume during pregnancy. J. Obstet. Gynaecol. Br. Commonw. 70:402-407, 1963.
128. Goodlin RC, Quaife MA, and Dirksen JW: The significance, diagnosis and treatment of maternal hypovolemia as associated with fetal/maternal illness. Seminar Perinatol. 5:163-174, 1981.

129. Csapo A: The four direct regulatory factors of myometrial function. In Progesterone: Its Regulatory Effect on the Myometrium, edited by GEW Wolstenholme and J Knight, pp. 13-42. London: Churchill, 1969.

130. Schwartz BE, Schultz PM, MacDonald PC, and Johnston JM: Initiation of human parturition. III. Fetal membrane content of prostaglandin E2 and F2 precursor. Obstet. Gynecol. 46:564-568, 1975.

131. Csapo AL and Herczeg J: Arrest of premature labor by isoxsuprine. Am. J. Obstet. Gynecol. 129:482-491, 1977.

132. Johnson JWC, Lee PA, Zachary AS, Calhoun S, and Migeon CJ: High risk prematurity--progestin treatment and steroid studies. Obstet. Gynecol. 54:412-418, 1979.

133. Cousins LM, Hobel CJ, Chang RJ, Okada DM, and Marshall JR: Serum progesterone and estradiol--17 B levels in premature and term labor. Am. J. Obstet. Gynecol. 127:612-615, 1977.

134. Hobel CJ: ABC's of perinatal medicine. In Major Mental Handicap: Methods and Costs of Prevention. Ciba Foundation Symposium 59(new series), pp. 53-76. Amsterdam: Elsevier-Excerpta Medica, 1978.

135. Lepage C, Sureau C, and Guillaume MF: La prevention de l'accouchement premature par l'acetate de chlormadione. Bull. Fed. Soc. Gynecol. Obstet. 22:404-406, 1970.

136. Johnson JWC, Austin KL, Jones GS, Davis GH, and King TM: Efficacy of 17 alpha hydroxyprogestrone caproate in the prevention of preterm labor. N. Engl. J. Med. 293:675-680, 1975.

137. Breart G, Lanfranchi M, Chavigny C, Rumeau-Rouquette C, and Sureau C: A comparative study of the efficiency of hydroxyprogesterone caproate and of chlormadinone acetate in the prevention of premature labor. Int. J. Gynaecol. Obstet. 16:381-384, 1979.

138. Food and Drug Administration: FDA Bull. 8:36-37. Public Health Service. Washington, D.C.: U.S. Government Printing Office, 1979.

139. Lesinski J: High-risk pregnancy: Unresolved problems of screening, management, and prognosis. Obstet. Gynecol. 46:599-603, 1975.

140. Hobel CJ: Recognition of the high-risk pregnant woman. In Management of the High Risk Pregnancy, edited by WN Spellacy, pp. 1-28. Baltimore: University Park Press, 1976.

141. Committee on Assessing Alternative Birth Settings: Review of obstetrical risk assessment methods. Appendix E, prepared by BJ Selwyn. In Research Issues in the Assessment of Birth Settings, pp. 149-170. Institute of Medicine. Washington, D.C.: National Academy Press, 1982.

142. Papiernik-Berkhauer E: Coefficient de risque d'accouchement prémature. Presse Med. 77:793-794, 1969.

143. Kaminski M and Papiernik E: Multifactorial study of the risk of prematurity at 32 weeks of gestation. II. A comparison between empirical prediction and a discriminant function analysis. J. Perinat. Med. 2:37-44, 1974.

144. Giffei JM and Saling E: First results and experiences with our prematurity and dysmaturity prevention program (PDP program). J. Perinat. Med. 2:45-53, 1974.
145. Sokol RJ, Philipson EM, and Williams T: Clinical detection of intrauterine growth retardation improved by sonographically diagnosed oligohydramnios. Presented at the Annual Meeting of the Society for Gynecological Investigation, Washington, D.C., March 1983.
146. Quaranta P, Currell R, Redman CWG, and Robinson JS: Prediction of small-for-date infants by measurement of symphysial-fundal-height. Br. J. Obstet. Gynaecol. 88:115-119, 1981.
147. Neilson JP, Whitfield CR, and Aitchison TC: Screening for the small-for-date fetus: A two-stage ultrasonic examination schedule. Br. Med. J. 280:1203-1206, 1980.
148. Belizan JM, Villar J, Nardin JC, Malamud J, and Sainz de Vicuna L: Diagnosis of uterine growth retardation by a simple clinical method: Measurement of uterine height. Am. J. Obstet. Gynecol. 131:643-646, 1978.
149. Ross M, Hobel CJ, Bragonier RJ, and Bear M: Prematurity: A simplified risk scoring system. Obstet. Gynecol. In press.
150. Creasy RK, Gummer BA, and Liggins GC: System for predicting spontaneous preterm birth. Obstet. Gynecol. 55:692-695, 1980.
151. Hall MH, Chng PK, and MacGillivray I: Is routine antenatal care worth while? Lancet II:78-80, 1980.
152. Rosenberg K, Grant JM, and Hepburn M: Antenatal detection of growth retardation: Actual practice in a large maternity hospital. Br. J. Obstet. Gynaecol. 89:12-15, 1982.
153. Wennergren M, Karlsson K, and Olsson T: A scoring system for antenatal identification of fetal growth retardation. Br. J. Obstet. Gynaecol. 89:520-524, 1982.
154. Kaminski M, Goujard J, and Rumeau-Rouquette C: Prediction of low birthweight and prematurity by a multiple regression analysis with maternal characteristics known since the beginning of pregnancy. Int. J. Epidemiol. 2:195-204, 1973.
155. Fedrick J: Antenatal identification of women at high risk of spontaneous pre-term birth. Br. J. Obstet. Gynaecol. 83:351-354, 1976.
156. Adelstein P and Fedrick J: Antenatal identification of women at increased risk of being delivered of a low birthweight infant at term. Br. J. Obstet. Gynaecol. 85:8-11, 1978.
157. Bennert HW, Davis V, and Bennert J: Identification of the high risk mother and fetus. J. Maine Med. Assoc. 10:345-349, 1977.
158. Herron MA, Katz M, and Creasy RK: Evaluation of a preterm birth prevention program: Preliminary report. Obstet. Gynecol. 59:452-456, 1982.
159. Stembera Z: Differentiated perinatal care for high-risk pregnancies. Zentralbl. Gynaekol. 99:1281-1285, 1977.
160. Papiernik-Berkhauer E: Development of risk during pregnancy. In Perinatal Medicine, edited by D Thalhammer, K Baumgarten, and A Pollak, pp. 118-125. Massachusetts: PSG Publishing Company, 1979.
161. Read MS, Catz C, Grave G, and McNellis D: Intrauterine growth retardation: Identification of research needs and goals. Seminar Perinatol. 8:2-4, 1984.

CHAPTER 3
Trends in Low Birthweight

This chapter analyzes changes in the rate of low birthweight and in the composition of the low birthweight population during the past 10 to 15 years. The proportion of low birthweight infants has declined, but only modestly--from 7.6 percent in 1971 to 6.8 percent in 1981. The decline has not been substantial, despite several favorable developments: the proportion of pregnant women starting prenatal care in the first trimester increased; educational attainment among women rose markedly; the proportions of pregnancies among teenagers and older mothers decreased; and the prevalence of cigarette smoking among women 20 to 44 years of age declined. Not all changes, however, were favorable. For example, the proportion of unmarried pregnant women increased during the same period.

The relatively small decline in the low birthweight rate contributed in only a minor way to the substantial decline in the overall infant mortality rate. Far more important were reductions in the mortality rates of low birthweight infants. Still, the low birthweight infant remains at very high risk of mortality.

This chapter attempts to understand the recent past in seeking means to reduce future low birthweight rates. Three categories of questions are examined.

1. Have larger reductions in the low birthweight rate begun to appear in recent years? Has a decline in the low birthweight rate been masked by a concomitant reduction in fetal mortality?

2. Is the composition of the low birthweight population changing? In particular, has the decline in low birthweight occurred among very low birthweight infants (1,500 grams or less), who are especially vulnerable to serious morbidity and mortality? Or has the decline occurred among moderately low birthweight infants (1,501-2,500 grams)? Are the changes concentrated in term deliveries (37 or more weeks gestation) or in preterm infants?

3. Has the differential in low birthweight rates between high-risk and low-risk women widened or narrowed? How large is the differential presently? What might be the effect on low birthweight rates of reducing or eliminating certain sociodemographic risk factors? What might be the impact of improvements in patterns of prenatal care?

To answer these questions, the committee analyzed data for the United States as a whole and for five states--California, Massachusetts, Michigan, North Carolina, and Oregon. Although analysis of data from all reporting states gives the broadest picture of trends in low birthweight, examination of the detailed experiences of selected states permits comparison of trends across different populations and jurisdictions. Accordingly, the states were chosen to reflect a wide variation in geography and demographic characteristics. The states also were selected because the vital records data collected in these states are believed to be of high quality, thus permitting additional consideration of U.S. data as a whole, which necessarily include data of widely varying quality.

The analysis of national trends and risk factors was based on published data and unpublished analyses performed by the National Center for Health Statistics. For California, Michigan, and Oregon, the analyses were derived from cross-tabulations performed by organizations within the respective states. For Massachusetts and North Carolina, the cross-tabulations were performed by the committee from public use tapes.

Birth records for the United States as a whole were analyzed for the period 1971-1981 and for individual, selected states by single year, as available, from 1968 to 1982. The salient results of the analyses are reported in Tables 3.1 through 3.13 in this chapter. More detailed tabulations are provided in Tables B.1 through B.13 in Appendix B.

The committee recognizes that entries on birth certificates, the original source of both the national and state data presented in this chapter, vary in their accuracy and completeness. Inferences based on reported gestational age, in particular, need to be qualified. Further, while birth records encode the month when prenatal care began and the total number of prenatal visits, the content and quality of care cannot be determined from such data alone. Nevertheless, the committee believes that important insights about trends in low birthweight rates and changes in the composition of the low birthweight population can be gained from information available on the birth record.

Overall Trends in Low Birthweight Rates

Table 3.1 shows changes in low birthweight rates in the United States and the five selected states from 1971 to 1981. Data by individual year for the United States are given in Appendix Table B.1 and for selected states in Appendix Table B.2. For some states, data are provided for the years 1968 to 1970 also.

Overall, from 1971 to 1981, the low birthweight rate for the United States declined by 11 percent. Although low birthweight rates declined by comparable magnitudes in the individual states studied, the decline was more marked for Massachusetts and less significant for North Carolina and Michigan. There is no clear indication, either in Table 3.1 or in the more detailed Tables B.1 and B.2, that low birthweight rates were declining more rapidly in the earlier or later portions of

TABLE 3.1 Low-Weight Births (2,500 Grams or Less) per 1,000 Live Births in the United States and Five States, 1971, 1976, and 1981

	1971	1976	1981	Percentage Decrease, 1971-1981[a]
United States	76	72	68	11
California	66	62	58	12
Massachusetts	71	66	59	17
Michigan	77	75	69	10
North Carolina	87	83	79	9
Oregon	57	54	50	12

NOTE: All data include both singleton and multiple births. For 1971 and 1976, low birthweight includes live births weighing 2,500 grams or less. Since 1979, the National Center for Health Statistics has defined low birthweight as less than 2,500 grams. Data presented in this table are derived from the sources described in reference no. 1.

[a]Computed from rates calculated to three significant figures.

the 1968-1982 period. (From the data in Table B.2 alone, it is not possible to determine if the apparent stagnation of low birthweight rates in Michigan and North Carolina from 1980 to 1982 is of longer-term significance.)

Table 3.2 and Tables B.3 and B.4 show trends in live births and late fetal deaths. If changes in medical practice or birth certification have moved increasing numbers of pregnancies from the fetal death category to the live birth category, then the computed trend in low birthweight rates among live births may understate the actual rate of decline in low-weight rates among all pregnancies. Because there is likely to be substantial undercounting of early fetal deaths, and because shifts in classification from fetal deaths to live births are much more likely in the late fetal death groups, only fetal deaths of 28 or more weeks gestation are included. The data in Table 3.2 suggest that the assessment of trends in low-weight births among live births alone may understate slightly the rate of decline in low birthweight rates. As Appendix Table B.4 shows, this conclusion is not altered when all fetal deaths of 20 or more weeks gestation are included. Hereafter, only data for live births are considered.

The Composition of Low-Weight Births

Table 3.3 depicts changes in very low birthweight (VLBW) and moderately low birthweight (MLBW) rates in the United States and five states. The data uniformly show that the decline in low birthweight

TABLE 3.2 Low-Weight Births and Late Fetal Deaths per 1,000 Live Births in Four States, 1971, 1976, and 1981

	1971	1976	1981	Percentage Decline, 1971-1981
California	71	66	61	14
Michigan	81[a]	77	72	11
North Carolina	93	87	82	12
Oregon	60	57	51	15

NOTE: For California, late fetal deaths are defined as fetal deaths weighing 500 grams or more. For other states, late fetal deaths include all fetal deaths of at least 28 weeks gestation. Data presented in this table are derived from the sources described in reference no. 1.

[a]Data are for 1972, the earliest year available.

rates was completely confined to the 1,501-2,500-gram group. With the exception of Massachusetts, there may have been a slight increase in the VLBW rate from 1971 to 1981.

Table 3.4 shows more detailed trends in low birthweight rates in relation to gestational age for the selected states. Interpretation of the results needs to be tempered by the uncertain quality of data on duration of pregnancy. Most states did not perform extensive editing to remove or revise implausible gestational age entries. Moreover, birth records with missing data on gestational age were excluded from the analysis. Because data on gestational age reported before 1975 were considered to be less reliable, only the experience from 1975 to 1981 is reported.

The results show some variation from state to state. For Massachusetts and Oregon, there was a slight decline in the rate of preterm births (those of less than 37 weeks duration), while there was no discernable decline in the preterm rate in North Carolina or Michigan. Concomitantly, Massachusetts and Oregon showed declines in preterm low-weight births, while Michigan and North Carolina did not. All states, however, showed a decline in the term low birthweight group. The larger absolute declines in low birthweight rates in Massachusetts and Oregon appear to be attributable to declines in preterm low-weight births.

Because the decline in low birthweight appears to be confined to the moderately low birthweight group (Table 3.3), the remaining two rows of Table 3.4 analyze trends in preterm and term moderately low-weight births. The results suggest that the decline in the proportion of 1,501-2,500-gram births reflects mostly a decrease in term infants.

These results are consistent with those reported nationally. For the United States during the period 1970 to 1980, Kessel et al.[2]

TABLE 3.3 Very Low Birthweight (VLBW) and Moderately Low Birthweight (MLBW) Rates per 1,000 Live Births in the United States and Five States, 1971, 1976, and 1981

	Weight Category[a]	1971	1976	1981
United States	VLBW	11	12	12
	MLBW	65	61	56
California	VLBW	9	9	10
	MLBW	57	52	49
Massachusetts	VLBW	10	9	9
	MLBW	61	57	50
Michigan	VLBW	12	13	13
	MLBW	64	62	57
North Carolina	VLBW	14	14	15
	MLBW	74	69	65
Oregon	VLBW	8	8	9
	MLBW	49	46	41

NOTE: Data presented in this table are derived from the sources described in reference no. 1.

[a]Very low birthweight defined as 1,500 grams or less; moderately low birthweight as 1,501 to 2,500 grams.

reported that the preterm low birthweight rate declined from 38 per 1,000 to 36 per 1,000. The term low birthweight rate declined from 36 per 1,000 to 28 per 1,000. Though declines in term low birthweight were predominant, the state data presented here suggest that those areas with more marked declines in low birthweight rates may be experiencing some additional decline in preterm births. Analysis based on a larger number of states is needed to assess this relationship further.

Sociodemographic Characteristics

Table 3.5 depicts the relationship between low birthweight rates and race in the United States and five states from 1971 to 1981. More detailed data are given in Tables B.1, B.5, and B.6 of Appendix B. For the United States as a whole, the relative decline in white low birthweight rates exceeded the corresponding relative decline in black low birthweight rates. Thus, white low birthweight rates declined by

TABLE 3.4 Preterm, Low-Weight Preterm, and Low-Weight Term Births per 1,000 Live Births of Known Gestational Age in Four States, 1975 and 1981

	Massachusetts		Michigan		North Carolina		Oregon	
	1975	1981	1975	1981	1975	1981	1975	1981
Preterm	71	67	95	94	92	93	66	61
Preterm LBW	33	30	42	42	42	42	29	25
Term LBW	34	29	33	28	38	32	27	22
Preterm MLBW	24	21			31	29	21	19
Term MLBW	33	28			38	31	25	22

NOTE: Data presented in this table are derived from the sources described in reference no. 1.

14 percent from 1971 to 1981, while black rates declined by only 6 percent. The absolute declines among whites and blacks, however, were more comparable. Although quantitative assessment of changes in the white-black differential depends on the measure used, there is no clear closing of the gap.

The numbers of black births in Massachusetts and Oregon were relatively small. Hence, the reported low birthweight rates in those states are subject to greater variability. For the remaining states studied, however, the trends accord with that observed nationally. It is noteworthy that both white and black low birthweight rates vary across states. Michigan's relatively high overall low birthweight rate, for example, appears attributable to the very high low birthweight rate among blacks in that state. North Carolina's relatively high overall low birthweight rate, by contrast, reflects elevated rates for both races. The trend in low birthweight among Spanish surnamed whites in California is comparable to that for other whites in the state.

For the United States as a whole from 1971 to 1981, Appendix Table B.7 depicts trends in low-weight births according to age of the mother for whites and blacks separately. To display more clearly the relative positions of the various age groups, Table 3.6 computes the relative risks of low birthweight. The relative risk is the ratio of the low birthweight rate for a particular category to the low birthweight rate for all births of the same race in the same year.* Thus, the low birthweight rate among all white births in 1971 was 65.5 per 1,000 (see Appendix Table B.7). Among white mothers under 15 years of age, the rate was 127.8 per 1,000, that is, 1.95 times the overall white rate in 1971 (see Table 3.6). For selected states, more detailed, absolute rates are given in Appendix Table B.8. As Table 3.6 shows, the highest

*This definition of relative risk is specific to this chapter and is not consistent with the usual use of the term or with its definition elsewhere in the report.

TABLE 3.5 Low-weight Births per 1,000 Live Births in Relation to Race in the United States and Five States, 1971, 1976, and 1981

	White			Black		
	1971	1976	1981	1971	1976	1981
United States	66	61	57	133	129	125
California[a]	51	46	44	111	108	101
Massachusetts	65	63	55	113	125	111
Michigan	64	61	57	144	140	137
North Carolina	70	64	61	135	130	124
Oregon	56	52	47	118	127	103

NOTE: Data presented in this table are derived from the sources described in reference no. 1.

[a]Multiple live births excluded. Data for white births exclude those with Spanish surnames. For Spanish surnamed births, rates per 1,000 were 53 in 1971, 47 in 1976, and 45 in 1981.

relative risks are found among births to teenage mothers, particularly among whites. However, a much greater proportion of black births are to teens. The gap in low birthweight rates between the high- and low-risk maternal age groups shifted only slightly from 1971 to 1981. No particular age group displayed a marked departure from the general pattern of small reductions in the low birthweight rate during the decade. Analysis of the individual state data produced a similar conclusion.

Table 3.7 shows trends in the relative risk of low birthweight according to maternal educational attainment for whites and blacks separately from 1971 to 1981. For both races, the relative risk of low birthweight declines sharply among mothers with at least 12 years of education. Moreover, the increased risk among mothers with less than 12 years education is more pronounced for whites. The relationship between education and low birthweight rates prevails among individual maternal age groups (Appendix Table B.9).

There is no indication of a narrowing gap in relative risk among births to mothers with disparate educational attainment. The trend, in fact, is toward a widening gap. Because the number of states reporting educational attainment varied during the 1971-1981 period, such a finding requires caution. Generally consistent findings, however, were obtained from analysis of individual selected states (Appendix Table B.10). Given the overall improvement in levels of educational attainment of mothers from 1971 to 1981, the finding of an increasing gap suggests that those who have remained poorly educated constitute an increasingly high-risk group.

TABLE 3.6 Relative Risk of Low Birthweight by Age of Mother and Race: United States, 1971, 1976, and 1981

Maternal Age (years)	Relative Risk[a]						Percent Distribution Total Live Births (1981)	
	White			Black				
	1971	1976	1981	1971	1976	1981	White	Black
Less than 15	1.95	1.91	1.84	1.43	1.31	1.33	0.1	0.9
15-19	1.26	1.32	1.36	1.13	1.17	1.12	12.7	24.4
15-17	--	--	1.54	--	--	1.17	4.2	10.5
18-19	--	--	1.27	--	--	1.09	8.6	13.9
20-24	0.93	0.98	1.02	0.96	0.97	1.00	33.3	35.4
25-29	0.91	0.86	0.88	0.88	0.87	0.91	32.5	23.7
30-34	0.98	0.94	0.88	0.89	0.89	0.90	16.7	11.5
35-39	1.20	1.14	1.10	1.02	1.01	0.99	4.0	3.4
40 or older	1.56	1.37	1.31	0.97	1.01	1.07	0.6	0.7

NOTE: Data presented in this table are derived from the sources described in reference no. 1.

[a]The base for calculating relative risks is the low birthweight rate for the total in each column.

Table 3.8 reports trends in the relative risk of low birthweight by marital status, maternal age, and race in the United States from 1976 to 1981. Unmarried mothers have a consistently higher risk of bearing a low birthweight infant than those who are married. The increased risk is not explained by age differences among married and unmarried women. The relative risk differential is more pronounced for whites than blacks; but the much larger proportion of unmarried mothers among blacks makes unmarried status a far more important risk factor for blacks than for whites.

Of even greater concern is the fact that births to unmarried women increased throughout the 1970s. Whereas 7 percent of white mothers and 51 percent of black mothers were reported unmarried in 1976, the proportions were 12 percent for whites and 56 percent for blacks in 1981.

It is difficult to discern a clear trend in relative risks from Table 3.8. Such a trend conceivably could be masked by changes in the number of reporting states and the relatively short period examined.

For two selected states, Table 3.9 presents trends in low birthweight rates in relation to a simple two-way classification of sociodemographic risk factors. "High-risk" mothers are defined as those who reported less than 12 years education, were unmarried, or were young (less than 20 years of age for Massachusetts, less than 18 years of age for North Carolina), or any combination of these risk factors. "Low-risk" mothers include all others. The data show that

TABLE 3.7 Relative Risk of Low Birthweight by Educational Attainment of Mother and Race: 1971, 1976, and 1981

Maternal Educational Attainment (years)	Relative Risk[a]						Percent Distribution Total Live Births (1981)	
	White			Black				
	1971	1976	1981	1971	1976	1981	White	Black
0-8	1.35	1.39	1.46	1.08	1.14	1.17	3.7	4.7
9-11	1.32	1.35	1.47	1.10	1.12	1.18	15.8	30.1
12	0.92	0.94	0.96	0.92	0.92	0.95	44.0	41.5
13-15	0.80	0.82	0.81	0.81	0.85	0.83	18.9	15.5
16 or more	0.74	0.73	0.74	0.74	0.72	0.71	16.2	6.5

NOTE: Includes 49 states and Washington, D.C., in 1981; 44 states and Washington, D.C., in 1976; 38 states and Washington, D.C., in 1971. Data presented in this table are derived from the sources described in reference no. 1.

[a]The base for calculating relative risks is the low birthweight rate for the total in each column.

declines in low birthweight rates have been concentrated in the low-risk groups. Such evidence supports the conclusion that the gap in low birthweight rates between low-risk and high-risk groups, at least as defined by maternal sociodemographic characteristics, is not closing.

Pregnancy History

Birth order is associated with smaller differentials in relative risk than is age, and here again the relative risk varies less among blacks than whites (Table 3.10 and Appendix Table B.11). The changes in relative risk have been small. Still, among whites there is a suggestion that first births are at increased relative risk for low birthweight.

The effect of the interaction between maternal age and birth order on low birthweight has been well documented in the past and these relationships persist to the present. Figure 3.1, based on 1981 data, indicates the high risk among women aged 15-19 bearing their second or later child; the sharp increase in risk among women having their first child as age advances past 25-29 years; and the lowered risk at third or higher birth orders when women are 25-34 years of age. Very similar patterns are found among white and black women.

Termination of last prior pregnancy with a fetal death elevates risk for low birthweight in the next pregnancy, but the increase is not dramatic (Table 3.10). The relationship is stronger for whites than

TABLE 3.8 Relative Risk of Low Birthweight by Marital Status, Age of Mother, and Race: 1976 and 1981

	Relative Risk[a]				Percent Distribution Total Live Births (1981)	
	White		Black			
	1976	1981	1976	1981	White	Black
Married	0.97	0.92	0.87	0.81	88.4	44.1
Unmarried	1.60	1.57	1.14	1.15	11.6	56.0
Married						
Less than 15	2.07	1.70	1.55	1.50	b	b
15-19	1.25	1.26	1.06	0.97	8.3	3.4
15-17	--	1.45	--	1.07	2.2	0.7
18-19	--	1.17	--	0.94	6.1	2.7
20-34	0.90	0.88	0.83	0.79	75.7	37.8
35 or older	1.36	1.06	1.02	0.87	4.4	2.9
Unmarried						
Less than 15	1.89	1.88	1.32	1.33	0.1	0.9
15-19	1.59	1.58	1.16	1.14	4.4	21.0
15-17	--	1.61	--	1.18	2.0	9.9
18-19	--	1.54	--	1.12	2.4	11.2
20-34	1.66	1.56	1.12	1.14	6.7	32.8
35 or older	1.97	1.82	1.13	1.32	0.3	1.2

NOTE: Includes total United states in 1981, 38 states and Washington, D.C., in 1976. Data presented in this table are derived from the sources described in reference no. 1.

[a]The base for calculating relative risks is the low birthweight rate for the total in each column.
[b]Less than 0.1 percent.

blacks. Differentials in relative risk between births preceded by a live birth and those preceded by a fetal death have decreased. The data related to the outcome of the last pregnancy need to be interpreted cautiously, however, because of likely problems in reporting accuracy and consistency, and variations in geographic coverage. Still, the narrowing of the gap observed is one of the few evidences of positive change in relative risk during the 1971-1981 period.

Special tabulations on 1981 live births, performed by the National Center for Health Statistics for this report, showed the relationship of birthweight to interval between termination of the last pregnancy and the first day of the last menstrual period before the current pregnancy. Analysis was confined to single births in which the prior pregnancy ended in a live-born infant. Table 3.11 shows a sharply elevated relative risk among both races when the interval is less than 6 months. (However, only 5-10 percent of births fall into this inter-pregnancy interval.) Risks decrease moderately thereafter to reach an optimum level at 2 to 3 years after the previous pregnancy in the white group and 2 to 4 years in the black group. The relative risk increases for births with longer interpregnancy intervals, especially in whites, reflecting, perhaps in part, impaired fecundity. Although the data are not shown here, the pattern of exceptionally high relative risk for a

TABLE 3.9 Trends in Low Birthweight Rates in Relation to Two-Way Classification of Maternal Risk, Massachusetts and North Carolina, 1971, 1976, and 1981

		1971	1976	1981
Massachusetts	High-risk	93	89	87
	Low-risk	61	57	49
North Carolina	High-risk	109	106	106
	Low-risk	62	58	55

NOTE: "High-risk" births defined as either maternal education less than 12 years, mother unmarried, or young maternal age (less than 20 for Massachusetts, less than 18 for North Carolina), or any combination of the above. "Low-risk" includes all others. Data presented in this table are derived from the sources described in reference no. 1.

TABLE 3.10 Relative Risk of Low Birthweight by Birth Order, Outcome of Prior Pregnancy, and Race: United States, 1971, 1976, and 1981

	Relative Risk[a]						Percent Distribution Total Live Births (1981)	
	White			Black				
	1971	1976	1981	1971	1976	1981	White	Black
Birth Order								
First birth	1.01	1.06	1.08	1.02	0.85	1.00	43.7	39.2
Second birth	0.93	0.89	0.90	1.01	0.98	0.96	32.5	29.3
Third birth	0.98	0.97	0.94	1.00	0.97	0.99	14.7	16.6
Fourth birth	1.09	1.10	1.08	0.99	1.02	1.06	5.2	7.6
Fifth and over	1.17	1.14	1.11	1.05	0.98	1.12	3.5	9.9
Outcome of Prior Pregnancy[b]								
Live birth	0.95	0.94	0.92	0.95	0.94	0.95	75.6	72.6
Fetal death	1.31	1.32	1.21	1.32	1.28	1.11	17.8	17.0
Unknown	1.37	1.38	1.30	1.31	1.22	1.17	6.5	10.5

NOTE: Data presented in this table are derived from the sources described in reference no. 1.

[a]The base for calculating relative risks is the low birthweight rate for the total in each column.

[b]Data are for second order births or higher. States reporting the information varied: 49 and Washington, D.C., in 1981; 43 and Washington, D.C., in 1976; 37 and Washington, D.C., in 1971.

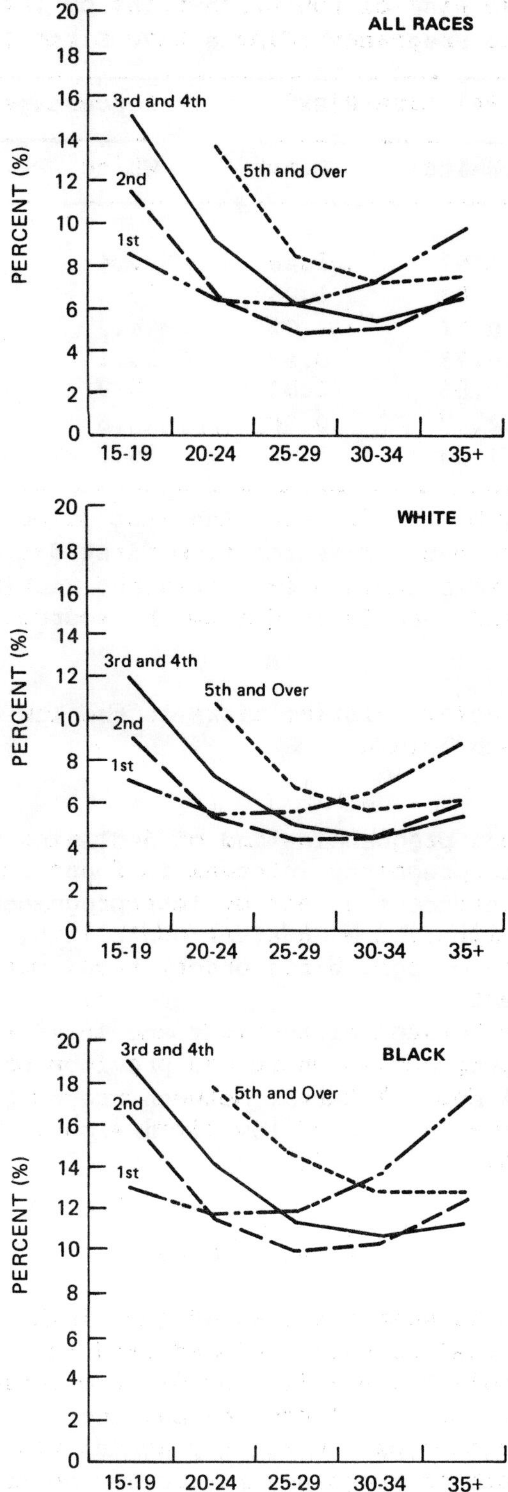

FIGURE 3.1 Percentage of low-weight births by age of mother, live birth order, and race: United States, 1981. Data presented in this figure are derived from the sources described in reference no. 1.

TABLE 3.11 Relative Risk of Low Birthweight by Interval Between Last Pregnancy and Current Pregnancy (Single Live Births), 1981

Interval (months)	Relative Risk[a]		Percentage of All Live Births	
	White	Black	White	Black
Less than 6	1.63	1.46	5.4	8.9
6-11	1.04	1.06	12.1	13.2
12-23	0.81	0.92	24.2	18.9
24-35	0.78	0.83	15.1	11.7
36-47	0.86	0.83	8.9	8.4
48 or more	1.07	0.90	17.6	23.0
Unknown	1.24	1.13	16.7	15.9

NOTE: Includes only births in which the last prior pregnancy terminated in a live birth. Pregnancy measured from first day of last menstrual period. Reporting areas include 49 states and Washington, D.C. Data presented in this table are derived from the sources described in reference no. 1.

[a]The base for calculating relative risks is the low birthweight rate for the total in each column.

short interval between pregnancies and of declining relative risk with increases in the interpregnancy interval is found at every age and birth order. An independent effect of interpregnancy interval on birthweight remains apparent even after controlling for the potentially confounding variables of age, birth order, race, marital status, and educational attainment.

The relationship between birthweight and interpregnancy interval is much different for pregnancies where the previous pregnancy terminated in a fetal death. A short interval between pregnancies is not associated with increased risk of low birthweight. In fact, the reverse is suggested.

Prenatal Care

The relationship between the risk of low birthweight and the timing and quantity of prenatal care is reviewed in detail in Chapter 6. Table 3.12 and Appendix Table B.12 provide information on this issue drawn from vital statistics. Among whites, there is an increase in relative risk as the time of the first prenatal visit advances from the first and second month of pregnancy to the second trimester. As other investigators have noted,[3] the risk of low birthweight appears reduced for mothers who begin care in their third trimester because such pregnancies already have reached more advanced gestational ages. Despite this bias, the relative risk remains high among the whites who

TABLE 3.12 Low Birthweight Relative Risk by Month Mother Began Prenatal Care and Race: 1971, 1976, and 1981

Start of Prenatal Care (month)	Relative Risk[a]						Percent Distribution Total Live Births (1981)	
	White			Black				
	1971	1976	1981	1971	1976	1981	White	Black
First-second	0.92	0.90	0.89	0.93	0.91	0.92	55.0	38.6
Third	0.94	0.95	0.95	0.93	0.97	0.94	24.4	23.9
Fourth-sixth	1.12	1.15	1.16	0.96	1.00	1.01	16.3	28.5
Seventh-ninth	1.08	1.10	1.12	0.86	0.93	0.94	3.2	6.2
No prenatal care	2.75	2.69	2.88	2.13	2.22	2.21	1.1	2.8
Seventh month or later or no care	1.42	1.48	1.56	1.24	1.31	1.35	4.3	9.1
Fourth month or later or no care	1.17	1.20	1.23	1.04	1.06	1.09	20.6	37.6

NOTE: Includes total U.S. in 1981; 44 states and Washington, D.C., in 1976; 39 states and Washington, D.C., in 1971. Data presented in this table are derived from the sources described in reference no. 1.

[a]The base for calculating relative risks is the low birthweight rate for the total in each column.

began care after the sixth month. For the no-care group, by contrast, many of the pregnancies may have terminated early, before such women would ordinarily have started prenatal care.

Analysis of trends in low birthweight rates in relation to prenatal care is complicated by variations over time in the number of states reporting data on such care. From reporting states (see Appendix Table B.12), it appears that low birthweight rates for all races combined declined in both early- and late-care groups, though the low birthweight rate for mothers with early care improved relatively more than the others.

For the individually selected states, analysis of the relationship between low birthweight rates and the timing of the first prenatal visit gave similar results (Appendix Table B.13). Except in North Carolina, the great bulk of the decline in low birthweight rates has occurred among the early-care group.

It is noteworthy that substantial increases occurred during the 1970s in the proportion of mothers reporting a first visit during the first trimester. Thus, for Massachusetts, mothers with early care comprised 79 percent of live births in 1970 and 87 percent of live births in 1980. For Michigan, the corresponding proportions for 1970 and 1980 were 69 percent and 78 percent, respectively. For North Carolina, the proportions were 67 percent and 78 percent, respectively; and for Oregon, the proportions were 71 percent in 1971 and 77 percent in 1980. For reporting states in the United States as a whole, the proportions with first trimester care were 79 percent of whites and 63 percent of blacks by 1980. The following year there was no decrease and in 1982, the figures were 79 and 61 percent, respectively, representing a departure from the steady increases during the decade 1970 to 1980.

Analysis of 1981 Single Live Births in the United States*

This section explores in more detail the relationship between low birthweight and certain maternal characteristics. The objective is to assess what fraction of current low-weight births might be eliminated by improvements in prenatal care and specific risk factors. This analysis ignores the finding of previous sections that past reductions in low birthweight were in some cases more pronounced among low-risk groups.

The upper part of Table 3.13 shows, for whites and blacks separately, the estimated effect on the 1981 low birthweight rate of eliminating all late prenatal care and the associated excess risk, as well as the estimated effect of eliminating late prenatal care and improving selected maternal risk factors (less than 12 years education, unmarried status, and high age of mother/birth order (ABO) risk, as defined in Table 3.13). The lower part of the table shows the same analysis, except that elimination of "nonadequate" care, rather than late care, is considered. "Late prenatal care" is defined as care begun after the first trimester of pregnancy or no care. "Nonadequate prenatal care" means either late start of prenatal care or a first trimester start with fewer prenatal visits than prescribed for the reported duration of pregnancy (an index adapted from the one developed by Kessner, et al.[4]).

The estimated effects in Table 3.13 correspond to what epidemiologists term "attributable risk" reduction; that is, they reflect both the relative risks of low birthweight among the maternal risk categories and the proportions of single live births in 1981 among the risk categories.

As the upper section of the table shows, late prenatal care by itself is a relatively minor factor in explaining the level of the low birthweight rate in 1981 for both racial groups; social and pregnancy history factors are far more important. The quantitative contribution of prenatal care increases appreciably when the measure of care takes into account the frequency of prenatal visits as well as the timing of the first visit (lower part of table). Eliminating excess risks among births with "nonadequate" care reduces the low birthweight rate by 15 percent among whites and 12 percent among blacks, in contrast to a 3 percent reduction for both races when prenatal care is gauged only by whether care started in the first trimester. The joint effect of eliminating nonadequate prenatal care and the other characteristics is substantial.

It is recognized that the preceding analysis controlled for only a limited number of risk factors. From the vital record data alone, the content of prenatal care could not be examined. Still, the results in Table 3.13 suggest that the pattern of prenatal care, rather than early initiation of care alone, may play an important role in determining birthweight.

---

*Based on special tabulations provided by Dr. Joel Kleinman, National Center for Health Statistics.

TABLE 3.13 Estimated Effects on Low Birthweight of Improvements in Prenatal Care and in Selected Maternal Risk Factors (Single Live Births), 1981

	White		Black	
	Rate (per 1,000)	Percent Reduction[a]	Rate (per 1,000)	Percent Reduction[a]
Original base rate	47	--	112	--
Estimated rate after elimination of excess risk among births with:[b]				
Late prenatal care	46	3	107	3
Late prenatal care and less than high school education, unmarried status, or high ABO risk[c]	38	20	84	24
Estimated rate after elimination of excess risk among births with:[b]				
Nonadequate prenatal care	40	15	97	12
Nonadequate prenatal care and less than high school education, unmarried status, or high ABO risk[c]	34	29	77	30

NOTE: United States, excluding births in California, New Mexico, Texas, and Washington, which did not report mother's education or number of prenatal visits. Data presented in this table are derived from the sources described in reference no. 1.

[a]Percent reduction determined from rates calculated to additional significant digit.

[b]Estimated rates are derived by adjusting data on live births cross-tabulated by the specified variables to eliminate associated excess risks.

[c]High ABO risk includes births to women under 18 years of age, second or higher order births to 18- and 19-year-old women, first order births to women 30 years of age or older, and all other births to those age 40 and older.

Conclusions

The committee investigated trends in the rate of low birthweight and the composition of low-weight births in the United States as a whole and in five selected states (California, Massachusetts, Michigan, North Carolina, and Oregon) during the past 10 to 15 years. For the United States, the proportion of low-weight births declined from 7.6 percent of live births in 1971 to 6.8 percent of live births in 1981. Although Massachusetts showed a more marked decline in low birthweight rates than the other states, the relative declines in all of the states and the United states were of the same order of magnitude (Table 3.1).

There is no clear indication that low birthweight rates were declining more rapidly during the earlier or later part of the 1968-1982 period. Moreover, inclusion of fetal deaths in the analysis of low birthweight trends results in only a slight to moderate increase in the rate of low birthweight decline (Table 3.2).

The decline in low birthweight rates was confined to the moderately low birthweight group (1,501-2,500 grams). No decline, or perhaps a slight increase, was observed in the very low birthweight group (1,500 grams or less) (Table 3.3). Although birth certificate data on gestational age are incomplete and of uncertain quality, the observed decline in low birthweight was apparently concentrated mostly in the full-term low birthweight group. However, in Massachusetts and Oregon, where overall declines in low birthweight rates were larger, a decline in preterm low birthweight rates also was observed. In each state, among moderately low-weight births, most of the decline was observed among term infants (Table 3.4).

Both white and black low birthweight rates have declined, but blacks remain at increased risk of low birthweight compared to whites. The data show no closing of the gap, although quantifying the white-black differential in low birthweight rates depends on the index used to measure the gap. Both white and black low birthweight rates vary appreciably across the states studied individually.

Teenage mothers and those aged 35 years or over have higher risks of low birthweight than mothers in their twenties or early thirties. Teenage mothers have the highest relative risk of low birthweight, especially among whites (although this elevated risk probably derives more from other characteristics of teenage mothers than from young age itself, as discussed in Chapter 2). Childbearing among teenagers is more prevalent among blacks, however. In both races, no particular age group showed a marked departure from the general pattern of small reductions in low birthweight from 1971 to 1981 (Table 3.6).

For both races, the risk of low birthweight declines sharply among mothers with at least 12 years of education. The relationship between education and low birthweight is independent of maternal age and race. The gap in low birthweight rates among mothers with disparate educational attainment is not closing, and may be widening. Because educational attainment of mothers has increased during the past 10 to 15 years, the finding of a widening gap in low birthweight among mothers with disparate education suggests that the poorly educated may constitute an increasingly high-risk group (Table 3.7).

Unmarried mothers have consistently higher risks of low birthweight. The elevated risk is not attributable to differences in age or race. No clear change in the low birthweight differential between married and unmarried births has been observed. However, the proportion of unmarried mothers appears to be increasing. Among blacks, 56 percent of mothers were reportedly unmarried in 1981 (Table 3.8).

A two-way measure of maternal sociodemographic risk was devised to reflect maternal educational attainment, marital status, and age. An analysis of trends in Massachusetts and North Carolina showed that the gap in low birthweight rates between high- and low-risk groups has been widening (Table 3.9).

There has been no clear change in the relationship between parity and the risk of low-weight birth. High-parity births continue to have slightly higher risks of low birthweight (Figure 3.1). Moreover, termination of the last pregnancy with a fetal death increases the risk of low birthweight in the subsequent pregnancy. However, the differential in low birthweight between those with a prior live birth and those with a prior fetal death appears to have narrowed (Table 3.10). Among mothers with a previous live birth, an interpregnancy interval of less than 6 months enhances the subsequent risk of low birthweight (Table 3.11).

The risk of low birthweight is reduced among mothers who initiate prenatal care during the first 3 months of pregnancy. The proportion of mothers with early prenatal care increased during the past 10 to 15 years. There was also a decline in low birthweight rates among mothers in the early care group (Table 3.12).

The committee performed a multivariate tabulation of single live births in the United States during 1981 according to educational attainment, marital status, age/birth order category, and the timing and quantity of prenatal care. With other factors controlled, a change in only timing of prenatal care starts was associated with a minor reduction in risk of low birthweight. The estimated contribution of prenatal care to a reduction in the low birthweight rate was more marked, however, when care was gauged by an index of "adequacy" that reflected both the start of care in the first trimester and number of visits. The tabulation suggested that the analyzed risk factors might account together for as much as 30 percent of the risk of low birthweight in both races. Moreover, the sensitivity of the estimated contribution of prenatal care to the method of measuring such care suggests that the pattern of care may be an important influence on the risk of low birthweight (Table 3.13). Chapter 6 explores this theme more fully.

In reaching these conclusions, the committee identified several issues for future analyses of low birthweight using vital statistics. First, as noted also in Chapter 2, pregnancy outcome measures need to be defined more precisely--e.g., very low birthweight, moderately low birthweight, and preterm and full-term low birthweight. And differential rates among white and black mothers, among those with higher and lower educational attainment, and among other high-risk and low-risk groups deserve careful scrutiny.

Future sources of information on low birthweight and other pregnancy outcomes also need to be more timely. Available data collection and reporting procedures, as well as terminology, need to be more uniform across states.

Vital record data alone may not gauge adequately the content and effectiveness of prenatal care; nor do such data characterize important aspects of maternal behavior (such as cigarette smoking) and medical history (such as maternal diabetes). Accordingly, high priority ought to be given to more detailed studies of selected cohorts of pregnant women. These should include new prospective designs and reanalysis of existing data. Further study is required on methods to measure more precisely the content and timing of prenatal care.

Greater attention should be given to analyses of the experiences of individual states and other jurisdictions. Geographic variations in pregnancy outcome or in the relationship between low birthweight and other risk factors could reflect differences in local public health programs and economic activity, as well as sociodemographic variations.

In making these observations, the committee recognizes that it is giving only limited attention to important problems in the nature, quality, and timeliness of the vital statistics data collected and analyzed in the United States. Limits of time and resources prevented the formulation of detailed suggestions in this area, aside from those above, and the committee's charge did not require an in-depth review of data collection issues. Nonetheless, Appendix D describes some important national vital statistics data sets that can help in studying the problem of low birthweight. The committee is also aware that several groups are already concerned with vital statistics issues (such as the National Committee on Vital and Health Statistics, the National Association of Vital Registrars, and the ad hoc Standard Terminology Group), and urges such groups to address the data problems highlighted in this chapter, Chapter 6, and elsewhere in the report.

References and Notes

1. All data for the United States are from published and unpublished data provided to the committee by the National Center for Health Statistics. For California, Michigan, and Oregon, the analyses were derived from cross-tabulations performed by organizations in the respective states. For Massachusetts and North Carolina, the cross-tabulations were performed by the committee from public use tapes.
2. Kessel SS, Villar J, Berendes HW, and Nugent RP: The changing pattern of low birthweight in the United States: 1970-1980. JAMA 251:1978-1982, 1984.
3. Harris JE: Prenatal medical care and infant mortality. In Economic Aspects of Health, edited by VR Fuchs, pp. 15-52. Chicago: University of Chicago Press, 1982.
4. Institute of Medicine: Infant Death: An Analysis by Maternal Risk and Health Care. Contrasts in Health Status, edited by DM Kessner, Vol. 1. Washington, D.C.: National Academy of Sciences, 1973.

PART II

Reducing the Incidence of Low Birthweight

CHAPTER 4

An Overview of Promising Interventions

A major conclusion that can be drawn from the data presented in Chapters 1 through 3 (Part I) of this report is that reducing the incidence of low birthweight holds great promise for improving the outcome of pregnancy and reducing infant mortality over the next decade. In Part II, summarized in this brief chapter, the committee explores various approaches to preventing low birthweight, based on current information and experience.

The committee reviewed many possible strategies, evaluating in particular interventions that could reduce the major low birthweight risk factors summarized in Chapter 2. The inquiry has been limited to interventions in the general domain of health services--an appropriate focus given the composition of the committee and its charge. The committee did not, for example, assess the relationship to pregnancy outcome of the majority of social welfare and income redistribution programs, although it is apparent that a variety of approaches well outside the purview of health services have much to contribute to reducing low birthweight. For example, the income maintenance experiment in Gary, Indiana, suggested a positive relationship between income supplementation and pregnancy outcome.[1] Also, research has suggested a link between high-quality early childhood education for economically disadvantaged children and lower pregnancy rates in the teenage years for the "graduates" of such programs--a significant finding because of the increased low birthweight risk among adolescent mothers.[2] Reducing poverty and improving education could do much to decrease low birthweight, given the strong associations among birthweight, socioeconomic status, and education (Chapter 3), but such perspectives are not explored in this report.

The committee's review of health-related strategies has led to the conclusion that, despite many unanswered questions regarding the causes of and risks associated with low birthweight, policymakers and health professionals know enough at present to intervene more vigorously to reduce the incidence of low birthweight in infants. Methods already available have demonstrated their value in reducing low birthweight. These and a few new measures, detailed in following chapters, merit additional support and investment. No single approach will solve the low birthweight problem. Instead, several types of programs should be undertaken simultaneously. These range from specific medical procedures to broad scale public health and educational approaches.

Promising Strategies

Activities that have been shown to reduce low birthweight or that have the potential for doing so can be grouped into five major areas. These clusters are:

1. Reducing risks associated with low birthweight in the interval before pregnancy by means of risk identification, counseling, and risk reduction; enlarging the content of general health education related to reproduction; and expanding and improving the provision of family planning services (Chapter 5).
2. Increasing the accessibility of early and regular high-quality prenatal care services to all women. Achieving this goal entails understanding the reasons why some women still obtain little or no prenatal care, and systematically removing major barriers (Chapter 7).
3. Strengthening and expanding the content of prenatal care for all women, and increasing the flexibility of such services to meet the varied needs of individual women. For women identified as being at elevated risk of delivering a low birthweight infant, certain components of care should be emphasized to lessen defined risks and to detect preterm labor or intrauterine growth retardation as early as possible to allow treatment of these conditions where feasible (Chapter 8).
4. Mounting a long-term, extensive public information program to convey a few well-chosen messages aimed at preventing low birthweight (Chapter 9).
5. Conducting a multifaceted program of research on low birthweight. Topics on which research is needed span many of the sciences--basic biomedical research, epidemiology, social and behavioral sciences, and health services research and evaluation.

The committee attaches great importance to this last strategy. As noted in earlier chapters, much remains to be learned about the etiology of low birthweight and the risks associated with it. In subsequent chapters, numerous research topics are highlighted, including issues in the content of prenatal care, how best to encourage high-risk, hard-to-reach women to enroll early in prenatal care, and how to decrease such behavioral risks as smoking during pregnancy. These and other research issues are noted throughout the report and are not confined to a single chapter.

Due to a lack of adequate data, the committee was not able to calculate the precise impact of the recommended interventions on the incidence of low birthweight, although both chapters 3 and 6 suggest the potential effects on the low birthweight rate of providing prenatal care to all pregnant women beginning in the first trimester. The committee believes, however, that if the interventions described in this report were implemented, it is reasonable to project that the nation would be able to meet the goal set by the Surgeon General for 1990: that low birthweight babies should constitute no more than 5 percent of all live births and that no county or racial/ethnic subpopulation should have a rate of low birthweight that exceeds 9 percent of all live births.[3]

The committee was not able to calculate the costs or cost-effectiveness of the recommended interventions because of problems in the quality and uniformity of available cost data, difficulties in delineating the specific services to be offered, and uncertainties about the definition of target populations. For example, estimates of the costs of measures that should be implemented in the period before pregnancy to reduce the risks associated with low birthweight are not available. Information does exist on the cost-effectiveness of family planning, but it does not include calculations of the economic impact of projected changes in the low birthweight rate resulting from family planning practices, and the committee did not undertake such an analysis. Lack of adequate data also prevented the committee from estimating the additional public expenditures that would be required to finance the recommended public information program and research efforts.

With regard to extending the availability of prenatal care, however, the committee found that a straightforward, common sense analysis could be performed regarding some of the financial implications involved in the provision of prenatal services to pregnant women (Chapter 10). The committee defined a target population of high-risk women (women with less than a high school education and on welfare) who often do not begin prenatal care in the first trimester of pregnancy. The current low birthweight rate in this group is about 11.5 percent. The committee estimated the increased expenditures that would be required to provide routine prenatal care to all members of the target population from the first trimester to the time of delivery. These expenditures were compared to savings that could be anticipated through a decreased incidence of low birthweight resulting from the improved utilization of prenatal care by the target population. The savings were estimated for a single year only and consisted of initial hospitalization costs, rehospitalization costs, and ambulatory care costs associated with general morbidity. The many assumptions that shaped these calculations are detailed in the chapter.

The analysis showed that if the improved use of prenatal care reduced the rate of low birthweight in the target population from 11.5 percent to only 10.76 percent, the increased expenditures for prenatal services would be approximately equal to a single year of cost savings in direct medical care expenditures for low birthweight infants in the target population. If the rate were reduced to 9 percent (the upper limit of the Surgeon General's goal described above), every additional dollar spent for prenatal care within the target group would save $3.38 in the costs of care for low birthweight infants because there would be fewer low birthweight infants requiring expensive medical care.

National Direction for a National Problem

Moving ahead in the directions advocated in this report will require that the issue of low birthweight become more widely understood and recognized as an important national problem. For too long this issue has been the concern only of those interested in maternal and child health. Low birthweight and its consequences merit the attention of Congress, state governments, professional groups, business and labor organizations, church and women's groups, schools, and the media. Each should become involved in addressing the problem of low birthweight.

The federal government, particularly the executive branch, is uniquely positioned to play a leadership role in stimulating necessary discussion and action. Its visibility and resources are great, and the public is attentive to its priorities.

> The committee urges that the Department of Health and Human Services define and pursue a variety of activities designed to focus attention on low birthweight--its importance, its causes and associated risks, and pathways for its prevention. Such leadership must include an increased commitment of resources to the low birthweight problem through approaches such as those outlined in this report.

Coupled with broad scale discussion in the private and public sectors, such federal leadership will increase the nation's awareness of the low birthweight challenge and help create the capacity to reduce its incidence.

References and Notes

1. Kehrer B and Wolin C: Impact of income maintenance on low birthweight: Evidence from the Gary experiment. J. Hum. Resourc. 14:434-462, 1979.
2. Weikart DP: The cost effectiveness of high quality early childhood education programs. Testimony prepared for the Select Committee on Children, Youth and Families. Washington, D.C.: U.S. House of Representatives, June 30, 1983.
3. Public Health Service: Promoting Health/Preventing Disease: Objectives for the Nation, pp. 17-18. Washington, D.C.: U.S. Government Printing Office, Fall 1980.

CHAPTER 5

Planning for Pregnancy

Much of the literature about preventing low birthweight focuses on the period of pregnancy--how to improve the content of prenatal care, how to motivate women to reduce risky habits while pregnant, how to encourage women to seek out and remain in prenatal care. By contrast, little attention is given to opportunities for prevention before pregnancy. Only casual attention has been given to the proposition that one of the best protections available against low birthweight and other poor pregnancy outcomes is to have a woman actively plan for pregnancy, enter pregnancy in good health with as few risk factors as possible, and be fully informed about her reproductive and general health. This chapter covers three courses of action applicable before conception to reduce the incidence of low birthweight:

1. Developing the notion of prepregnancy consultation to identify and reduce risks associated with poor pregnancy outcomes, including low birthweight; emphasizing the importance of risk reduction in the period between pregnancies, particularly for women who have had a poor outcome in a previous pregnancy; and making health professionals more aware of the possibilities in the periods before and between pregnancies for improving the outcome of pregnancy by providing appropriate services, education, and referrals.
2. Enlarging the content of health education related to reproduction, particularly in schools and in family planning settings.
3. Recognizing the contribution of family planning to reducing the incidence of low birthweight and continuing to expand such services where unmet need remains; and emphasizing the special needs of teenagers and the importance of publicly subsidized family planning services.

Prepregnancy Risk Identification and Reduction

Many of the risks associated with low birthweight can be recognized in a woman before pregnancy occurs and specific interventions can be instituted to decrease the risk. Such factors include:

- certain chronic illnesses;
- smoking;
- moderate to heavy alcohol use and substance abuse;
- inadequate weight for height and poor nutritional status;
- susceptibility to rubella and other infectious agents;
- age (under 17 and over 34);
- the likelihood of a very short interval between pregnancies; and
- high parity.

For some of these factors, risk reduction before conception may offer more protection than risk reduction during pregnancy. For example, the importance of an adequate diet during the period immediately before pregnancy was made evident by the famine studies of World War II.[1] Many major maternal chronic illnesses, especially hypertension and diabetes, present a more serious risk to both mother and fetus if the condition is not adequately under control before pregnancy. For example, Fuhrmann et al. found that strict metabolic control initiated before conception in insulin-dependent diabetic mothers was associated with significantly fewer congenital malformations than metabolic control begun after conception.[2] Similarly, it is possible that reducing high levels of tobacco consumption before conception exerts more of a protective effect with regard to low birthweight than reduction after conception. And finally, the risk factors of childbearing at extremes of the reproductive age span, brief interpregnancy interval, and high parity can be managed by family planning to prevent, or more carefully time, the occurrence of pregnancy.

Such considerations have led some experts to suggest that more attention be given to preconception counseling aimed at detecting risk factors and intervening, where possible, to reduce them.[3,4] Anecdotal and small area reports indicate that informal prepregnancy consultation already occurs in some settings[5] and is used as an opportunity to gather relevant information including historical, physical, and laboratory data; to discuss potential risks before conception occurs; and to refer for specific services ranging from treatment of medical problems to behavioral risk reduction programs, such as smoking cessation activities. These consultations also provide an opportunity to explain the importance of prompt pregnancy diagnosis and early prenatal care and to help ensure that a woman knows where to obtain such services.

Prepregnancy consultation and risk reduction are especially important during the interval between pregnancies for women who have experienced a prior reproductive casualty. In Chapters 2 and 3, the associations between certain elements in an obstetric history and subsequent low birthweight deliveries are described. Researchers have found, for example, that the relative risk that a second birth will be premature (less than 36 weeks gestation) is 4.4 if the first birth was premature.[6] Accordingly, health professionals in contact with women who have such obstetric histories should give careful attention to risk identification and reduction to help increase the chances of better outcomes in future pregnancies.

Prepregnancy consultations should be available from a variety of health care providers in different settings. Certainly this counseling is in the practice domain of obstetricians and gynecologists, nurse-midwives, family planning personnel, and family practitioners who provide obstetric and gynecologic services. Not all women of reproductive age are in touch with such personnel, however, so referral for prepregnancy consultation should be offered by a wide variety of health care providers to reach more women at risk. Education will be required to sensitize these providers to the importance of counseling in the interval before pregnancy.

Pediatricians, in particular, have an important role to play. In caring for families that have experienced a previous reproductive loss or low-weight birth, pediatricians and other primary care providers can offer counseling about risk reduction if a future pregnancy is anticipated. Also, in working with adolescent girls, pediatricians and related health professionals have an opportunity to reduce selected risks (for example, by immunizing against rubella) and to introduce basic concepts of planning for pregnancy. In urging that pediatricians give more attention to risk identification and reduction among adolescents, the committee recognizes that physician counseling of teenagers is not always successful. However, if such counseling were supported by the many other strategies outlined in this report--particularly the health education priorities described later in this chapter and in Chapter 9--it is reasonable to believe that effective communication would increase. It addition, more research is needed in the area of adolescent health and behavior generally to improve our understanding of how best to work with young people to protect and promote their health, and to instill concepts of risk reduction and planning for pregnancy.

The committee concludes that identifying and reducing risks before pregnancy can help reduce the incidence of low birthweight. Realizing the benefits of this strategy will require:

- further elaboration and discussion by the relevant professional groups of the content and timing of such counseling, with particular attention to data on the risks associated with low birthweight (and other poor pregnancy outcomes) that can be identified and modified before conception;
- incorporation of such consultations into a wide variety of settings to reach as many women as possible;
- development of written materials for professionals and for women themselves;
- health services research to monitor the costs and results of such consultations;
- willingness of third party payers to reimburse such services, once defined and evaluated;

- education of health care providers and other professionals in touch with women of reproductive age about these concepts;
- determination of the adequacy of health services resources in a given setting to manage problems that are identified through prepregnancy assessment; and
- additional research on how best to influence the health-related behavior of individuals, particularly teenagers.

It should be noted that the approach outlined here assumes a degree of coordination and free flow of information throughout the health care sector that rarely exists. For example, laboratory tests ordered as part of a consultation before pregnancy probably would be repeated once pregnancy is diagnosed if different providers were involved, resulting in significant overall cost increases. Practices of this type should be given explicit attention in the development of programs for risk counseling before pregnancy. The experience of regional perinatal care systems should be reviewed in this context; methods for coordinating data collection and avoiding duplication of effort are an important part of these systems.

The committee recognizes that emphasis on risk counseling and reduction before conception raises two troublesome issues. First, it is probably true that the women most likely to benefit from such counseling are those least likely to be in a service system sufficiently organized to provide it. For example, very poor women and the very young often fall completely outside of the health care system. Rather than providing an argument against prepregnancy counseling, this reality lends support to the provision of such counseling and education in multiple settings and by a wide range of health care providers to increase the potential points of contact. Moreover, even if only one segment of the population obtains such consultations initially, the practice could help set a trend that might be adopted widely over time.

The second issue raised by the notion of consultation before pregnancy involves the implication that women are always "almost pregnant," or "probably pregnant in the future." For couples desiring pregnancy, such a view may be acceptable, but for a woman not contemplating pregnancy, it could be exceedingly offensive. Such considerations underscore the need for sensitivity and tact in pursuing preconception risk reduction, with regard both to content and timing.

Enlarging the Content of Health Education

A second strategy in the period before pregnancy is concerned with health education related to reproduction. Education about reproduction, contraception, pregnancy, and associated topics is already provided in a variety of ways: through public information campaigns; in school-based classes, group sessions, lectures, and related printed materials; and in various health care settings. Available data regarding both the etiology and risks of low birthweight suggest that in all such settings health education related to reproduction should be expanded to include the following six topics:

1. the major factors that place a woman at risk of a poor pregnancy outcome, including low birthweight;
2. the general concept of reducing specific risks before conception and the advisability of consultation before pregnancy to identify and reduce risks associated with low birthweight;
3. the importance of early pregnancy diagnosis and of early, regular prenatal care, and where to obtain such services;
4. the importance of immunizing against rubella and of identifying other infection-related risks to the fetus;
5. the value of altering behavior to reduce a range of risks associated with low birthweight, including smoking, poor nutrition, and moderate-to-heavy alcohol consumption and substance abuse; and
6. the heightened vulnerability of the fetus to environmental and behavioral dangers in the early weeks of pregnancy, often before pregnancy is suspected or diagnosed. This fact points to the importance of avoiding x-rays, alcohol and drug use, selected toxic substances and similar threats especially in the first trimester.[7] Bringing up such topics at the time of pregnancy confirmation--typically well into the first trimester--is often too late, because fetal development is already well under way.

These topics should be incorporated into reproduction-related health education as major themes, not minor addenda. Although the individual topics suggested here probably could be expanded and refined, the central message remains--education about ways to increase the chances of a good pregnancy outcome should not be delayed until after conception.

These health education themes should be included in a variety of health care settings, including family planning clinics where many women of reproductive age receive care. Although no comprehensive data exist on the precise content of the education provided in these clinics, anecdotal information suggests that the major--often exclusive--emphasis is on contraception. Such education should be expanded to include the themes noted above, and national organizations of family planning providers should promote the use of educational materials encompassing these themes, particularly for their clients who are considering becoming pregnant. Private providers also should offer comprehensive health education related to reproduction, incorporating these same topics.

Of equal importance are the sex education and family life curricula of schools. Although these issues may be discussed in some settings, the little information available on school-based health education suggests that they are of low priority. Two recent surveys have been conducted on the content of sex education in public secondary schools, but it is difficult to discern whether the issues detailed above were covered. The topic "pregnancy and childbearing" was frequently included in the curricula surveyed, but the precise content of this topic is not known. Moreover, not all schools have such courses. According to a 1982 survey of almost 200 districts in large U.S. cities conducted by the Urban Institute, one out of four school districts with junior and/or senior high schools offered no sex education in any of its schools.[8 9]

The committee recognizes that the subject of family life and sex education is controversial in some communities, but asserts nonetheless that the need is great for young people to understand fully and accurately human reproduction and family planning, as well as the topics highlighted above. Further, recent polls have demonstrated clear majority support for public school instruction in sex education.[10] Such education must focus on the role of men as well as women in choices about reproduction. Family planning should be a shared responsibility, and education about pregnancy should not be confined to women.

A last caveat on this topic of health education. It is well known that mere provision of information frequently is insufficient to change behavior. A full literature review on this subject was not attempted, but several summaries suggest that: (1) educational programs tend to attract those who already have information and are motivated; (2) acquisition of information is not always accompanied by changes in behavior or other outcome measures; and (3) educational programs would be more successful if attention were paid to factors such as support of family, friends, culture, and providers.[11] Health education alone is likely to be of only limited value, but when joined with the other suggestions in this report for reducing the incidence of low birthweight, including the public information approaches described in Chapter 9, the probability of benefit from such education increases.

> The committee concludes that health education should be an important component of low birthweight prevention. To be more helpful in this regard, the content of such education should be expanded to include discussion of the major risk factors associated with low birthweight and the importance of early pregnancy diagnosis and prenatal care. Health education should be provided in a variety of settings, particularly in family planning clinics and schools, and be strengthened in the private sector as well.

The Role of Family Planning in Reducing Low Birthweight

The committee examined the data relating use of family planning services to poor pregnancy outcome, both infant mortality and low birthweight. The close relationship between the two measures (Chapter 1) justifies examination of both sets of data to determine the utility of family planning in reducing low birthweight.

Several studies suggest strongly that the reduction in infant mortality in the United States over the past 20 years is due in part to effective family planning. For example, Morris et al. analyzed data from the United States 1960 Live Birth Cohort Study and found that 27 percent of the reduction in infant mortality between 1965 and 1967 was due to changes in the age and parity of the mother. They attributed this shift to individual family planning.[12] Similarly, Grossman and Jacobowitz used variations in infant mortality rates among counties in 1971 to study the probable impact of public policies and programs. They found that the increase in the use of organized family planning services by low-income women was the second most important factor, after abortion, in reducing nonwhite neonatal mortality. The authors believe they may have underestimated the impact of all family planning services because their analyses did not include a measure of services delivered by private physicians.[13] Thorne and Green also found a relationship between availability of family planning services and declining perinatal mortality in Maryland, particularly among nonwhites.[14]

The evidence that family planning services reduce low birthweight is less complete than for infant mortality, but compelling nonetheless. It derives in part from the notion that family planning has averted a number of high-risk pregnancies, some of which would have resulted in low birthweight infants. For example, family planning services, as well as abortion and sterilization, have decreased childbearing among women with high-risk characteristics such as grand multiparity, chronic severe hypertension, and appreciable heart and renal disease, as well as such demographic risks as age (under 17 and over 34).

Better documentation exists to show that family planning has been especially useful to two populations at increased risk of low birthweight, low-income women and teenagers. Dryfoos has estimated that 2.4 million low-income women and 1.7 million teenagers in 1978 used the most highly effective reversible methods of contraception and successfully avoided an unplanned pregnancy.[15] Zelnik and Kantner have suggested that up to 680,000 pregnancies among unmarried, sexually active teenagers between 15 and 19 years of age were averted in 1976 by use of contraceptives.[16] Forrest et al. calculated that in 1979 an estimated 417,000 unintended teenage pregnancies were prevented by enrollment in publicly financed family planning programs.[17]

Family planning also increases the interval between births for many women. Because a very short interval between pregnancies is a risk factor for low birthweight, family planning practices that reduce this risk contribute to the prevention of low birthweight. Spratley and Taffel reported that 19.2 percent of the 1977 births occurring within 1 year of a previous live birth were of low birthweight, about 3 to 4-1/2 times the proportion observed for longer interbirth intervals. The percent of infants of low birthweight was lowest when the interval between live births was between 2 and 4 years.[18] The importance of pregnancy interval also is discussed in Chapter 3.

The committee explored the notion that family planning could reduce low birthweight by increasing the proportion of pregnancies that are intended and wanted at the time of conception. It is apparent, for example, that both teenagers and unmarried women experience higher than average rates of low birthweight; they also report higher rates of unintended pregnancies. It has been suggested that a woman who has planned for and welcomes her pregnancy probably will adhere to the health practices necessary to increase the chances of a successful pregnancy outcome.[19] Recent data from the 1980 National Natality Survey support this thesis. In that survey of married women, wantedness of pregnancy had a strong relationship to seeking prenatal care. Women who wanted a child at the time they became pregnant were more likely to receive care early in pregnancy than were those who would have preferred to have had a child at a later time. Women who had not planned to have another child showed the most delay in seeking prenatal care. These factors accounted for about a third of the black/white differential in the number of prenatal visits reported.[20] Nonetheless, concepts of intendedness and wantedness of pregnancy, and the relationship of such factors to pregnancy outcome, remain unclear. Problems of definition and methods in conducting research on this topic are large.[21]

In sum, although the exact mechanisms and magnitude of effect are not well defined, there does seem to be general agreement that family planning has had a positive impact on infant mortality and probably also on low birthweight.

> The committee concludes that family planning services should be an integral part of overall strategies to reduce the incidence of low birthweight in infants.

Closely related to family planning as a means of fertility regulation is induced abortion. It seems reasonable to examine whether abortion has helped to decrease the overall incidence of low birthweight by, for example, increasing intervals between births and averting childbearing in high-risk individuals. Several studies have tried to assess directly the impact of abortion availability on a range of reproductive outcomes, including low birthweight.[22-25] These studies suggest that the significant increase in the availability of abortion between the late 1960s and the mid-1970s contributed to the gradual decline in low birthweight rates over the same period, although the magnitude of the influence has not been well-defined. The issue of the effect of a previous induced abortion on subsequent pregnancy outcome is discussed in Chapter 2.

Unmet Need for Family Planning

The widely recognized value of family planning notwithstanding, it is apparent that such services are not always used for reasons ranging from service inadequacies to the knowledge, attitudes, and practices of women themselves. Three types of evidence can be used to document this assertion: the number of unintended pregnancies, the percentage of women at risk for unintended pregnancies who do not use contraception or obtain family planning services, and the number of abortions.

With regard to unintended pregnancies, Dryfoos estimates that 4.4 million women in the United States experienced unintended pregnancies in 1978. These pregnancies resulted from contraceptive failure despite an effective method, use of fewer or ineffective methods, or lack of a method. Her figures also show that during this period about 4 million sexually active, fecund women were at high risk of an unintended pregnancy because they were using no method or methods with high failure rates. About 1 million of these women were from low-income families and almost 900,000 were teenagers.[15]

Evidence of the failure to use contraceptives includes a report by Torres and Forrest in which they estimate that in 1981 almost 9.5 million low-income women were at risk of unintended pregnancy, but only 58 percent were obtaining family planning services from clinics (about two-thirds) or private physicians (about one-third). The corresponding figure for the other high-risk, underserved group--women under age 20--was over 5 million at risk and only 57 percent served, almost equally by clinics and private physicians.[26]

Because induced abortions often signal the end of an unintended pregnancy, the increasing number of abortions obtained in the United States (more than 1.5 million in 1980) suggests a failure of family planning. Almost 30 percent of those abortions were to women under age 20. Henshaw and O'Reilly estimate that 30 percent of pregnancies in 1980 terminated in abortion.[27] Westoff et al. found that almost 73 percent of women under age 20 and 52 percent of women 20 and over who obtained abortions in Illinois in 1980 were using no contraceptive method at the time of conception.[28]

Clearly, large segments of the population apparently are still in need of contraceptive services. The unmet need is largest among those at particularly high risk for low birthweight, the poor and the young. In 1981, the Alan Guttmacher Institute (AGI) estimated that "9.5 million low income women and 5 million sexually active teenagers needed subsidized (that is, supported at least in part by public funds) family planning care, but over 40 percent of both groups did not obtain medically supervised contraceptive care."[29]

In this regard, the committee calls attention to the special role of Title X of the Public Health Service Act, the Family Planning Assistance Program. Title X authorizes project grants to public and private nonprofit organizations for the provision of family planning services to all who need and want them, including sexually active adolescents, but with priority given to low-income persons. The service program is buttressed by a training program for clinic personnel, limited community-based education activities, and evaluation requirements designed to ensure program accountability.

In 1981, more than 4.5 million women received family planning services in clinics supported at least in part by Title X money. AGI estimated that more than 800,000 unintended pregnancies--about 425,000 of them among teenagers--were averted as a direct result of the federally funded family planning program in 1981. AGI suggests that if these unplanned pregnancies had occurred, there would have been an estimated 282,000 additional births and 433,000 more abortions that year (the remaining pregnancies would have ended in miscarriages); and further, during the 1970s, 2.3 million unintended births were averted because of the federally supported family planning program.[29]

The merits of the Title X program are reviewed periodically by the U.S. Congress, often as part of the reauthorization process. In such reviews, the committee urges that the following perspective be kept clearly in mind:

> The need for subsidized family planning remains significant and federal funds should be made generously available to meet documented needs. With regard to the particular relationship of family planning and low birthweight, it is important to stress that both young teenage status and poverty are major risk factors for low birthweight and that Title X is specifically targeted at low income women, including adolescents. As such, the program should be regarded as an important part of public efforts to prevent low birthweight.

By highlighting Title X, the committee recognizes that it appears to underrepresent the enormous contribution made by the private sector and by other public financing and service programs to the provision of family planning to low-income women. The latter category includes Medicaid, the Maternal and Child Health Services Block Grant, the Social Services Block Grant, and state and local government revenues. Several of these sources of public funds are discussed elsewhere in this report.

Emphasis in any family planning program should be given to the prevention of unwanted pregnancies in sexually active teenagers, particularly those under 18 who are unmarried. (As noted in Chapter 2, childbearing in early adolescence carries an increased risk of low birthweight, even though such risk appears to derive less from young age itself than from the other risk factors that accompany teenage childbearing, such as poor educational attainment, low socioeconomic status, and late receipt of prenatal care.) It is well known that more than 50 percent of girls in the United States engage in sexual intercourse before they reach their nineteenth birthdays and that effective contraceptive use in this population is poor.[30] Young teenage mothers and their infants are at high risk for a number of medical and social problems, one of which is low birthweight (Chapters 2 and 3). The vulnerability of the infants of teenagers recently has been examined by McCormick et al. They found that infants born to mothers age 17 and under and to 18- and 19-year-old multiparas had substantially higher low birthweight, neonatal mortality, and postneonatal mortality and morbidity rates than infants born to mothers in their 20s.[31]

Such findings underscore the recommendation made above about the value of Title X funds and call further attention to the importance of providing family planning services to teenagers in a manner that is acceptable to this group and therefore used by them. Despite much attention to this issue by groups such as the Planned Parenthood Federation of America, the high rates of teenage pregnancy, abortion, and childbearing in the United States attest to the complexity of the problem. Surveys conducted by Zelnik and Kantner found that, although more teenagers reported using contraceptives in 1979 than in 1976, more than a quarter of premaritally sexually active women 15 to 19 years old never used contraceptives and almost two-fifths used them inconsistently. Moreover, the use of the most effective methods, the pill and the IUD, had declined between the two study years.[16]

The committee did not study carefully the issue of how to increase effective contraceptive use among sexually active teenagers; it is a complicated problem around which a large literature and body of program experience have developed. For example, Chamie et al. studied counties in which a high proportion of teenagers at risk of unintended pregnancy obtained birth control services in clinics. They found that the clinics in these counties, in contrast to those in low-met-need counties, more often had special activities designed to recruit adolescents and engaged in follow-up and outreach activities to adolescent clients. All five special adolescent clinics were in high-met-need counties. Such clinics were better able to retain teenage clients and more likely to provide services without charge, and to see adolescents without a formal appointment.[33] Zabin and Clark found that the three most important reasons given by teenagers for choosing a family planning clinic were confidentiality, a staff perceived to care about teens and relate well to them, and proximity.[34]

Effective use of contraceptives by sexually active teenagers is likely to increase as a result of family planning services organized along the lines suggested by such studies. Complementary strategies, some of which are noted in this chapter and elsewhere, include absence of financial barriers to care; widely available family life and sex education in schools and communities, beginning in junior high school at the latest; public information and education directed at concepts of family planning and avoiding unintended pregnancies; and increased efforts to involve boys and young men in family planning.

The committee realizes, however, that the problem of adolescent pregnancy will not be completely solved by increasing access to family planning services. Peer pressure toward early initiation of sexual activity is not balanced by societal incentives to delay childbearing. An improved educational system, increased opportunities for interesting employment for young women and men, and economic assistance for youth who seek advanced training and/or education will likely be essential components of a campaign to reduce pregnancy among adolescents.

Summary

Numerous opportunities exist before pregnancy to reduce the incidence of low birthweight, yet these are often overlooked in favor of interventions during pregnancy. In a fundamental sense, healthy pregnancies begin before conception. The committee emphasizes, therefore, the importance of prepregnancy risk identification, counseling, and risk reduction; health education related to pregnancy outcome generally and to low birthweight in particular; and full availability of family planning services, especially for low income women and adolescents.

References and Notes

1. Stein Z, Susser M, Saenger G, and Marolla F: Famine and Human Development: The Dutch Hunger Winter of 1944-1945. New York: Oxford University Press, 1975.
2. Fuhrmann K, Reiher H, Semmler K, Fischer F, Fischer M, and Glockner E: Prevention of congenital malformations in infants of insulin-dependent diabetic mothers. Diabetes Care 6:219-223, 1983.
3. Chamberlain G: The prepregnancy clinic. Br. Med. J. 281:29-30, 1980.
4. Queenan JT: Prepping your patients for pregnancy. Contemp. Obstet. Gynecol. 21:11, 1983.
5. Alexander Burnett, M.D., Obstetrician-Gynecologist, Chevy Chase, Md. Personal communication.
6. Bakketeig LS, Hoffman HJ, and Harley EE: The tendency to repeat gestational age and birthweight in successive births. Am. J. Obstet. Gynecol. 135:1086-1103, 1979.
7. Cefalo RC and Moos MK: Preconceptional health and fitness to prevent reproductive casualties. Unpublished paper. Department of Obstetrics and Gynecology, Division of Maternal and Fetal Medicine, University of North Carolina School of Medicine, Chapel Hill, 1984.
8. Orr MT: Sex education and contraceptive education in U.S. public high schools. Family Plan. Perspect. 14:304-313, 1982.
9. Sonenstein FL and Pittman KJ: The availability of sex education in large city school districts. Family Plan. Perspect. 16:19-25, 1984.
10. The Alan Guttmacher Institute: School sex education in policy and practice. Public Policy Issues in Brief 3:1-6, February 1983.
11. Select Panel for the Promotion of Child Health: Behavioral aspects of maternal and child health: Natural influences and educational intervention. Prepared by PD Mullen. In Better Health for Our Children: A National Strategy. Vol. IV, pp. 127-188. DHHS No. (PHS) 79-55071. Public Health Service. Washington, D.C.: U.S. Government Printing Office, 1981.
12. Morris NM, Udry JR, and Chase CL: Shifting age-parity distribution of births and the decrease in infant mortality. Am. J. Public Health 65:359-362, 1975.
13. Grossman M and Jacobowitz S: Variations in infant mortality rates among counties of the United States: The roles of public policies and programs. Demography 18:695-713, 1981.
14. Thorne MC and Green LW: The contribution of family planning programs to health: From correlations to causal inference. 1977 revision of paper presented at the Annual Meeting of the Population Association of America, Montreal, Canada, 1976.
15. Dryfoos JG: Contraceptive use, pregnancy intentions and pregnancy outcomes among U.S. women. Family Plan. Perspect. 14:81-94, 1982.
16. Zelnik M and Kantner JF: Contraceptive patterns and premarital pregnancy among women aged 15-19 in 1976. Family Plan. Perspect. 10:135-142, 1978.
17. Forrest JD, Hermalin AI, and Henshaw SK: The impact of family planning clinic programs on adolescent pregnancy. Family Plan. Perspect. 13:109-116, 1981.

18. National Center for Health Statistics: Interval between births: United States, 1970-1977. Prepared by E Spratley and S Taffel. Vital and Health Statistics, Series 21, No. 39. DHHS No. (PHS) 81-1917. Public Health Service. Washington, D.C.: U.S. Government Printing Office, August 1981.
19. Select Panel for the Promotion of Child Health: Better Health for Our Children: A National Strategy. Vol. I. DHHS No. (PHS) 79-55071. Public Health Service. Washington, D.C.: U.S. Government Printing Office, 1981.
20. Kleinman JC, Machlin SR, Cooke MA, and Kessel SS: The relationship between delay in seeking prenatal care and the wantedness of the child. Paper presented at the Annual Meeting, American Public Health Association, Anaheim, Calif., November 11-15, 1984.
21. Klerman LV and Jekel JF: Unwanted pregnancy. In Perinatal Epidemiology, edited by MB Bracken, pp. 283-300. New York: Oxford University Press, 1984.
22. Kreipe RE, Roghmann KJ, and McAnarney ER: Early adolescent childbearing: A changing morbidity? J. Adolesc. Health Care 2:127-131, 1981.
23. Lanman JT, Kohl SG, and Bedell JH: Changes in pregnancy outcome after liberalization of the New York State abortion law. Am. J. Obstet. Gynecol. 118:485-492, 1974.
24. Quick JD: Liberalized abortion in Oregon: Effects on fertility, prematurity, fetal death and infant death. Am. J. Public Health 68:1003-1008, 1978.
25. Rovinsky JJ: Impact of a permissive abortion statute on community health care. Obstet. Gynecol. 41:781-788, 1973.
26. Torres A and Forrest JD: Family planning clinic services in the United States, 1981. Family Plan. Perspect. 15:272-278, 1983.
27. Henshaw SK and O'Reilly K: Characteristics of abortion patients in the United States, 1979 and 1980. Family Plan. Perspect. 15:5-16, 1983.
28. Westoff CF, DeLung JS, Goldman N, and Forrest JD: Abortions preventable by contraceptive practice. Family Plan. Perspect. 13:218-223, 1981.
29. The Alan Guttmacher Institute: Questions and answers about Title X and family planning. Public Policy Issues in Brief 4:1-4, March 1984.
30. The Alan Guttmacher Institute: Eleven Million Teenagers: What Can Be Done About the Epidemic of Adolescent Pregnancies in the United States? New York, 1976.
31. McCormick MC, Shapiro S, and Starfield BH: High-risk young mothers: Infant mortality and morbidity in four areas in the United States, 1973-1978. Am. J. Public Health 74:18-23, 1984.
32. Chamie M, Eisman S, Forrest JD, Orr MT, and Torres A: Factors affecting adolescents' use of family planning clinics. Family Plan. Perspect. 14:126-139, 1982.
33. Zabin LS and Clark SD Jr: Institutional factors affecting teenagers' choice and reasons for delay in attending a family planning clinic. Family Plan. Perspect. 15:25-30, 1984.

CHAPTER 6

The Effectiveness of Prenatal Care

Inadequate or absent prenatal care is often cited as a risk factor for low birthweight and other poor pregnancy outcomes. The value of prenatal care, however, cannot be determined solely on the basis of the association of its absence with increased risk. It is possible that it is not prenatal care itself that increases the chances of a normal birthweight infant, but rather the other characteristics usually found in women who obtain such care, including optimal childbearing age, high level of education, being married, and income above the poverty line. Conversely, women who do not receive adequate prenatal care may deliver infants of low birthweight because they are characterized by other risk factors, such as extreme youth or age, poor education, being unmarried, or low income (Chapter 2).

This chapter deals with the issue of whether inadequate prenatal care is an independent risk factor for low birthweight. Clearly, unless the committee could be convinced that prenatal care makes a separate contribution to birthweight, it could not claim that increasing access to prenatal care would help to reduce the incidence of low birthweight, or expect others to share its views. The committee believes that the studies reviewed in this chapter provide substantial evidence that high quality prenatal care begun early in pregnancy can lower the incidence of low birthweight.

The committee reached this conclusion after looking for answers to three questions:

1. Why is it difficult to obtain valid information on the value of prenatal care in the prevention of low birthweight?
2. What factors might account for the differences in findings among studies?
3. Given the present state of knowledge, can any conclusions be reached about the value of prenatal care in the prevention of low birthweight?

Issues in Studying the Effects of Prenatal Care

The positive impact of prenatal care on pregnancy outcome tends to be assumed in the American health-care literature. The Select Panel for the Promotion of Child Health concluded that prenatal care was one of the services "for which there is such a clear consensus regarding their effectiveness and their importance to good health, that it should no longer be considered acceptable that an individual is denied access to them for any reason. . . ."[1] The Public Health Service report, Promoting Health/Preventing Disease--Objectives for the Nation, was somewhat more cautious, stating that the "relative effectiveness of various interventions to improve pregnancy outcome and infant health is not without controversy."[2] Nevertheless, it listed as one of several objectives in the area of pregnancy and infant health an increase in the proportion of women obtaining prenatal care in the first trimester of pregnancy.

Although there have been questions raised in the British literature about the effectiveness of prenatal care, particularly routine care for symptom-free women,[3-5] most physicians and public health experts in the United States would agree with the sentiments expressed by the Select Panel and incorporated in the Public Health Service's objective. Researchers are aware, however, that the task of determining the effectiveness of prenatal care in the prevention of low birthweight, as well as other poor pregnancy outcomes, is complicated by a variety of problems.

Research Design

The first problem is the ethical barrier to conducting randomized clinical trials, which are considered the best source of evidence on the efficacy of a medical procedure. In the absence of a truly experimental model, researchers have been forced to rely on analyses of birth certificates and other large data sets and on analyses of interventions in selected populations, most frequently using comparison groups or before-after analyses. Positive findings from early studies often are difficult to interpret because significant variables were not controlled; because certain historical events have affected the availability of services (e.g., the passage and implementation of Medicaid); and because medical care has changed (e.g., improvements in managing certain high-risk conditions such as diabetes and innovations in obstetrical practice such as electronic fetal monitoring). More thorough understanding of confounding variables, as well as the application of more discriminating statistical techniques, have overcome these difficulties to some extent.

Defining Prenatal Care

The Select Panel's statement and the Public Health Service's objective both regard prenatal care as if it were a uniform entity. However, as the following review and subsequent chapters make clear, the quantity and the content of prenatal care vary widely. Although some prenatal care is clearly better than none, it also is likely that some types of prenatal care are more effective than others.

Research studies vary in the precision with which they define prenatal care. Quantitative definitions based on the number and timing of prenatal visits are more prevalent than those based on content. A few studies are limited to measuring care versus no care, but most employ more sensitive indicators of month or trimester when care was initiated or number of visits. These indicators may be misleading, however. Women who deliver prematurely have fewer prenatal visits than those who deliver at full term, even if they follow the recommended visit schedule until delivery; they also make a disproportionately lower number of visits because the usual schedule calls for more frequent visits later in pregnancy, by which time they have already delivered. Thus, unless a statistical adjustment is made, early deliveries are almost always associated with fewer prenatal visits, although the early delivery has not necessarily been caused by lack of visits. This confounding of cause and effect has been addressed in a number of ways. Kessner, most notably, developed a prenatal care index based on number of prenatal visits in relation to duration of pregnancy, the interval to the first visit, and type of hospital delivery service (private or general). Care was classified as adequate, intermediate, or inadequate.[6] Many other investigators have used adaptations of this index, usually omitting the delivery service factor.

Similarly, a report of more prenatal visits than the number recommended may be neither an indicator of excellent prenatal care nor a predictor of positive outcome. Rather, a greater-than-recommended number of visits usually indicates a high-risk pregnancy, which may have an adverse outcome despite a large number of visits.

Although most current research tries to solve the quantitative issue, the problem of defining the content of prenatal care--probably of equal or greater importance--is addressed less frequently. Kleinman stated, "Rather than one specific intervention, prenatal care consists of a myriad of interventions that are (or should be) tailored to the individual woman and her pregnancy."[7] Few studies measure those interventions, however, although some employ proxy variables, such as Kessner's use of delivery in a private versus a general hospital service as a measure of continuity of care. An exception is Morehead's 1970 study of health care providers.[8] She developed a six-component obstetrical score for judging the quality of care based on a review of records. Although several of her components were the same quantitative ones described above, i.e., month of registration and the number of prenatal visits, the greatest number of points (50 out of a possible 100) was given to prenatal work-up, including history, laboratory procedures, measurements of weight and blood pressure, nutrition discussion, and dental care. The content of the postpartum visits, including family planning, also was scored. Research of this type is very expensive, however, because it is labor-intensive, but may be necessary in order to obtain information about the relationship between the content of prenatal care and pregnancy outcomes.

Validity of Data

The largest source of data on prenatal care and low birthweight consists of vital statistics reports, but the validity of the information recorded on the source documents, birth certificates, has been questioned by several researchers. In a study of North Carolina birth certificates from 1975 through 1979, David found that birthweight was almost always recorded and was usually correct. Gestational age, however, was omitted in almost a fifth of the records and the values given were at times inconsistent with other information. Information about the father also was missing in almost a fifth of the records.[9] Whether these state findings are representative of the nation is not known.

Other serious problems attend the data on the timing and quantity of prenatal care. At present, all 50 states* include month in which prenatal care began, and 49 states* include number of prenatal visits. Anecdotal reports suggest, however, that the methods by which these data are collected may be unreliable, especially for those receiving publicly funded care. For example, if a woman changes her source of care during pregnancy, only the date when she started care at the site used immediately before delivery will likely be reported, thus ignoring early care visits; and in some instances, the date of a pregnancy test is used as the date of initiation of prenatal care, which may or may not accurately reflect when actual care began. The existence of such problems is substantiated by a 1972 National Natality Survey study in which reporting of the number of prenatal visits on birth certificates was compared with survey data.[10] Perfect agreement was found in only 16 percent of the cases. Land and Vaughan reviewed Missouri 1980 birth certificate data completed in hospitals using different sources of data.[11] They found that hospitals that obtained information on prenatal care exclusively from the mother reported earlier prenatal care and more prenatal visits than those using the prenatal record only or the prenatal record and the mother.

Moreover, many researchers drop from their analyses certificates on which the timing or amount of prenatal care is missing. If the number of such cases is large, this procedure may bias the results, because these women are unlikely to have the same prenatal care experiences as those for whom data are recorded, i.e., they are more likely to have little or no care; and they are unlikely to be of the same socioeconomic status. The implications of these problems are discussed by Harris[15] and by Showstack et al.[14]

A comprehensive study of the validity of the prenatal care items on birth certificates is essential for further high-quality research on prenatal care. Such a study should include women from a range of socioeconomic levels who receive care in a variety of settings.

---

*Plus Washington, D.C.

Control Variables

Some of the same variables that influence receipt of prenatal care also can influence pregnancy outcome (including complications in a prior pregnancy or low socioeconomic status); therefore, to determine the independent effects of prenatal care, it is essential to try to control for as many of these variables as possible. Most studies control for age and race at a minimum, because these clearly are associated both with receipt of prenatal care and pregnancy outcome. Other sociodemographic variables considered important include income level, education of mother and father, and marital status. Obstetrical variables also are influential, and many studies control for parity, single/multiple births, and previous pregnancy history. Although multivariate statistical measures enable more factors to be considered simultaneously than was previously feasible, it is impossible to know or include all possible confounding variables.

Selection Bias

The overriding problem in nonrandomized studies assessing the impact of prenatal care is selection bias. The initiation of prenatal care requires action on the part of the pregnant woman. Women who take this action early usually differ from those who delay it, and in ways that can be inherently associated with risk. Seeking prenatal care early may be a result of a woman's perception that she is at-risk. For example, high-risk women may seek prenatal care in disproportionate numbers because they may be worried about their pregnancies or their health, or feel ill early in their pregnancies. They may be more likely than women without anxiety or symptoms to seek early care. In many cases, the woman's anxiety may be based on family or personal experiences that place her at higher risk. Similarly, the symptoms that lead some women to seek care early may be caused by problems associated with low birthweight. Selection bias can also affect studies of prenatal care effectiveness when low-risk women seek early care disproportionately. Seeking prenatal care is a "good health habit." Women who seek care relatively early usually know more about health and have better general health habits than women who delay. Their knowledge and good health habits may help to protect their babies from low birthweight.

Similarly, delay in seeking care suggests selection bias as well. For example, women who never seek care or only come for care near the end of their pregnancies may know little about health and have poor health habits. Some women may delay initiation of care because they are dealing with one or more stressful situations, and this stress may increase their risk of low birthweight.

All studies are flawed to some extent by their inability to control for selection bias, although proxies such as maternal education may be used. Despite this bias and the other problems in studying prenatal care noted above, policymakers must proceed on the basis of the available evidence, because it is not possible to conduct randomized trials to assess the efficacy of prenatal care.

Review of Studies of Prenatal Care Effects

The committee reviewed two groups of studies that have attempted to determine the value of prenatal care in the prevention of low birthweight. The first group is composed of research involving large data bases, usually a year of live births for a large city, state, or county, and, in one case, information from the 1980 National Natality Survey (NNS). The advantage of such studies is that the large number of cases they analyze enhances the general applicability of the results and makes it possible to control for many of the variables discussed earlier and, potentially, to isolate the impact of the prenatal care. The disadvantage is the lack of precision in the measurement of prenatal care. These studies rely exclusively on data recorded on birth certificates (or the survey instruments in the NNS) for information on initiation of care and number of visits; the problems associated with these data have been noted above. Similarly, such studies provide no information on the quality or the content of the prenatal care. Women who receive inadequate care are counted in exactly the same way as those who receive high-quality care.

The second group of studies analyzed by the committee includes evaluations of the impact on pregnancy outcome, and particularly on birthweight, of specific programs offering prenatal care. The advantages and disadvantages of such studies are the opposite of those described above for the large data base studies.

The major disadvantage is that most of them involve a small number of births, which limits the number of variables that can be controlled. Several other possible problems with the second group of evaluations also must be noted. Most, though not all of them, focus on low income, largely minority populations. Women in these populations are at elevated risk of delivering a low birthweight infant; but no effort has been made to determine whether programs judged ineffective for these high-risk women might be effective in reducing low birthweight in a low-risk population. Moreover, the positive effects reported in these studies may be influenced by the quality of inpatient care or other undocumented local conditions, making it difficult to generalize their findings to other settings.

The advantage of these program-specific studies, however, is their greater precision in assessing the critical variable, prenatal care. A few of these studies obtain information about initiation of care and number of visits from clinic or hospital records, usually a more valid source of data than birth certificates. Most of them evaluate programs whose objective is to offer prenatal care appropriate to the needs of the population served. Although the content and quality of care is not usually substantiated by record reviews or other methods, there seems little doubt that most of the investigators believe they are evaluating programs offering high-quality prenatal care. Although not every women in these programs may receive outstanding care, the range of quality and content is probably narrower than in the large data base studies.

The results of the committee's analyses of both types of studies are summarized in the following sections. The review is limited to studies published since 1978, with the exception of the 1973 Kessner study,[6] because this report has been cited so frequently and because its prenatal care index has been adopted by other studies. Restricting the range of articles reviewed in this way allowed the committee to focus on studies reflecting the recent improvements in prenatal care and the expansion of availability of care in the 1960s and 1970s.* More recent reports also are more likely to use stronger statistical techniques to separate the multiple effects of socioeconomic factors, medical risks, and other variables from the effects of prenatal care alone.

Results of Studies Using Large Data Bases

The analyses presented in Chapter 3 are the most recent in a long history of studies using local, state, and national data bases. This review begins with Kessner's study of New York City births in 1968.[6] He found a significant association between adequacy of prenatal care, using variables described earlier, and the percentage of newborns weighing 2,500 grams or less in each of his sociodemographic and medical-obstetric risk groups, controlling for ethnicity. Mean birthweights also varied positively with care. The strongest associations between care and birthweight were for those mothers with sociodemographic or medical risk factors. Gortmaker reanalyzed the same data in 1979, excluding the foreign born, and reached the same conclusion using a more discriminating analytic technique that considered sociodemographic factors, gravidity, and pregnancy complications.[12] He also found a significant relationship between adequacy of care and incidence of low birthweight. In addition, he noted that inadequate care was more frequently associated with low birthweight for white mothers who delivered in a general (nonprivate) service and for all black mothers. Another study of New York City was reported by Lewit in 1983 using 1970 birth certificates.[13] After controlling for sociodemographic factors, gravidity, and prior pregnancy loss, he reported a 140-gram increase in birthweight if care was started in the first trimester and a 13.6-gram increase for each visit, corrected for duration of gestation.

Although no other city has been studied as intensively as New York, the data from several large counties and states have been analyzed. Showstack et al. analyzed all births in 1978 to mothers who resided in Alameda and Contra Costa counties in California.[14] Prenatal care was judged as adequate, intermediate, or inadequate on the basis of a

---

*Even using the 1978 cut-off date, several of the studies reviewed include data from births that occurred more than 10 years ago.

modification of the Kessner criteria. Controlling for sociodemographic factors, multiple births, pregnancy complications, whether the birth took place in a Kaiser-Permanente hospital, and gestational age, they found that adequate prenatal care added 197 grams to birthweight when all infants were considered. Because birthweight increased with length of gestation only until about 40 weeks, the analysis was repeated for infants of 280 or fewer days gestation. In this analysis, the association between adequate prenatal care and birthweight continued to be significant, but the impact was reduced to 100 grams for the total group and 126 grams for black infants. Harris analyzed 1975 and 1976 data from Massachusetts, focusing particularly on blacks and taking into account sociodemographic factors, gravidity, and prior pregnancy loss.[15] He found that early initiation of care was associated with increased birthweight and that the effect was primarily through lengthening the duration of gestation. Elster examined all Utah birth certificates from 1974 to 1979 for white women experiencing single births who had fewer than three previous live births.[16] He found that early entry into prenatal care significantly reduced the risk of having a small-for-gestational age infant among primiparous women under age 15.

Data on trends in low birthweight for four states, mentioned in Chapter 3 and documented in Appendix Table B.13, show a decrease over the last 10 to 15 years in the rate of low-weight births regardless of the trimester in which prenatal care was initiated. In three of the states, however, the percent decline was greater for those who began care in the first trimester.

Many studies have used national data to examine these issues. Eisner et al. analyzed 1974 U.S. births controlling for sociodemographic factors, gravidity, interpregnancy interval, and reproductive history.[17] They found that the absence of prenatal care was associated with an increased incidence of low birthweight; in fact, the authors labeled it as the greatest risk factor for low birthweight in their study. Taffel studied 1976 U.S. data controlling for educational attainment in age-race groups.[18] She found that the incidence of low birthweight was higher in women with no prenatal care and that the proportion of low birthweight infants decreased with the frequency of visits. Greenberg analyzed 1977 U.S. birth certificates, controlling for race and maternal education, and found a significant relationship between no prenatal care and the incidence of low birthweight.[19] The absence of prenatal care had the greatest effect among black, less-educated women. Unfortunately, neither Eisner et al., Taffel, nor Greenberg controlled for gestational age in their analyses.

Instead of using birth certificate data, Rosenzweig and Schultz used information from the 1967-1969 National Natality Survey (NNS) of births to married women.[20] They included the usual birth certificate variables, plus NNS information on husband's income and employment, and also added variables descriptive of the health facilities and socioeconomic characteristics of the study areas. They found that delay in seeking care reduced weight and gestational age at birth and that this effect was more pronounced among younger women and women of higher parity.

The multivariate analysis of national data reported in Chapter 3 examined the effect of prenatal care, education, marital status, and an index of age/live birth order risk on 1981 single live births. When the timing of the first visit was used as a measure of care, elimination of late care reduced the risk of low birthweight by only 3 percent among both whites and blacks. When a modified version of the Kessner measure of the adequacy of care was used, elimination of non-adequate care reduced the low birthweight risk by 15 percent among whites and by 12 percent among blacks. The sensitivity of the results to differences in the method of measuring prenatal care suggests that the pattern of care is more significant than merely when care begins.

All of these studies based on analyses of birth certificates (and in one study, data from the National Natality Survey) report one or more of these conclusions related to birthweight:

- some prenatal care is better than none;
- early prenatal care is better than late; and
- adequate prenatal care is better than intermediate or inadequate care (whether adequacy is defined in terms of the time of the first visit, the number of visits in relation to gestational age, or the service setting).

Finally, international data confirm the value of prenatal care. A recent report of an international maternity care monitoring project found a positive impact of prenatal care on birthweight.[21] Six countries were studied and in four--Chile, Honduras, Sweden, and Thailand--there was a significant positive relationship between the number of prenatal visits and birthweight after other factors were controlled. However, the study was limited to term deliveries.

Results of Program Evaluations

The studies reviewed in this section assess the effectiveness of special programs to provide prenatal care by comparing the pregnancy outcomes of women enrolled in the programs with the pregnancy outcomes of other women. The committee was particularly interested in programs for women at high risk because of poverty, minority status, or age, but it did not ignore programs for women generally. The latter are reviewed first.

<u>The UCSF Prematurity Prevention Program</u> One program that is of current interest is based at the University of California at San Francisco. The program includes (1) screening to detect women at high risk for preterm labor, who then receive special care; (2) education about the symptoms of preterm labor and the importance of reporting it; (3) tocolytic therapy when indicated; and (4) staff training. Herron et al. reported a reduction in the incidence of preterm deliveries at their hospital between 1977 and 1979 (the program was initiated in 1978).[22] The only comparison group was another affiliated institu-

tion, which did not report a similar decline in preterm deliveries. The concept of a prematurity prevention program is being replicated in several sites using an improved research design and is described more completely in Appendix C.

Health Maintenance Organizations Several studies have examined the effectiveness of care in a health maintenance organization (HMO). They were intended to test the assumption that HMOs can reduce the incidence of low birthweight by encouraging early prenatal care (no financial barriers, educational programs, etc.) and by providing high-quality care. Quick et al. found, however, that despite the absence of financial barriers, members of an HMO in Portland, Oreg., began prenatal care 1 month later and had three fewer visits than the general population of the city.[23] This is particularly surprising because the HMO mothers tended to be older, better educated, and more often married--generally characteristics of early and frequent care seekers. For the entire cohort of 1973 and 1974 white births in the Portland area, as well as for the HMO group, the percent of infants with low birthweight increased as the level of adequate prenatal care (measured by a modification of the Kessner index) decreased. The impact of prenatal care was higher for women at elevated medical-obstetric risk. When sociodemographic and medical-obstetric risk factors and prenatal care were considered, HMO members had better pregnancy outcomes than did the general population. The predicted birthweight of infants born to HMO members was 29 grams greater than that of the general population. The relatively small size of this effect is probably due to the fact that the study population was a very healthy one.

Another HMO study was conducted by Wilner et al. in Boston.[24] The HMO population in this study had a higher percentage of high-risk patients (nonwhites, primigravidas, grand multiparas, and younger women) than the comparison fee-for-service group. Enrollment for prenatal care in the first trimester was the same in both groups, but a significantly higher percentage of HMO patients had 11 or more visits. Although the two groups had no statistically significant differences in outcomes, including low birthweight infants, the findings suggest a positive impact of prenatal care since the HMO group had a higher proportion of high-risk women. In the Showstack et al. study cited earlier,[14] delivery in a Kaiser-Permanente hospital was associated with a small but statistically significant increase in birthweight among infants of all gestations, but the difference was not significant when only the shorter gestation infants were considered.

Another HMO study suggests that the content of prenatal care may be a critical factor in its potential impact on low birthweight. In a small demonstration project, Ershoff et al. reported higher mean birthweights and fewer low-weight infants among HMO mothers who received individual nutritional counseling and a smoking cessation program, compared to a control group of HMO women who did not receive such services.[25]

Maternity and Infant Care Projects The federal government has assisted the states in developing several program models whose objective is to improve access to and the quality of the prenatal care received by low-income women. This section reviews two studies of the Maternity and Infant Care (MIC) model; the next describes one study of the Improved Pregnancy Outcome Project (IPO) model.

Grants for MIC projects were first awarded in 1963, but later legislation required that each state have at least one such project by 1976. They are now optional. MICs were originally intended to reduce the incidence of mental retardation and other handicapping conditions associated with childbearing. In 1967, an explicit goal of reducing infant mortality was added to the legislation. The working hypothesis was that accessible and attractive project services would encourage women to receive early and regular prenatal care which, in turn, would contribute to fewer prenatal complications, low birthweight infants, and fetal and neonatal deaths. Projects were to be located in low-income areas and to provide a wide array of medical and supportive services.

Two major evaluations of MICs have been published in the past 5 years. Sokol et al. compared MIC patients to women from neighborhoods not served by the project, but who were of similar socioeconomic and medical risk status and received prenatal care in a teaching hospital clinic.[26] Both groups delivered in the same hospital and received the same intrapartum and neonatal care. MIC participants had a lower incidence of preterm deliveries and of infants weighing under 2,500 grams than women in the control group. The authors observed: "The key finding of this study is that with similar social and medical-obstetric risks, patients who received care from the MIC project experienced a significantly lower perinatal mortality than those who did not. Given that all study patients received the same care during labor and delivery, it is reasonable to infer that the observed differences in outcome may have been related to differences in care during the antepartum period. . . . The major difference in antepartum care lies in the ancillary services of the MIC project. Thus, the authors consider it more likely that the entire MIC ancillary support system, which includes paramedical services such as patient education, home visitation, nutrition assessment and counselling, social service assessment and intervention, and dental care, plays an important role in achieving these results" (p. 155-156).[26]

Peoples and Siegel used more discerning methods of data analysis to study the impact of the North Carolina MIC Project.[27] Controlling for a variety of sociodemographic and obstetric risks, they found a reduction in the percentage of low birthweight infants among high-risk subpopulations registered for MIC care, particularly nonwhite teenagers, but not among low-risk subgroups in the MIC program. The authors suggest two alternative explanations for their findings: (1) that high-risk clients are more responsive to MIC services; or (2) that MIC services are provided differentially to high- and low-risk clients; MICs were designed for high-risk populations.

Improved Pregnancy Outcome Projects The federal government took another approach to infant health problems in 1976, when it initiated the Improved Pregnancy Outcome (IPO) Projects. The IPOs were to improve maternal care and pregnancy outcome in states that had contributed heavily to the incidence of infant mortality. While the federal maternal and child health agency specified many of the components of MIC projects, the states were encouraged to devise their own methods for using IPO funds. Regionalization, professional education, interorganizational arrangements, and other administrative approaches were emphasized, rather than direct service provision. Eventually, 34 states received IPO funds. Many difficulties were encountered in evaluating these projects.[28]

In North Carolina, IPO funds were used to develop a comprehensive care program in two counties with inadequate maternity services. Certified nurse midwives provided maternity care with assistance from local obstetricians. The local health departments provided nutritional counseling, social services, and health education. Interdisciplinary teams planned, coordinated, and monitored patient care. Peoples et al. evaluated the effects for the period July 1, 1979, to August 30, 1981, by comparing the pregnancy outcomes of (1) all black women in the two counties served by the IPO program with those of all black women in two neighboring counties of similar socioeconomic composition; (2) all black women in the IPO counties who actually registered in the IPO program with those of all black women in the comparison counties; and (3) all black teenage IPO registrants with those of all black teenagers in the comparison counties.[29] On the basis of data from vital statistics, the investigators reported that the adequacy of prenatal care, as measured by an adaptation of the Kessner index, was significantly improved in all three IPO groups. They did not, however, find a corresponding decrease in the incidence of low birthweight. They suggest that this may be because (1) the program did not include specific protocols for managing high-risk women (such as education of women at high-risk for preterm delivery about the early signs and symptoms of preterm labor, or interventions to decrease smoking); (2) the intensity of care was inadequate to the degree of risk; or (3) the comparison group women were at less risk and this was not completely controlled in the analysis.

Community Health Centers Another federal initiative with a potential for influencing pregnancy outcome is the Community Health Center. This program evolved from the War on Poverty initiative in the mid-1960s. Today, Community Health Centers (CHCs) are private, nonprofit medical practices established by community groups receiving federal grants to provide primary health care services at reduced rates to the poor and near poor. As of mid-1984, there were a total of 586 grantees located in all of the states and territories of the United States. Data are not available on how many of these centers provide prenatal care, nor on its content when provided, nor on how many refer pregnant women elsewhere. Of the estimated 4.5 million people currently using CHCs, however, about 29 percent are women of childbearing age (15 to 44).

Unfortunately, the published literature evaluating the effects of CHCs on low birthweight is scant. Two unpublished reports suggest that CHCs have an important impact on pregnancy outcome. Grossman and Goldman estimated that between 1970 and 1978, CHCs reduced the black infant mortality rate by one death per thousand live births, or 12 percent of the total decline during that period.[30] Unfortunately, Grossman and Goldman did not collect data on low birthweight so it is not known whether the CHCs achieved their effect on infant mortality via birthweight improvement or other means.

Schwartz and Poppen specifically analyzed the impact of CHCs on pregnancy outcomes in Baltimore in 1981.[31] Women who used Baltimore CHCs as their primary source of care were matched with women who received some care at another institutional source (excluding no care or care from a private physician). Both groups were limited to women who lived in specific census tracts, who delivered in one of seven hospitals, who were black, and who had single births. The investigators were able to show a significant effect of adequate prenatal care on birthweight and gestational age. They were unable to show any effect of receiving care at a CHC.

Programs Using Nurse-Midwives The introduction of nurse-midwives into many service settings has provided a special opportunity to study the impact of prenatal care on underserved populations. Evaluations of the impact of such service programs include those described above by Sokol et al.[26] and Peoples et al.;[27] a 1971 study by Levy et al. that showed a decrease in prematurity;[32] a 1979 study by Reid and Morris;[33] and several studies focusing on programs serving pregnant teenagers, such as that by Piechnick and Corbett.[34] Most of these studies are discussed in Chapter 7.

Reid and Morris compared women who delivered at Glynn-Brunswick Memorial Hospital in Georgia after the initiation of a nurse-midwife program in July 1972 with those who delivered earlier. They found a reduced incidence of low birthweight in the group served by nurse-midwives, but were uncertain whether this effect was due to the program per se. Moreover, because the nurse-midwives were providing care in an area that had a growing lack of providers generally, the study is more an anlysis of the effect on pregnancy of some care versus no care.[33]

OB Access The Obstetrical Access Pilot Project (OB Access) was an attempt to improve the delivery of prenatal care to low-income, high-risk women in California. In the late 1970s, an increase in physicians refusing to accept Medi-Cal patients, coupled with increases in the number of Medi-Cal-eligible and other pregnant women reporting difficulties in obtaining prenatal care, led to the development of OB Access, funded and administered jointly by California's Medi-Cal and Maternal and Child Health programs.[35] The project's goals were (1) to provide better access to comprehensive obstetrical services for Medi-Cal-eligible mothers in areas with inadequate obstetrical care resulting from the lack of a resident obstetrician or from the decision of resident providers not to participate in Medi-Cal; and (2) to reduce perinatal mortality and morbidity rates and the percentage of pregnancies with complications. The OB Access services included eight or more prenatal visits; nutritional and psychosocial assessments, with counseling provided to those women judged to be high risk; 16 hours of childbirth education classes; prenatal vitamins; and over 30 possible diagnostic tests, some of which (like urine testing) were done at most or all prenatal visits. By contrast, the prenatal care financed by Medi-Cal in the comparison group was limited to routine prenatal visits, with no reimbursement for nutritional, educational or psychosocial services or for prenatal vitamins. Some routine diagnostic screening was financed, but not to the extent offered in the OB Access project.

Evaluators of the OB Access Project compared project participants with a group of women whose prenatal care was reimbursed through the Medi-Cal program, matched by race/ethnicity, maternal age, parity, plurality, sex of infant, and county of residence.[36] They reported that the incidence of low birthweight was 4.7 percent for OB Access births and 7.1 percent for the Medi-Cal births. The rate of very low birthweight (less than 1,500 grams) was 61 percent lower in the OB Access group (1.3 percent versus 0.5 percent).

Other Projects A variety of other demonstration projects have been or are being evaluated for their impact on pregnancy outcome, including birthweight. These include projects that emphasize home visiting, such as the Prenatal/Early Infancy Project in Elmira, N.Y.; a group of 10 rural infant care programs funded by the Robert Wood Johnson Foundation; and a much larger group of projects targeted specifically at pregnant teenagers, including demonstrations funded and/or evaluated by the federal Office of Adolescent Pregnancy Programs, the Ford Foundation (especially Project Redirection), the Mott Foundation through its Too-Early Childbearing Network, the Ounce of Prevention Fund in Chicago, and other public and private organizations.

The committee has chosen not to discuss these projects in its review of prenatal care effects for several reasons: some are ongoing programs that have not yet been evaluated; some have sample sizes that are too small; and some utilize research designs that are poorly described, weak, or constructed in a way that will not provide valid estimates of the independent impact of prenatal care on birthweight. Over the next several years, evaluations of many of the projects will be completed and will probably yield new information about how to draw women into prenatal care, the effectiveness of prenatal services generally, and how best to care for selected groups of pregnant women once they are in a prenatal system.

Conclusions

This chapter reviews both the difficulties faced in assessing the value of prenatal care and two types of studies that attempt to overcome these difficulties. After considering this material carefully, the committee concludes:

• Although a few studies have not been able to demonstrate a positive effect of prenatal care, the overwhelming weight of the evidence is that prenatal care reduces low birthweight. This finding is strong enough to support a broad, national commitment to ensuring that all pregnant women, especially those at medical or socioeconomic risk, receive high-quality care.*

• Because content of prenatal care is not defined carefully in many of the studies reviewed, it is not possible to trace the benefits of care to specific aspects of the total care package.

• A major theme of virtually all the studies reviewed is that prenatal care is most effective in reducing the chance of low birthweight among high-risk women, whether the risk derives from medical factors, sociodemographic factors, or both. Thus, differences in the risk status of various study populations may partially explain variations in the prenatal care effects observed across studies.

• All of the studies reviewed that are based on large numbers of cases, particularly those using vital statistics data, show that prenatal care exerts a positive effect on birthweight. More variation exists among the results of studies evaluating special programs, although the majority show that prenatal care is associated with improved birthweight. Those special programs that have shown a positive impact on birthweight usually offer prenatal care that goes beyond more routine services to include flexible combinations of education, psychosocial and nutritional services, and certain clinical interventions such as low threshhold for hospitalization, careful screening for medical risks, and a rapid response to the first signs of early labor. The successful projects also typically offer a package of services that is carefully defined and often described in written standards.

• The limited impact of prenatal care suggested by some of the special programs may result from the fact that the care was not organized to address what is now known about the causes and risks of low birthweight. For example, the care may not have focused on such factors as smoking reduction, adequate weight gain, reducing alcohol and other substance abuse, patient and provider education about prevention of prematurity, or specific medical risks associated with low birthweight, such as bacteriuria.

• Unfortunately, evaluations of the smaller, more specialized programs suffer from the usual problems of studies based on quasi-experimental designs, such as self-selection and problems in obtaining suitable comparison groups. A few of these studies also have relatively small sample sizes, which can make it more difficult to detect program effectiveness.

---

*Steps to achieve this goal are outlined in Chapter 7, and a discussion of what high-quality prenatal care should emphasize to reduce the incidence of low birthweight appears in Chapter 8.

The committee believes that little will be accomplished by further efforts to document the value of prenatal care generally. Instead, more studies should be undertaken to determine the effectiveness of different approaches to delivering prenatal care and of different, flexible packages of care. This issue is elaborated further in Chapter 8.

References and Notes

1. Select Panel for the Promotion of Child Health: Better Health for Our Children: A National Strategy. Vol. I, p. 192. DHHS No. (PHS) 79-55071. Public Health Service. Washington, D.C.: U.S. Government Printing Office, 1981.
2. Public Health Service: Promoting Health/Preventing Disease: Objectives for the Nation, p. 17. Washington, D.C.: U.S. Government Printing Office, Fall 1980.
3. Hall MH, Chng PK, and MacGillivray I: Is routine antenatal care worthwhile? Lancet II:78-80, 1980.
4. Oakley A: The origins and development of antenatal care. In Effectiveness and Satisfaction in Antenatal Care, edited by M Enkin and I Chalmers, pp. 1-21. Philadelphia: Spastics International Medical Publications, 1982.
5. Enkin M and Chalmers I: Effectiveness and satisfaction in antenatal care. In Effectiveness and Satisfaction in Antenatal Care, edited by M Enkin and I Chalmers, pp. 266-290. Philadelphia: Spastics International Medical Publications, 1982.
6. Institute of Medicine: Infant Death: An Analysis by Maternal Risk and Health Care. Contrasts in Health Status, Vol. 1., edited by DM Kessner. Washington, D.C.: National Academy of Sciences, 1973.
7. National Center for Health Statistics: Trends and variations in birthweight, p. 12. Prepared by JC Kleinman. In Health, United States, 1981. DHHS No. (PHS) 82-1232. Public Health Service. Washington, D.C.: U.S. Government Printing Office, 1981.
8. Morehead MA, Donaldson RS, and Seravalli MR: Comparisons between OEO neighborhood health centers and other health care providers of ratings of the quality of health care. Am. J. Public Health 61:1294-1306, 1971.
9. David RJ: The quality and completeness of birthweight and gestational age data in computerized birth files. Am. J. Public Health 70:964-973, 1980.
10. National Center for Health Statistics: Comparability of Reporting Between the Birth Certificate and the National Natality Survey. Prepared by LJ Querec. Vital and Health Statistics, Series 2, No. 83. DHEW No. (PHS) 80-1357. Public Health Service. Washington, D.C.: U.S. Government Printing Office, April 1980.
11. National Center for Health Statistics: Birth certificate completion procedures and the accuracy of Missouri birth certificate data. Prepared by G Land and B Vaughan. In Priorities in Health Statistics: Proceedings of the 19th National Meeting of the Public Health Conference on Records and Statistics, August 1983, pp.

263-265. DHHS No. (PHS) 81-1214. Public Health Service. Washington, D.C.: U.S. Government Printing Office, December 1983.

12. Gortmaker SL: The effects of prenatal care upon the health of the newborn. Am. J. Public Health 69:653-660, 1979.
13. Lewit E: The demand for prenatal care and the production of healthy infants. In Research in Human Capital and Development, Vol. 3, edited by D Salkever, I Sirageldin, and A Sorkin. Greenwich, Conn.: JAI Press, 1983.
14. Showstack JA, Budetti PP, and Minkler D: Factors associated with birthweight: An exploration of the roles of prenatal care and length of gestation. Am. J. Public Health 74:1003-1008, 1984.
15. Harris JE: Prenatal medical care and infant mortality. In Economic Aspects of Health, edited by VR Fuchs, pp. 15-52. Chicago: University of Chicago Press, 1982.
16. Elster AB: The effect of maternal age, parity, and prenatal care on perinatal outcome in adolescent mothers. Am. J. Obstet. Gynecol. 149:845-847, 1984.
17. Eisner V, Brazie JV, Pratt MW, and Hexter AC: The risk of low birthweight. Am. J. Public Health 69:887-893, 1979.
18. National Center for Health Statistics: Prenatal Care: United States, 1969-1975. Prepared by S Taffel. Vital and Health Statistics, Series 21, No. 33. DHEW No. (PHS) 78-1911. Public Health Service. Washington, D.C.: U.S. Government Printing Office, September 1978.
19. Greenberg RS: The impact of prenatal care in different social groups. Am. J. Obstet. Gynecol. 145:797-801, 1983.
20. Rosenzweig MR and Schultz TP: The behavior of mothers as inputs to child health: The determinants of birth weight, gestation, and rate of fetal growth. In Economic Aspects of Health, edited by VR Fuchs, pp. 53-92. Chicago: University of Chicago Press, 1982.
21. Donaldson DJ and Billy JOG: The impact of prenatal care on birth weight: Evidence from an international data set. Med. Care 22:177-188, 1984.
22. Herron MA, Katz M, and Creasy RK: Evaluation of a preterm birth prevention program: Preliminary report. Obstet. Gynecol. 59:452-456, 1982.
23. Quick JD, Greenlick MR, and Roghmann KJ: Prenatal care and pregnancy outcome in an HMO and general population: A multivariate cohort analysis. Am. J. Public Health, 71:381-390, 1981.
24. Wilner S, Schoenbaum SC, Monson RR, and Winickoff RN: A comparison of the quality of maternity care between a health maintenance organization and fee-for-service practices. N. Engl. J. Med. 304:784-787, 1981.
25. Ershoff DH, Aaronson NK, Danaher BG, and Wasserman FW: Behavioral, health and cost outcomes of an HMO-based prenatal health education program. Public Health Rep. 98:536-547, 1983.
26. Sokol RJ, Woolf RB, Rosen MG, and Weingarden K: Risk, antepartum care, and outcome: Impact of a maternity and infant care project. Obstet. Gynecol. 56:150-156, 1980.

27. Peoples MD and Siegel E: Measuring the impact of programs for mothers and infants on prenatal care and low birthweight: The value of refined analyses. Med. Care 21: 586-605, 1983.
28. Strobino DM: Is it Possible to Evaluate the IPO Project? Am. J. Public Health 74:541-542, 1984.
29. Peoples MD, Grimson RC, and Daughty GL: Evaluation of the effects of the North Carolina improved pregnancy outcome project: Implications for state-level decision-making. Am. J. Public Health 74:549-554, 1984.
30. Grossman M and Goldman F: An Economic Analysis of Community Health Centers: Final Report. New York: National Bureau of Economic Research, 1982.
31. Schwartz R and Poppen P: Measuring the Impact of CHCs on Pregnancy Outcomes: Final Report. Cambridge, Mass.: ABT Associates, 1982.
32. Levy BS, Wilkinson FS, and Marine WM: Reducing neonatal mortality rate with nurse-midwives. Am. J. Obstet. Gynecol. 109:50-58, 1971.
33. Reid ML and Morris JB: Prenatal care and cost-effectiveness: Changes in health expenditures and birth outcome following the establishment of a nurse-midwife program. Med. Care 17:491-500, 1979.
34. Piechnik SL and Corbett MA: Adolescent pregnancy outcome: An experience with intervention. J. Nurse-Midwifery, in press.
35. Maternal and Child Health Branch: Final Evaluation of the Obstetrical Access Pilot Project, July 1979 to June 1982. Sacramento, Calif.: Department of Health Services, 1984.
36. Korenbrot CC: Risk reduction in pregnancies of low-income women: Comprehensive prenatal care through the OB Access Project. Mobius 4:34-43, 1984.

CHAPTER 7

Ensuring Access to Prenatal Care

An earlier chapter called for more emphasis on reducing risks associated with low birthweight before pregnancy occurs--a relatively new perspective in discussions of low birthweight prevention. This chapter, by contrast, takes up a long-standing issue--ensuring the availability of prenatal care to all pregnant women.

The importance of ensuring access to prenatal care has been highlighted forcefully in recent years by various groups,[1] including the Public Health Service, through the Surgeon General of the United States. The 1980 report, Objectives for the Nation, set specific goals for reducing the number of women who receive inadequate prenatal care and for eliminating variations among groups in access to such services.*

The committee concurs with these statements. The weight of the evidence is that prenatal care reduces low birthweight among all women and that it conveys particular benefit to socioeconomically and medically high-risk women (Chapter 6). Efforts to reduce the nation's incidence of low birthweight must include a commitment to enrolling all pregnant women in prenatal care, particularly because many of the women who receive inadequate prenatal care are those at greater than average risk of a low birth- weight delivery. Moreover, participation in a system of prenatal care is a prerequisite for undertaking many individual interventions that help reduce the risk of low birthweight, ranging from medically oriented procedures such as hypertension management to counseling against smoking (Chapter 8).

If prenatal care is to become available to all pregnant women, the population of women who receives inadequate or no prenatal care must be defined, circumstances analyzed to reveal why such women receive insufficient care, and then ways found to remove the barriers identified. The balance of this chapter takes up these matters in three sections. The first presents data on prenatal care utilization, including recent trends. The second section describes some reasons

---

*The Surgeon General's objective states: "By 1990, the proportion of women in any county or racial or ethnic groups who obtain no prenatal care during the first trimester of pregnancy should not exceed 10 percent."[2]

why prenatal care is not sufficiently accessible and discusses ways to reduce the barriers. The chapter concludes with a proposal for a broad reaching commitment to making prenatal care fully available.

Who Receives Inadequate Prenatal Care?

The Advance Report on the 1981 natality statistics[3] states that almost 24 percent of all births were to women who began prenatal care after the first trimester of pregnancy. An additional 5 percent delayed care until the third trimester or received no care. Blacks were more likely (9 percent) than whites (4 percent) to delay care until the third trimester of pregnancy or to receive no care.

Women between the ages of 25 and 34 were more likely (over 82 percent) to receive care in the first trimester than were younger women, especially those under 20 (15 years of age, 34.2 percent; 15-19 years of age, 53 percent). Mothers under 20 were also more than three times as likely to have received delayed or no care. The median number of visits by women receiving any prenatal care was 11.4 (whites, 11.7; blacks, 10.2).

A report from the federal Division of Maternal and Child Health provides a further analysis by race and ethnic group of initiation of care.[4] Data from 1980 show that 41 percent of Native Americans, 40 percent of Hispanics (based on 22 states only), 37 percent of blacks, and 21 percent of whites registered after the first trimester. All four groups showed increases in the 1978-1980 period in the percentage registering early. A comparison with data from 1970 shows that the overall percentage registering after the first trimester decreased by 26 percent (whites, 25 percent; blacks, 31 percent).

The latest detailed analysis of receipt of prenatal care by the National Center for Health Statistics was conducted using 1969-1975 data.[5] In addition to race and age factors, it showed that women pregnant with their first child were less likely to receive care in the first trimester than those pregnant with their second child, but that for subsequent births the proportion starting care early decreased. Unmarried mothers, those who did not complete high school, and those living in nonmetropolitan areas received less care than those who were married, had more education, and lived in metropolitan areas.

Time Trends

The Advance Report on the 1980 natality statistics stated that the proportion of births to mothers who began prenatal care in the first trimester of pregnancy continued to increase in 1980, as it had over the past 11 years for which this information is available.[6] Unfortunately, the 1981 Advance Report noted that no change occurred in this indicator between 1980 and 1981, and that 1981 was the first year since 1969 in which no increase was found in the precentage of black mothers initiating care in the first trimester.[3] Unpublished natality data for 1982 suggest that the erosion in early prenatal care starts is continuing. Also between 1980 and 1981, a smaller proportion of women between 15 and 29 received first trimester care, with teenagers showing the greatest decline.[3]

Final federal statistics on patterns of prenatal care utilization are not available after 1981. In their absence, the committee reviewed reports from two advocacy groups and several state organizations to assess patterns of prenatal care use since 1981. These data must be interpreted with caution because of the brief time period involved and because of normal year-to-year variations in such rates in small geographic areas.

In January 1984, the Children's Defense Fund (CDF) released a report, American Children in Poverty, which found that over the past 3 years there had been a disturbing nationwide decrease in the percentage of women receiving prenatal care during the first 3 months of pregnancy and a rise in the percentage of women receiving late or no prenatal care. CDF listed 26 states (out of 33 reporting) that had increased percentages of late or no prenatal care in 1982 and 20 that documented decreased percentages of early care. Sixteen states (out of 20 with racial data) had an increase in late or no care among nonwhite women and a similar number had a decrease in first trimester care. Some states showed particularly sharp increases in late or no care among nonwhite women between 1978 and 1982, e.g., Florida, 63 percent; New York, 34 percent; and South Carolina, 29 percent.[7]

The Food Research and Action Center (FRAC) also released a report in January 1984, entitled The Widening Gap: The Incidence and Distribution of Infant Mortality and Low Birth Weight in the United States, 1978-1982.[8] FRAC described increases between 1981 and 1982 in inadequate prenatal care (defined as care initiated in the third trimester, no care, or 0 to 5 visits) in seven states and several cities and urban counties.

The Kentucky Coalition for Maternal and Child Health and Kentucky Youth Advocates, Inc., studied prenatal care and perinatal outcomes in Lexington and Fayette counties.[9] They found that the rate of women not receiving prenatal care had gone from 36 per 1,000 births in 1979 to 32 in 1980, to 33 in 1981, and then to 55 in 1982.

The Oregon Center for Health Statistics' analysis of inadequate prenatal care (no care, care begun in the third trimester, or less than five prenatal visits) showed that the marked improvement observed throughout the 1970s had been reversed.[10] The increase in inadequate care was greatest among teenagers, unwed mothers, and blacks. The Children's Defense Fund in Ohio reported that the percentage of all women reporting third trimester or no care fluctuated only slightly from 1978 through 1981, but for nonwhite mothers the percentages were substantially higher by 1981.[11]

The uniformity among the trends--the halting of declines in the proportion receiving inadequate care and the beginning of increases at the national, state, county, and city levels--strongly suggests that the numbers reflect a real change in the use of prenatal care rather than a statistical artifact. The timing of the changes, coinciding with increased unemployment, reductions in Medicaid eligibility and benefits, and decreases in the number of public prenatal services point to a decrease in access to prenatal care, with the greatest impact on minorities and other high-risk groups.

The committee views with deep concern the possibility that the nation's progress in extending prenatal benefits to all women might be arrested or reversed. Seen in this context, the suggestions made in this chapter for enrolling more women in care are of heightened significance.

Why Do Some Women Obtain Inadequate Prenatal Care?

There are several possible reasons why an individual woman does not enroll in prenatal care early or at all, but the literature that could help in understanding this problem is not extensive. From those studies and programs reviewed, however, the committee has defined several types of barriers related to the poor utilization of prenatal care:

- financial constraints, including inadequate insurance or public funds such as Medicaid to purchase adequate prenatal care;
- inadequate availability of maternity care providers, particularly providers willing to serve socially disadvantaged or high-risk pregnant women;
- insufficient prenatal services in some sites routinely used by high-risk populations such as Community Health Centers, hospital outpatient clinics, and health departments;
- experiences, attitudes, and beliefs among women that make them disinclined to seek prenatal care;
- transportation and child care services that are poor or absent; and
- inadequate systems to recruit hard-to-reach women into care.

In the following sections, each of these barriers is described and suggestions made for improvement.

Financial Constraints

The availability of funds to cover the costs of prenatal care, as well as hospitalization for labor and delivery, undoubtedly influences many women's decisions about seeking care. Direct evidence of the importance of financing was reported by Chao et al. in a recent study of a group of poor, urban women who had obtained no prenatal care by the time of delivery. When asked why they had not received prenatal care, over half mentioned a money problem.[12]

Similar findings have been reported from a very different population in the rural Southwest. Berger studied a group of low-income pregnant women who had obtained virtually no prenatal care. Though some community physicians felt that factors such as cultural practices and lack of information explained the absence of care, it was found that 87 percent of the 400 women interviewed stated that the reason they had not obtained prenatal care was that they could not afford it.[13]

Additional evidence of the impact of financial barriers on the receipt of prenatal care is indirect, based on associations between the care-seeking behavior of certain groups and the presence of insurance, personal funds, free or low price clinics, or Medicaid. The CDF and FRAC reports and those of several state organizations cited earlier explore these issues. Many of them stress decreases in Medicaid eligibility. Some describe declines in private insurance coverage because of unemployment; others note increasingly restrictive eligibility or increased cost-sharing requirements in health department clinics and Community Health Centers. These reports also cite hospital clinics or delivery services that are turning away women who can not pay for care. It seems reasonable to assume that such circumstances discourage women from seeking prenatal care early or at all.

Easing such financial barriers can be approached from many perspectives. For example, ways could be explored to make private health insurance more affordable for those who currently have no coverage but do not qualify for Medicaid. The problem of the uninsured poor is especially relevant to the low birthweight problem because young adults in their childbearing years are particularly likely to be without health insurance and because minorities are disproportionately represented in the uninsured group. A 1977 survey supported by the National Center for Health Services Research found that 12 percent of the total population had no health insurance coverage of any type, public or private. For persons age 18 to 24, however, the proportion was close to 22 percent.[14] Data from the 1980 National Medical Care Utilization and Expenditure Survey suggest that the situation has changed little, if at all, in the intervening years.[15] Health Interview Survey data from 1978 and 1980 also show that Hispanic and black people are more likely than whites to have no health insurance of any type. Twenty-six percent of Hispanics, 18 percent of blacks, and 9 percent of whites had no coverage.[16]

Having private health insurance does not, however, guarantee that prenatal services are covered adequately. Insured individuals may still find that out-of-pocket expenses for maternity services are high. Thus, removing financial barriers to prenatal care involves not only increasing the number of individuals covered by private health insurance, but also assuring that the maternity benefits of such policies are adequate.

Another approach to lowering financial barriers to prenatal care is to increase support of public agencies that serve groups most likely to receive inadequate maternity services. Such an approach is developed more fully later in this chapter.

In this section the committee has chosen to focus on the Medicaid program, the largest public program financing prenatal care. The significance of the Medicaid program for reducing low birthweight derives from its capacity to reduce financial barriers to care generally and thereby increase the proportion of low-income women receiving prenatal care, which in turn is associated with improved pregnancy outcome. National Center for Health Statistics data show that the number of visits to physicians per year by the poor has increased since the passage of Title XIX of the Social Security Act in 1965 (the Medicaid program), and it is reasonable to assume that visits for prenatal care are among them. Also, the marked increase in those seeking first trimester care from 1967 to 1980, especially among blacks, who are more likely to be Medicaid recipients, suggests a probable cause and effect relationship.[6 17]

Specific studies supporting such a relationship include that of Norris and Williams, who found that between 1968 and 1978, Medi-Cal (the California Medicaid program) greatly increased access to early prenatal care. In 1968, Medi-Cal was the financing mechanism for 13 percent of California deliveries. By 1978, the proportion had more than doubled to 27 percent. During the same period, the proportion of women receiving early prenatal care increased for all subpopulations surveyed (both Medi-Cal and non-Medi-Cal covered populations), but the increase was consistently larger for Medi-Cal births in all racial groups.[18]

Other data suggest that enrollment in Medicaid is associated with better pregnancy outcomes, though more often in terms of improved mortality rates than improved birthweight distributions. The same Norris and Williams study found that low-income women not covered by Medi-Cal had a greater risk of poor pregnancy outcome. They found that "among all three ethnic subpopulations studied [white, non-Spanish surname; white, Spanish surname; and black], the perinatal mortality rates for most birthweight groups were lower for Medi-Cal babies, especially in 1978. Decreases in birthweight specific mortality rates for all race-ethnicity groups were generally largest in the Medi-Cal group" (p. 1114).[18]

Similarly, Schwartz and Poppen noted that women who received Medicaid had better pregnancy outcomes than similar women without it. They suggested that women with Medicaid coverage do not need to rely on free care or worry about the cost of care and thus have better access to care.[19]

The program is also of great significance to the low birthweight problem because of the characteristics of the recipients themselves. By the mere fact of their eligibility for Medicaid, they are at high risk for delivering a low birthweight infant. Medicaid-eligible pregnant women are typically poor and single and often have other risk factors. For example, Missouri data on the characteristics of Medicaid recipients who gave birth in 1980 show that 78 percent were unmarried, as compared with 18 percent of all Missouri mothers; that these Medicaid mothers were more likely to smoke during pregnancy, to be underweight, to space births less than 18 months apart, and to have four or more children. Medicaid mothers living in Missouri had a 75 percent greater low birthweight rate than the state's overall low birthweight rate.[20] While these data may not be generalizable to other states, they do highlight the high-risk characteristics of many Medicaid-eligible women.

Another body of data indicates the cost-effectiveness of Medicaid maternity benefits. For example, expanding improved Medicaid benefits to more low-income women was found to be cost-effective in the OB Access Project, which was conducted in 13 counties in California from 1979 to 1982. Cost savings were achieved by decreasing low birthweight (4.7 percent incidence of low birthweight in the study population versus 7.1 percent in a Medi-Cal comparison group) and by reducing associated costs of infant hospital care. Korenbrot found that for every dollar Medi-Cal reimbursed for prenatal care, the state would save $1.70 in reimbursements for newborn intensive care. She suggested that additional cost savings of unknown magnitude might be achieved from reduced need for Crippled Children's Services, Developmentally Disabled Programs, and other high-risk infant follow-up services.[21] Chapter 6 describes the content of care offered in the OB Access project and Chapter 10 discusses the cost-effectiveness of prenatal care in more detail.

The committee does not mean to suggest that in all instances a simple, direct link can be shown between participation in Medicaid and reduced low birthweight. Our assessment of available data, however, leads to the conclusion that:

> Medicaid increases participation in prenatal care by lowering financial barriers to such services. And because participation in prenatal care is associated with improved birthweight, efforts to expand and strengthen the Medicaid program should be part of a comprehensive program to reduce the nation's incidence of low birthweight. Decreasing the participation of pregnant women in the Medicaid program by such means as changing welfare or Medicaid eligibility criteria serves only to undermine the purpose of the program and, among other things, threatens appropriate use of prenatal care and increases costs for low birthweight infant care. Changes in the program should be dedicated to enrolling more, not fewer, indigent, eligible women in the program and to providing them with early and regular prenatal care of high quality.

The committee did not undertake a detailed review of the 52 Medicaid programs in the United States or the many ways that have been suggested for revising the programs' maternity policies. It is apparent, though, that defining the population of Medicaid-eligible pregnant women is a controversial topic both in Congress and in state governments. In that context, the committee recommends that:

> The Health Care Financing Administration (HCFA), in collaboration with the Division of Maternal and Child Health (DMCH), should establish a set of generous eligibility standards that maximize the possibility that poor women will qualify for Medicaid coverage and thus be able to obtain prenatal care. All Medicaid programs should be required to use such standards. In particular, eligibility standards should provide Medicaid coverage for pregnant,

indigent women, regardless of their family composition or the employment status of the chief breadwinner in the family unit.

Medicaid policies and reimbursement rates also should reflect the high-risk nature of the Medicaid-eligible population. Pregnant women enrolled in the program often are at elevated risk of a poor pregnancy outcome, including low birthweight, and may need more frequent prenatal visits and care of a more specialized, intense nature than low-risk women.

To reflect the high-risk status of many Medicaid-eligible pregnant women, program policies should not set a limit on the number of prenatal visits a Medicaid-eligible woman may have, and reimbursement rates should reflect the fact that such women often need more services and more specialized care than low-risk women.

In Chapter 8, the committee urges that DMCH define a model of prenatal care for use in publicly financed facilities providing prenatal care. Building on that recommendation, the committee also urges that:

HCFA should adopt the prenatal care model developed by DMCH as its standard of care for Medicaid recipients and should require its use in all Medicaid programs. HCFA and appropriate state agencies should monitor the adequacy of adherence to such a standard of care.

Maternity Care Providers

A second barrier is the lack of prenatal care providers. The problem of inadequate numbers of private physicians providing prenatal care in some areas is well documented. For example, as part of a 1983 needs assessment, the Oklahoma Department of Health administered questionnaires and interviews to public health providers throughout the state. Respondents in 66 counties reported "an insufficient number of physicians who will provide any prenatal or delivery care. Almost one-third of the physicians who were providing maternity services were not taking new patients."[22] Similarly, a survey of Kentucky obstetricians and gynecologists found that in Lexington and Fayette counties none accepted Medicaid patients, even though these counties have the highest concentration of physicians in the state.[9]

Increasing the availability of prenatal care providers in various locales is a complicated issue, in part because the participation of several provider groups must be considered in addition to obstetrician-gynecologists, who perform about 80 percent of deliveries in the United States. In 1977, for example, family physicians and general practitioners performed almost 20 percent of all deliveries (6 percent and 12 percent, respectively); and certified nurse-midwives managed approximately 2 percent of deliveries,[23] many of which involved socially disadvantaged women. Moreover, a substantial amount of prenatal care (as distinct from deliveries) is managed by nurse-midwives, nurse practitioners, and public health nurses. Nonetheless, in this section only two of the provider groups are discussed: obstetrician- gynecologists, who offer the majority of prenatal services, and a combined group consisting of certified nurse-midwives and obstetrical nurse practitioners, because they often care for socioeconomically disadvantaged women who are at elevated risk of low birthweight.

Obstetrician-Gynecologists

The major role played by obstetrician-gyncologists in providing prenatal care is obvious. In recent years, however, several developments in the obstetric community have restricted the capacity of the specialty to provide prenatal care to more pregnant women.

Of special concern is the fact that the participation rate of obstetrician-gynecologists in the Medicaid program is relatively low and may be decreasing. In California, for example, the number of obstetrician-gynecologists accepting Medicaid patients for maternity care dropped by 30 percent between 1974 and 1977 (from 65 percent to 46 percent).[24] A 1983 Oklahoma report stated that one-third of Oklahoma physicians providing maternity care will not accept Medicaid as a method of payment.[22] It seems reasonable to assume that such poor participation in Medicaid results in an overall lack of available prenatal care.

In one of the few detailed studies of Medicaid participation among obstetrician-gynecologists, Mitchell and Schurman studied a sample of more than 1,800 office-based physicians to assess the factors influencing Medicaid participation decisions by physicians in three specialities: obstetrics-gynecology, pediatrics, and general surgery. They found that obstetrician-gynecologists had substantially smaller Medicaid patient loads (8 percent) than either pediatricians or general surgeons (more than 13 percent). Moreover, almost 36 percent of the obstetrician-gynecologists saw no Medicaid patients whatsoever, in contrast to 23 percent of pediatricians and about 10 percent of general surgeons.[25]

Massachusetts Department of Public Welfare data from 1983 support these findings. Ten welfare service areas had no participating obstetrician-gynecologist for more than a thousand Medicaid women under 65, and 13 welfare service areas had only one obstetrician-gynecologist.[26]

Mitchell and Schurman's study found that obstetrician-gynecologists, along with general surgeons, receive unusually low Medicaid reimbursement rates. Among the physicians they surveryed, they found that Medicaid often paid less than 60 percent of the usual office visit fee. California, for example, reimbursed participating obstetrician-gynecologists in 1982 at only one-third of the private fee paid for normal prenatal care and delivery. These relatively low reimbursement rates account for some of the differences found in physician participation rates, as documented in other studies.[24, 27]

Another reason for differentials in provider participation is the fact that obstetricians are paid by Medicaid for a "package" of services that usually includes 10 to 12 patient care visits, plus delivery and postpartum care. In many Medicaid programs, billing for all of these services cannot occur until after the delivery, so that by the time the physician is paid, 10 to 18 months may have elapsed, further reducing the reimbursement amount in real dollars because of inflation. Also, the fixed Medicaid fee for prenatal care does not allow for the large number of high-risk pregnancies in this population. These women often need more intensive care than low-risk women. Finally, in some states, the entire Medicaid fee goes to the health professional attending the delivery, whether or not that individual provided the majority of the prenatal care. Thus, the incentives are directed more toward managing the deliveries of Medicaid-eligible women than toward their prenatal care.[28] Consistent with such findings, Mitchell and Schurman reported that factors that appeared to increase physician participation in Medicaid included higher Medicaid fees, more efficient processing of Medicaid claims, and fewer benefit restrictions, such as prior authorization and service limitations.

In short, one reason that prenatal care is not fully accessible to poor populations is the relative lack of private obstetrical services for women relying on Medicaid. To ease this problem the committee recommends that:

> HCFA should develop a series of demonstration/evaluation projects aimed at increasing the participation of obstetrician-gynecologists in Medicaid. Approaches should include reducing delays in reimbursement, increasing reimbursement rates, and increasing the number of prenatal visits reimbursed by Medicaid. The results of these projects should be vigorously disseminated to policy leaders and others in a position to modify Medicaid policies.
>
> To the extent that provider attitudes are found to impede Medicaid participation, local and national professional societies, including the American College of Obstetricians and Gynecololgists, should undertake appropriate education to urge members to increase their Medicaid patient loads.

The increased risk of a poor pregnancy outcome among high-risk women, discussed above, creates an additional disincentive to caring for these groups. Poor outcomes raise the possibility of a malpractice suit, and indeed, the threat of malpractice has emerged as a serious barrier to expanding obstetric care to women at risk of low birthweight and related problems. In response to increasing malpractice insurance premiums and other factors, obstetrician-gynecologists are revising their practices. A 1983 survey of obstetrician-gynecologists revealed that almost 18 percent of those surveyed had decreased their level of obstetric care to high-risk women, 10 percent had decreased the number of deliveries, and 9 percent no longer practiced obstetrics at all.[29] Because prevention of low birthweight requires fully available prenatal care and, more important, specialized care for high-risk women, these survey findings are of major concern.

Nurse-Midwives and Obstetrical Nurse Practitioners

The committee also considered whether access to prenatal care could be extended by greater reliance on the use of nurse-midwives and nurse practitioners. Certified nurse-midwives (CNMs) are health professionals trained to manage the care of essentially normal women and their newborns during pregnancy, childbirth, and the postpartum/neonatal period. They work in conjunction with physicians, with whom they consult and to whom they refer patients who develop complications or high-risk medical conditions. Although nurse-midwives currently deliver only about 2 percent of the babies born in the United States, they are more active in many other industrialized nations. In Norway, almost 96 percent of pregnant women receive prenatal care and delivery services from midwives; in England, 70 percent do.[30] Nurse practitioners (NPs), quite similar in most respects to nurse-midwives, do not manage intrapartum and immediate postpartum care; their training places greater emphasis on gynecology, but they also provide substantial amounts of prenatal care.

The relevance of such providers to low birthweight prevention derives from the fact that CNMs and NPs have been shown to be particularly effective in managing the care of pregnant women who are at high risk because of social and economic factors.[31] These women often have difficulty communicating effectively with authority figures and may need a great deal of education and support during pregnancy. CNMs and NPs are particularly well-suited to meet such needs. They tend to relate to their patients in a nonauthoritarian manner and to emphasize education, support, and patient satisfaction. Many anecdotal reports suggest that nurse-midwives and nurse practitioners spend more time with their patients than do physicians and are more likely to include counseling and education in their interactions--components of care that are central to prevention of low birthweight (Chapter 8). This general impression is confirmed by a 1981 study that analyzed the content and process of prenatal care provided by CNMs and found significant time spent on teaching during each visit. The mean length of the prenatal visit with the CNM was 23.7 minutes.[32] The 1975 National Ambulatory Medical Care Survey found that prenatal visits with office-based physicians tended to be brief (about 10 minutes) and usually did not include counseling. Thirty-two percent of the patients' visits included no more than 5 minutes with the physician.[33]

One manifestation of the special skills of nurse-midwives and nurse practitioners is the finding of increased "compliance"--i.e. keeping appointments and following specified treatments--among women served by nurse-midwives. For example, in 1976, Slome et al. reported on a randomized clinical trial of nurse-midwifery care as compared to care by the obstetric house staff at the University of Mississippi Medical Center. Nurse-midwifery patients kept a sigificantly greater proportion of appointments for prenatal care. [34]

An older study described the impact on prenatal care, prematurity, and neonatal mortality rates of a 3-year demonstration program employing nurse-midwives. From 1960 to 1963, two nurse-midwives managed most normal pregnancies in a county hospital in rural California and delivered 78 percent of the patients. Until the arrival of these CNMs, the area had a major undersupply of maternity care providers. Their presence was associated with an increase in the frequency and regularity of prenatal care visits and a decrease in prematurity and neonatal mortality rates. The discontinuation of the program after 3 years was associated with a reversal of these trends, even though more physicians had by then moved into the area, thereby alleviating the earlier deficit in care providers.[35]

With specific regard to low birthweight, Piechnik and Corbett found a significantly lower incidence of low birthweight among the infants of pregnant adolescents cared for by a multidisciplinary team (medicine, nurse-midwifery, nutrition, social work, and nursing, with CNMs managing the case load and seeing each patient at every prenatal visit), than among a matched control group who received prenatal care through state-supported maternal and child care clinics. Patients in both groups were of low socioeconomic status. The low birthweight rate of the nurse-midwife group was 28 percent less than that of the control group. Among adolescents under age 15, the nurse-midwife patients' low birthweight rate was 50 percent lower than that of the control group.[31]

CNM services are important to low birthweight prevention for another reason. In the United States, CNMs serve disproportionate numbers of women who are poor, adolescent, members of minority groups, and residents of inner cities or rural areas,[36] the same groups in which low birthweight rates are often elevated. In selected communities, they have developed specialized maternity care services to meet the needs of socially and economically high-risk women. In recognition of such factors, the committee recommends that:

> More reliance should be placed on nurse-midwives and nurse practitioners to increase access to prenatal care for hard-to-reach, often high-risk groups. Maternity programs designed to serve socioeconomically high-risk mothers should increase their use of such providers; and state laws should be supportive of nurse-midwifery practice and of collaborations between physicians and nurse-midwives/nurse practitioners.

Insufficient Prenatal Care Services

Closely related to the issue of financial barriers and poor provider availability is the possibility that there are an inadequate number of organized facilities, often publicly financed, providing prenatal care to those unable or unwilling to use the private care system. Often these are women who traditionally have relied for care on facilities such as Community Health Centers, Maternity and Infant Care Projects, hospital outpatient departments, and health departments.

The importance of these facilities derives not only from their capacity to provide prenatal care to groups often receiving inadequate services, but also from the fact that there are populations that may be better served by public facilities offering a range of services than by physicians in private practice who traditionally provide only medical care. The poor and the very young, as well as those not yet part of the mainstream culture, such as recent immigrants and Native Americans, benefit from the outreach activities, the social work, the nutritional counseling, and other nonmedical services that are often provided in such settings. Other sections of this chapter and portions of Chapters 6 and 8 discuss the significance of such expanded prenatal services for low birthweight prevention.

Unfortunately, information is lacking on the extent of prenatal services in such settings. Moreover, the issues of financial barriers, indequate numbers of providers, and inadequate service sites are highly interrelated, which makes it difficult to study the problems separately. Nonetheless, the committee has identified a number of studies and reports that bear directly on the topic of service availability. A few of these are summarized below.

The Ohio Department of Health, for example, reports that maternal and child health services are nonexistent in 11 counties that have the greatest primary care need. The Department also reports that in counties with clinics, waiting time for a prenatal care appointment may be 2 months.[11] Similarly, the Children's Defense Fund estimates that in Ohio 35,000 low-income women delivering babies each year need subsidized services; yet only 13,000 are served by existing clinics. In a 1983 review of prenatal services, CDF Ohio reports that only 28 of the state's 88 counties have state or federally funded prenatal clinics.[11]

A 1983 study of prenatal care in Kentucky found that in order to reduce deficits, the University of Kentucky Medical Center has had to reduce the amount of money spent for "uncompensated care" (e.g., care for indigent patients not reimbursed by federal, state, or local funds). One consequence has been a reduction in services that do not typically generate profits for the hospital, such as prenatal and obstetrical services.[9]

An April 1984 report by Statewide Youth Advocacy, Inc., in Rochester, N.Y., documents the lack of service sites as a significant barrier to obtaining prenatal care in upstate New York: "In 39 of the 57 upstate counties, there are no service providers other than private doctors. . . . It is estimated that in 1981 nearly 20 percent of New York State's population resided in federally designated medically underserved areas. This means that for many upstate New Yorkers neither clinics nor private doctors are easily accessible."[37]

In the absence of adequate data on prenatal service availability, both state and national, the committee is unable to determine how widespread such service gaps are, what the overall trends in availability are, or whether other systems have been able to meet changing needs. However, the data presented earlier on inadequate numbers of obstetric care providers accepting Medicaid, and on the number of women who still do not begin prenatal care in the first trimester, are consistent with the view that prenatal services in organized settings such as hospital out-patient departments and Community Health Centers are insufficient.

In many communities, increased support of health departments in particular could help improve the availability of prenatal services. The committee highlights health departments for several reasons. They are numerous and ubiquitous; virtually every person in the United States lives in an area that is served by a health department, usually organized at the local level. Moreover, health department clinics are known to be active providers of prenatal care. The Association of State and Territorial Health Officials (ASTHO) Foundation has estimated that in 1982, state health department agencies provided, purchased, or arranged prenatal services for over 13 percent of all pregnant women in the United States receiving prenatal care. Although this estimate is based on only 37 of the 50 states, the ASTHO Foundation believes that the figure is a reasonable estimate for the nation.[38]

ASTHO Foundation data also indicate that reliance on health departments for maternity care has been increasing. Whereas in 1981 about 11.7 percent of pregnant women obtained their prenatal services through a health department, by 1982 this figure had increased to 13.4 percent,[38] as noted above. This trend is consistent with recent economic events. The recession in the early 1980s, imposing high unemployment rates and loss of health insurance, and service cutbacks such as those noted above, probably caused some women who previously obtained care from private sources to turn to local health departments for prenatal care. For example, the health department in Guilford County, N.C., reported an 11 percent increase in maternity visits from 1982 to 1983, a change that health department personnel attributed not to population growth but rather to a switch from private to public care. The Multnomah County Health Department in Oregon also reported great increases in demand for prenatal care. In 1978, 100 clients received prenatal care through the health department; in 1982, the figure had grown to 900, some of whom were channeled into care by private physicians under contract with the health department. These and other reports of long waiting lists for care and increased prenatal care patient loads in selected health departments are consistent with an overall increase in the demand for prenatal care through health departments.[39]

Relying on health departments to address the unmet needs for prenatal care will, of course, require greater resources. But it should not be assumed that in all instances, greater reliance on health departments will be the preferred way to fill gaps in services. In some communities, additional support of Community Health Centers, Maternity and Infant Care Projects, hospital outpatient departments, or related settings may be a better way to provide an adequate network of prenatal services.

The committee believes, however, that while support of individual programs or service systems is important and clearly desirable, gaps in care probably will remain until a stronger commitment is made nationally to providing full access to prenatal care. This chapter concludes with a proposal along these lines.

Women's Experiences, Attitudes, and Beliefs

Access to prenatal services depends not only on adequate providers, facilities, and funds. It is also affected by a woman's perceptions of whether such care is useful, supportive, and pleasant; by her general fund of knowledge about prenatal care; and by her cultural values and beliefs. In particular, a perceived lack of "caring" in prenatal care, especially as provided to poor and socially disadvantaged women, may be an important cause of late registration, poor continuation in care, unsuccessful communication with providers, and, consequently, heightened risk for a poor pregnancy outcome. This has been confirmed by numerous studies of reasons given for not seeking prenatal care, including those of Herzog and Bernstein,[40] the Perinatal Association of Michigan,[41] and Chao et al.[12] Economic and health care system-related reasons are quoted often in these reports (which span two decades), but there is also considerable emphasis on reasons related to women's attitudes and beliefs.

For example, women may fail to seek prenatal care early because they lack information about the symptoms of pregnancy, the facilities that could assist them, or the importance of early care in averting the complications of pregnancy. The very young are particularly likely to fall into this category, as are the foreign born and those with limited formal education. Women who have experienced previous pregnancies may be unaware of their high-risk status or believe that they know enough and do not need early care or frequent visits. Additionally, some women may harbor fears about examinations, labor and delivery, and pregnancy generally to the extent that they avoid contact with health care providers.

Some women may be aware of their need for prenatal care but be indifferent or resistant to seeking it. Often this is related to previous unfortunate experiences with medical care. Several studies have noted frequent consumer dissatisfaction with prenatal services and the desire for more personal care.[42-45] In a 1968 report on factors affecting perinatal mortality in England, Vaughan noted that "many mothers who delayed [prenatal care] had had previous pregnancies during which they had gained the impression that there is no value in prenatal care. They supported their arguments from their experience, with complaints of long waits, rushed examinations, and an impersonal approach which did not encourage them to ask questions or seek advice" (p. 144).[46] More recent studies from the United States reveal the same themes. A 1976 study based on interviews with almost 300 women who had recently delivered babies in hospitals in the midwestern United States reported that only 69 percent were satisfied that their doctors understood their feelings during pregnancy, and only about 60 percent thought that their physicians' explanations of procedures and medications were satisfactory.[47]

Cultural, religious, or family beliefs also may impede acceptance of prenatal care or compliance with provider recommendations. For example, in discussion sessions held before the initiation of a federal information and education campaign to improve the outcome of pregnancy (the Healthy Mothers, Healthy Babies Coalition), women reported dietary patterns that made it difficult to follow selected nutritional guidelines. A more common cultural barrier to prenatal care is the view among some groups that women should receive prenatal care only from other women. Thus, some Hispanic, Southeast Asian, and Middle Eastern immigrants, accustomed to receiving health care from women practitioners, are reluctant to seek prenatal care from male physicians.

A further cultural difference that impedes access to care is language incompatibility. The scarcity of health care providers who serve non-English speaking clients in their own language presents a serious obstacle to many pregnant women. Inability to communicate with a health care practititioner effectively renders health care inaccessible.

Women who are aware that their life styles are not conducive to a healthy pregnancy also may delay seeking care. These would include drug abusers, heavy smokers or drinkers, the obese, and those with poor eating habits. Delay also may be related to psychological factors, such as an unwanted pregnancy. A desire to conceal the pregnancy also may keep women from seeking care. This situation is found more often among very young or unmarried women and it may be related to denial or a wish not to be pregnant. Intrapsychic factors such as depression and denial also may be major reasons for failure to seek out prenatal care, particularly among teenagers.[48]

The strategies available to overcome such barriers to participation in prenatal care fall generally into two categories. The first, and most often discussed, is general education about prenatal care, provided in a variety of settings and through multiple media (Chapters 5 and 9). The second strategy concerns the nature and atmosphere of prenatal care itself. A personal, caring environment has been a key ingredient of several prenatal care programs designed specifically to reduce low birthweight and infant mortality in high-risk groups, especially teenagers.[49] Although programs differ, some common elements of a "caring environment" can be defined and should be incorporated into prenatal services to make them more accessible, particularly for socioeconomically disadvantaged women:

- respect for patients--their questions, their problems, and their time; conveyance of the expectation that they can, with support and education, assume increasing responsibility for their own health and that of their babies;
- accessibility--institution of a system by which patients can always reach a provider who is known to them and who will respond to their concerns; this involves an increased capacity for telephone consultation;

• continuity of care--no more than two or three primary care providers for each woman; missed appointments should be followed up by a telephone call or home visit;

• restricted size (or decentralization into teams of limited size) so the woman does not have to deal with a large, impersonal bureaucracy--a program designed to be sensitive to local conditions and the schedules of the women themselves;

• responsiveness through individual education and communication to the concerns that are most salient to women in early pregnancy, such as first trimester nausea and other discomforts of pregnancy, and recognition of the need for emotional support and acceptance;

• flexibility that allows providers to help women obtain benefits other than prenatal care, such as welfare and housing services, and enrollment in the Special Supplemental Program for Women, Infants and Children (WIC); and

• understanding of cultural barriers such as language incompatibility and preferences for certain types of providers.

Transportation and Child Care

Difficulty in getting to a prenatal care facility, particularly in rural areas, contributes to the problem of access. For the poor, distance appears to be a significant deterrent to seeking preventive care.[50] Where health care services exist but are difficult or impossible to reach because people lack adequate transportation, transportation services are a necessary component of care.

Further, many women who would seek prenatal services have difficulty in arranging babysitting for other children at home and may put off getting care except in acute or emergency situations.

Health care programs must intervene on behalf of their patients in circumstances such as these by providing transportation and child care services. For socially disadvantaged populations, these services should be viewed as important elements in overall maternity care.

Increasing the Capacity for Outreach

Sometimes health care programs must do more than provide an open door. They must take the initiative to find, educate, and help bring women in to receive care. Two principal strategies to do so are the use of outreach personnel and the forging of referral relationships among various service systems.

Outreach Personnel

Over the last two decades, many health and social service programs have used trained personnel, sensitive to the needs and backgrounds of target populations, to recruit individuals into service programs. The tasks performed by these workers vary from setting to setting. In the field of maternity services, their activities generally include some of the following: identifying women requiring services and enrolling them in prenatal care; acting as an advocate for women to ensure access to needed services; and establishing links with other social services to address the housing, nutrition, income, and related needs of pregnant women.

A recent report from the Harvard School of Public Health suggested that declining visits for prenatal care in a group of Boston neighborhood health centers could be attributed in part to the decrease in outreach workers resulting from financial cutbacks.[51] The committee shares the belief that these workers are an effective way to improve access to care for difficult-to-reach populations. However, support for the role of outreach personnel stems mainly from anecdotal reports and program descriptions. Little information exists, for example, on the comparative advantages of various case-finding approaches; the costs of different outreach systems and workers and their effectiveness; the types of personnel best suited to various program goals and target groups; the utility of adjuncts to typical outreach programs, such as financial incentives or links to other programs; and how to meet the security needs of outreach personnel in some settings. This partial list of unanswered questions about such an important topic leads the committee to urge that:

> Research and analysis should be supported on the nature and value of outreach to increase access to prenatal care. Efforts should be made to assemble and integrate existing information about outreach approaches and to identify additional research needs. Both costs and effectiveness should be considered.

Outreach Through Program Links

Bringing hard-to-reach women into care also can be accomplished by forging strong referral relationships between prenatal services and other programs that are in touch with potential clients. The Special Supplemental Food Program for Women, Infants and Children (WIC) is a case in point. Several features of WIC facilitate increased prenatal care utilization. First, all WIC prenatal participants must document their pregnancy status, an act that encourages a formal prenatal visit and thereby increases the likelihood of early entry into a prenatal care network. Second, many WIC sites are located in neighborhood or county health centers--a fact that facilitates use of adjoining or coexisting prenatal clinics. And third, the WIC nutrition staff actively encourages prenatal care during nutritional counseling.

Research on WIC's impact on enrollment in prenatal care is slim. Kotelchuck et al. showed that WIC prenatal participation is associated with increased prenatal care utilization. Based on birth certificate data in Massachusetts in 1978, they found that fewer WIC participants obtained inadequate prenatal care (measured by number of visits) than a matched high-risk control group (3.8 percent versus 7 percent). This was particularly true for teenage mothers in the WIC program, only 5.8 percent of whom obtained inadequate prenatal care, compared with 11 percent of the control group.[52]

In South Carolina, health department prenatal clinics and WIC clinics were integrated in 1981. WIC enrollment is now closely tied to prenatal services. Health department officials report that as a result of this change, the 21,000 pregnant women enrolled in WIC, representing 40 percent of all South Carolina births, are more assured of receiving prenatal care beginning at the time of certification for WIC. A trend over the last 2 years for pregnant women to enroll earlier in WIC has been paralleled by an increase in early starts in prenatal care.[53]

In sum, WIC appears to increase early enrollment in prenatal care by serving as a "recruiter." When WIC and prenatal care are closely tied, their mutual benefits may be enhanced. This particular set of findings illustrates the importance of program links as a source of outreach to clients in need of prenatal services.

A System of Accountability and Responsibility

The six preceding sections explore reasons why some women obtain inadequate prenatal care, but it is the committee's conclusion that problems of access also reflect the nation's patchwork, nonsystematic approach to making such services available. Although numerous programs have been developed in past years to extend prenatal care to more women, no institution bears responsibility for assuring that such services are genuinely available in some very fundamental, practical sense. That is, no local, state, or federal entity can be held accountable for inadequate care. Without such responsibility or accountability, it should not be surprising that gaps in care remain and that efforts to expand prenatal services often face enormous organizational and administrative difficulties.

The federal government has long been on record as supporting prenatal care and urging that all women secure such care early in pregnancy. This support must be accompanied by specific actions:

- providing funds to state and local agencies in amounts sufficient to remove financial barriers to prenatal care (through channels such as the Maternal and Child Health Services Block Grants, Medicaid, health departments, Community Health Centers, and related systems);
- providing prompt, high-quality technical consultation to the states on clinical, administrative, and organizational problems that can impede the extension of prenatal services;
- defining a model of prenatal services for use in public facilities providing maternity care; and
- funding demonstration and evaluation programs, and supporting training and research related to these responsibilities.

States should take a complementary leadership role in extending prenatal services, backed by adequate federal money, support, and consultation. One way to do so is for each state to designate an organization--probably the state health department--as responsible for ensuring that prenatal services are reasonably available and accessible in every community. This would involve the state in:

- assessing unmet needs--e.g., surveying existing prenatal services and identifying the localities and populations that have inadequate prenatal services;
- serving as a broker to contract with private providers to fill gaps in services; and
- in some instances, providing prenatal services directly through facilities such as Community Health Centers and health department clinics.

In addition, the committee suggests that in each community a single organization be designated by the state as the "residual guarantor" of prenatal services. These organizations should be provided with sufficient funds to care for pregnant women who still remain outside of the prenatal care system. Local health departments could meet this responsibility in many ways: through contracts with private providers; through special programs; through arrangements with local hospitals, medical schools, and nurse-midwifery services; and through direct provision of care.

In order to develop these concepts more fully, the committee recommends that:

> The Secretary of the Department of Health and Human Services should convene a task force charged with defining a system for making prenatal services fully available to all pregnant women. Such a group must include representatives from the Congress, the Public Health Service, the Health Care Financing Administration, state governments and health authorities, maternity care providers, and consumers.

This task force should define concrete ways for both federal and state leaders to assume responsibility for the tasks outlined above. In so doing, the group should focus on four specific issues in the development of a workable system. First, the system must incorporate mechanisms at both federal and state levels to bring together the knowledge and general goals of maternal and child health programs with the "dollar power" of the Medicaid program. The clinical and health expertise of the one is rarely related to the financial power of the other. The committee did not define how such links might be made, but wishes to highlight this as a central issue.

Second, existing experience with regionalization of perinatal services should be reviewed for lessons applicable to prenatal care. The regionalization of perinatal services has been shown to reduce neonatal mortality,[54] and some aspects of the process probably could contribute to a decrease in low birthweight. In particular, regionalization could help to:

• assess unmet needs, define available resources, and specify high-risk target populations;
• disseminate new data in an orderly way to practitioners;
• rationalize the system of health care services and facilties, and help to limit inappropriate dissemination of technology;
• monitor selected health indices and patterns of practice; and
• arrange early referral/transport for high-risk women to a facility providing an appropriate level of obstetrical care.

A third topic that the task force should address is the lack of adequate state and national data for assessing unmet need for prenatal services and available resources to meet these needs. Regionalized networks of perinatal care may provide a model for collecting such data. The Alan Guttmacher Institute has developed a workable, well-respected system for estimating unmet family planning needs; a similar effort should survey prenatal care. In so stating, the committee wishes to highlight the more general problem of inadequate data on a wide range of health indicators and health services. Lack of sufficient and timely data hamper efforts to monitor maternal and child health on a population basis and, in particular, to assess the impact of public programs such as Medicaid and various private initiatives on specific health outcomes. Efforts such as the Child Health Outcomes Project of the University of North Carolina are important in addressing this concern and in helping to increase available data. The professional societies concerned with maternal and child health (such as the American Academy of Pediatrics and the American College of Obstetricians and Gynecologists) also are involved in developing and refining various outcome measures that are useful in judging the impact of clinical and programmatic interventions. Additional observations on data systems are contained in Appendix D.

Fourth, the task force should consider the long-term prospects for ensuring that prenatal care is financed adequately in times of cost containment. Preventive services, of which prenatal care is a prime example, often have been poor competitors for dollars. In part, this results from the fact that such services lie in the domain of low technology, labor-intensive services, and are often provided on an ambulatory basis. Such services traditionally have not been incorporated into insurance plans and are considered to be services for which individuals can and will pay from their own resources. For those unable to pay, preventive services are often supported by chronically underfunded municipal and county resources.

In view of the general underfunding of such preventive services, the committee is concerned about the effects of current efforts at cost containment, which include the reimbursement of hospitals for publicly funded care on a per-case basis (diagnosis-related groups or DRGs); "preferred provider options," under which care is payed for only if provided by approved providers; and "prepaid managed health care," which restricts the use of care by publicly funded patients to specific, limited provider systems that are paid prospectively. Each of these mechanisms has the potential to reduce costs and improve care, especially by increasing accountability among providers and improving continuity. However, in certain situations these alternatives also may have serious disadvantages, such as disruption of existing patient-provider relationships, decreased access to services in the name of cost-saving for high-risk patients known to require such services, and changes in established referral patterns in regionalized systems. They also may threaten the roles traditionally played by health departments, nurse-midwives, Community Health Centers, and hospital outpatient departments. Thus, where such changes in the delivery of care are introduced, the committee urges that adequate resources be made available to monitor the access to and adequacy of care, particularly prenatal care, provided under the new arrangements.

In sum, the committee believes that, in the long run, full access to prenatal care requires a fundamental assumption of responsibility by the public sector for making such services available. In many instances, arrangements with private providers will be able to fill gaps in care; in others, governmental agencies may need to provide care directly. Federal leadership will be critical to this policy goal, but states also must attach high priority to prenatal care. At both levels, full support of the private sector and a greater commitment of public funds will be required.

References and Notes

1. Select Panel for the Promotion of Child Health: Better Health for Our Children: A National Strategy. Vol. I, p. 192. DHHS No. (PHS) 79-55071. Public Health Service. Washington, D.C.: U.S. Government Printing Office, 1981.
2. Public Health Service: Promoting Health/Preventing Disease: Objectives for the Nation, p. 18. Washington, D.C.: U.S. Government Printing Office, Fall 1980.
3. National Center for Health Statistics: Advance Report of Final Natality Statistics, 1981. Monthly Vital Statistics Report, Vol. 32, No. 9 (supplement). DHHS No. (PHS) 84-1120. Public Health Service. Washington, D.C.: U.S. Government Printing Office, December 1983.
4. Division of Maternal and Child Health: Statistical Update on Progress, Pregnancy and Infant Health Objectives. Progress Review, Rockville, Md., March 29, 1983.
5. National Center for Health Statistics: Prenatal Care: United States 1969-1975. Prepared by S Taffel. Vital and Health Statistics, Series 21, No. 33. DHHS No. (PHS) 78-1911. Public Health Service. Washington, D.C.: U.S. Government Printing Office, September 1978.
6. National Center for Health Statistics: Advance Report of Final Natality Statistics, 1980. Monthly Vital Statistics Report, Vol. 31, No. 8 (supplement). DHHS No. (PHS) 83-1120. Public Health Service. Washington, D.C.: U.S. Government Printing Office, November 1982.
7. Children's Defense Fund: American Children in Poverty. Washington, D.C., 1984.

8. Food Research and Action Center: The Widening Gap: The Incidence and Distribution of Infant Mortality and Low Birthweight in the United States, 1978-1982. Washington, D.C., 1984.
9. Kentucky Coalition for Maternal and Child Health, Kentucky Youth Advocates Inc.: Healthy Mothers and Babies: Pay Now or Pay Later. Lexington, Ky., 1983.
10. Oregon State Health Division: Prenatal Care in Oregon, 1982. Eugene, Oreg.: Center for Health Statistics, 1982.
11. Lazarus W: Right From the Start: Improving Health Care for Ohio's Pregnant Women and Their Children. Columbus, Ohio: Children's Defense Fund-Ohio, 1983.
12. Chao S, Imaizumi S, Gorman S, and Lowenstein R: Reasons for absence of prenatal care and its consequences. Unpublished paper. Department of Obstetrics and Gynecology, Harlem Hospital, New York, 1984.
13. Berger LR: Public/private cooperation in rural maternal child health efforts: The Lea County, New Mexico Perinatal Program. Unpublished paper, 1983.
14. National Center for Health Services Research: Who are the uninsured? Data Review #1. Prepared by JA Kasper, D Walden, and G Wilensky. Hyattsville, Md.: National Center for Health Services Research, 1981.
15. National Center for Health Statistics: Health care coverage and insurance premiums of families, United States, 1980. Prepared by M Dicker. National Medical Care Utilization and Expenditure Survey, Preliminary Data Report, No. 3. DHHS No. (PHS) 83-20000. Public Health Service. Washington, D.C.: U.S. Government Printing Office, May 1983.
16. National Center for Health Statistics: Health insurance coverage and physician visits among Hispanic and non-Hispanic people. Prepared by FM Trevino and AJ Moss. In Health, United States, 1983, pp. 45-48. DHHS No. (PHS) 84-1232. Public Health Service. Washington, D.C.: U.S. Government Printing Office, December 1983.
17. National Center for Health Statistics: Vital Statistics of the United States, Vol. I, Natality. Individual years: 1967 through 1979. Public Health Service. Washington, D.C.: U.S. Government Printing Office.
18. Norris FD and Williams RL: Perinatal outcomes among Medicaid recipients in California. Am. J. Pub. Health 74:1112-1117, 1984.
19. Schwartz R and Poppen P: Measuring the Impact of CHCs on Pregnancy Outcomes: Final Report. Cambridge, Mass.: ABT Associates, 1982.
20. Missouri Monthly Vital Statistics. Provisional Statistics from the Missouri Center for Health Statistics. Vol. 16, No. 9. Jefferson City, Mo.: Missouri Division of Health, November 1982.
21. Korenbrot CC: Risk reduction in pregnancies of low income women: Comprehensive prenatal care through the OB Access Project. Mobius 4:34-43, 1984.
22. Task Force on Perinatal Care in Oklahoma: Caring for Pregnant Women and Their Infants in Oklahoma: A Needs Assessment, p. 54. Oklahoma City, Okla., 1983.

23. American College of Obstetricians and Gynecologists and the Liaison Committee for Obstetrics and Gynecology: Manpower Planning in Obstetrics and Gynecology, 1977. Supported, in part, by MCH Grant MC R-170397.
24. California Department of Consumer Affairs: Pregnant Women and Newborn Infants in California: A Deepening Crisis in Health Care. March 26, 1982.
25. Mitchell J and Schurman R: Access to OB-GYN services under Medicaid. Discussion paper. Chestnut Hill, Mass.: Center for Health Economics Research, June 30, 1982.
26. Boston Globe: Many obstetricians refusing to take patients on Medicaid, pp. 1, 28. December 4, 1983.
27. Davidson S, Simon M, and Connelly J: Interstate variation in Medicaid coverage of newborns. Unpublished paper prepared for the American Academy of Pediatrics, 1984.
28. Committee to Study the Prevention of Low Birthweight: The role of Medicaid in delivering prenatal care to low income women. Unpublished paper prepared by MA McManus. Washington, D.C.: Institute of Medicine, November 1983.
29. American College of Obstetricians and Gynecologists: Professional liability insurance and its effects: Report of a survey of ACOG's membership. Unpublished report prepared by Porter, Novelli and Associates. Washington, D.C., August 31, 1983.
30. Judith Rooks, President, American College of Nurse-Midwives, Washington D.C. Personal communication, 1984.
31. Piechnik SL and Corbett MA: Adolescent pregnancy outcome: An experience with intervention. J. Nurse-Midwifery, in press.
32. Lehrman E: Nurse-midwifery practice: A descriptive study of prenatal care. J. Nurse-Midwifery 26:27-41, 1981.
33. National Center for Health Statistics: Office Visits by Women: The National Ambulatory Medical Care Survey. Prepared by BK Cypress. Vital and Health Statistics, Series 13, No. 45. DHHS No. (PHS) 80-1976. Public Health Service. Washington, D.C.: U.S. Government Printing Office, March 1980.
34. Slome C, Wetherbee H, Daly M, Christensen K, Meglen M, and Thiede H: Effectiveness of CNMs: A prospective evaluation study. Am. J. Obstet. Gynecol. 124:177-182, 1976.
35. Levy BS, Wilkinson FS, and Marine WM: Reducing neonatal mortality rates with nurse-midwives. Am. J. Obstet. Gynecol. 109:50-58, 1971.
36. Adams C: Nurse-Midwifery in the United States: 1982. Washington, D.C.: American College of Nurse-Midwives, 1984.
37. Statewide Youth Advocacy, Inc.: Prenatal Care in Upstate New York, pp. 3-4. Rochester, N.Y.: Statewide Youth Advocacy, 1984.
38. Association of State and Territorial Health Officials Foundation: Public Health Agencies, 1982. Services and Activities, Vol. 2. Kensington, Md., 1984.
39. Data summarized by CA Miller for the committee based on data supplied by the Guilford County Health Department, N.C., by the Multnomah County Health Department, Oreg., and by the Commonwealth of Massachusetts.

40. Herzog E and Bernstein R: Health Services for Unmarried Mothers. Children's Bureau No. 425-1964. U.S. Department of Health, Education, and Welfare, Washington, D.C., 1964.
41. Perinatal Association of Michigan: Barriers to Early Prenatal Care in Michigan. Pub. No. H-837-MDPH. Lansing, Mich., May 5, 1983.
42. Enkin M and Chalmers I: Effectiveness and satisfaction in antenatal care. In Effectiveness and Satisfaction in Antenatal Care, edited by M Enkin and I Chalmers, pp. 266-290. Philadelphia: Spastics International Medical Publications, 1982.
43. Garcia J: Women's views of antenatal care. In Effectiveness And Satisfaction in Antenatal Care, edited by M Enkin and I Chalmers, pp. 81-91. Philadelphia: Spastics International Medical Publications, 1982.
44. Hall MH, Chng PK, and MacGillivray I: Is routine antenatal care worthwhile. Lancet II:78-80, 1980.
45. Reid ME and McIlwaine GM: Consumer opinion of a hospital antenatal clinic. Soc. Sci. Med. 14A:363-368, 1980.
46. Vaughan DH: Some social factors in perinatal mortality. Br. J. Prev. Soc. Med. 22:138-145, 1968.
47. Light HK, Solheim JS, and Hunter GW: Satisfaction with medical care during pregnancy and delivery. Am. J. Obstet. Gynecol. 125:827-831, 1976.
48. Joyce K, Diffenbacker G, Green J, and Sorokin Y: Internal and external barriers to obtaining prenatal care. Social Work in Health Care 9:91-96, Winter 1983.
49. Georgetown University School of Nursing: Community of Caring: 1983 Annual Report. Washington, D.C.: Georgetown University, January 9, 1984.
50. Select Panel for the Promotion of Child Health: Children's health care: The myth of equal access. Prepared by D Dutton. In Better Health for Our Children: A National Strategy. Vol. IV, pp. 357-440. DHHS No. (PHS) 79-55071. Washington, D.C.: U.S. Government Printing Office, 1981.
51. Feldman PH and Mosher BA: Preserving Essential Services: Effects of the MCH Block Grant on Five Inner City Boston Neighborhood Health Centers. Executive Summary. Boston: Harvard School of Public Health, June 1984.
52. Kotelchuck M, Schwartz JB, Anderka MT, and Finison KS: WIC participation and pregnancy outcomes: Massachusetts statewide evaluation study. Am. J. Public Health 74:1086-1092, 1984.
53. Committee to Study the Prevention of Low Birthweight: How to encourage disadvantaged women to enroll in prenatal care early and remain in care. Unpublished paper prepared by M Meglen. Washington, D.C.: Institute of Medicine, 1984.
54. McCormick MC, Shapiro S, and Starfield BH: The regionalization of perinatal services: Summary of the evaluation of a national demonstration program. JAMA, in press.

CHAPTER 8

Improving the Content of Prenatal Care

The data reviewed in Chapters 3 and 6 demonstrate that participation in prenatal care in its current form is associated with a reduced incidence of low birthweight. The data also raise the possibility that the capacity of prenatal services to prevent low birthweight could be increased by emphasizing certain elements of its content. Prenatal care undoubtedly has contributed to the recent reduction in neonatal mortality (Chapter 1). The challenge now is to build on this success and on new developments in maternity services to increase the capacity of prenatal care to prevent low birthweight.

This perspective forms the basis of the four conclusions explored in this chapter:

1. Increased prominence should be given to certain elements of prenatal care, many of which are relatively low in technological complexity; and further, prenatal care should be increasingly tailored to meet the widely varying needs and risk profiles of individual pregnant women.
2. Interventions closely associated with prenatal services can help to reduce low birthweight, particularly programs aimed at smoking reduction and better nutrition. Stress alleviation approaches also may prove valuable.
3. Strategies are available to encourage provision of improved, more flexible prenatal care, particularly for women at elevated risk of low birthweight. (Revision of professional practice standards, federal leadership, provider education, and changes in reimbursement practices are discussed.)
4. Over the longer term, the full promise of prenatal care for preventing low birthweight lies in research on its content, including the effectiveness of its individual components and the value of various combinations of interventions.

Based on the information summarized in Part I, the committee calls attention in this section to selected elements of prenatal care that are particularly important to the detection and prevention of low birthweight. Most of the care components discussed below are mentioned in the Standards for Obstetric-Gynecologic Services, published by the American College of Obstetricians and Gynecologists (ACOG),[1] and also in the Guidelines for Perinatal Care, developed jointly by the American Academy of Pediatrics and ACOG.[2] By highlighting them in this report, the committee hopes to increase their prominence in prenatal services and to strengthen the consensus among maternity care providers that these components of care are essential, not marginal elements of good prenatal services, and are especially important in preventing low birthweight. The following section outlines areas for increased emphasis in the services provided to all pregnant women; to women at elevated risk of preterm delivery; and to women at elevated risk of intrauterine growth retardation (IUGR).

Care for All Pregnant Women

The committee has identified seven components of the prenatal care offered to all pregnant women that merit increased emphasis in the effort to improve pregnancy outcome generally and to prevent both preterm delivery and IUGR in particular.

1. Establishing Explicit Goals Greater efforts to organize prenatal care around explicit goals can help focus the attention of the patient on the purposes of the prenatal visits and engage her more in her own care; the process of establishing goals also can help the practitioner to structure appropriate interventions. Reducing the risks of preterm delivery and intrauterine growth retardation are two such goals; other important ones include the prevention of perinatal mortality and fetal anomalies, and preparation for labor and delivery.

Defining the prevention of low birthweight as an explicit goal of prenatal care may require adjustments in clinical practice. For example, more prenatal visits early in pregnancy may be appropriate. At present, prenatal care seems particularly oriented toward the prevention, detection, and treatment of problems that are manifested in the third trimester, particularly preeclampsia--thus the emphasis on blood pressure monitoring, screening for proteinuria, attention to possible edema, and increased frequency of prenatal visits toward the end of pregnancy. By contrast, the goal of preventing low birthweight requires additional attention during the first and second trimesters especially to screening, diagnosis, and treatment, as early as possible, of conditions that predispose to preterm labor or IUGR, such as smoking and poor nutritional status. These problems should be addressed earlier in pregnancy (or, ideally, before conception, as discussed in Chapter 5), and in a more concentrated fashion, than the current schedule of visits permits.

2. Risk Assessment Prenatal care should include formal evaluation of risk, which may be facilitated by using risk assessment scoring systems such as those described in Chapter 2. Risk assessment must be a dynamic process--assessment should begin at the first visit early in

pregnancy and be followed by repeated evaluations to identify developing problems. Once patients are identified as high risk, a specific plan must be made to reduce the risk conditions where possible.

Screening for elevated risk of low birthweight typically involves consideration of sociodemographic factors, such as age, race, educational level, marital status, and income, as well as characteristics of the woman's personal and physical environment, and possible sources of psychosocial stress. Assessments also focus on obstetric history, general medical history (including the presence of genetic risks), and behaviors known to increase the risk of a poor pregnancy outcome, such as smoking and alcohol or other substance abuse.[3]

Risk assessment can help to increase the flexibility of prenatal care. A review of each patient's history and current situation enables health care providers to design individualized prenatal care plans. This flexibility is particularly important for women in socially disadvantaged, high-risk groups; set packages of prenatal care often are not flexible enough to manage their multiple problems.

The importance of risk assessment is underscored by evidence suggesting the need for more careful diagnosis of problems during the prenatal period. For example, Hall et al. reviewed the records of 2,186 women from the city district of Aberdeen who delivered in 1975 and found that less than half the cases of intrauterine growth retardation were detected by the clinician antenatally; related problems of misdiagnosis and overdiagnosis are also described by the authors.[4] Similarly, it has been suggested that in a significant proportion of pregnancies, hypertension is underdiagnosed; or even if diagnosed, is not treated adequately.[5] Pregnancies burdened by hypertension are more likely to culminate in growth-retarded infants and are more difficult to manage during labor. Infections, too, may go unrecognized and untreated during pregnancy. For example, some data point to asymptomatic bacteriuria as a potential cause of low birthweight (Chapter 2), yet in many prenatal settings, no attention to detecting asymptomatic bacteriuria occurs. Risk assessment can help to focus attention on such risk factors.

3. Pregnancy Dating Accurate dating of pregnancy is a cornerstone of good prenatal care. Without it, a clinician is less able to detect intrauterine growth retardation, to determine if labor is premature or how premature it might be, or to avoid iatrogenic prematurity that can be associated with elective induction of labor and nonemergency cesarean section.

The minimum data required to determine gestational age include the date of the beginning of the last menstrual period, uterine size by pelvic exam during the first trimester, date of quickening, date on which the fetal heart tones are first heard by ascultation, and serial fundal height measurements after 20 weeks gestation. When a uterine size-date discrepancy exists early in pregnancy, ultrasound can help to establish gestational age.

4. Ultrasound Imaging Ultrasonography has become a highly developed technology capable of detecting many problems associated with both preterm delivery and with infants that are small for gestational age. In particular, ultrasonography can help to date pregnancies accurately and to monitor fetal growth and development. It has therefore become an important component of prenatal care directed at preventing low birthweight and other poor outcomes.

In February 1984, the National Institutes of Health and the Food and Drug Administration sponsored a consensus development conference to assess the use of diagnostic ultrasound imaging in pregnancy.[6] The conference concluded that routine ultrasound examination of all pregnancies is not supported by available data. Almost 30 specific indications for ultrasound examination were identified, however; many of these are relevant to planning care for women at risk of low birthweight. Selected indications include estimation of fetal weight or fetal presentation in premature rupture of membranes or premature labor; evaluation of fetal condition in late registrants for prenatal care; evaluation of fetal growth when there is an identified cause of uteroplacental insufficiency, such as severe preeclampsia, or when other medical complications of pregnancy predisposing to fetal malnutrition are suspected; significant uterine size/clinical dates discrepancy as determined by serial fundal height measurements; and serial evaluation of fetal growth in multiple gestation.

5. Detection and Management of Behavioral Risks Prenatal care, and particularly periodic risk assessment, should include explicit attention to detecting behavioral risks associated with low birthweight, especially smoking, nutritional inadequacies such as poor weight gain, and moderate to heavy alcohol use (and substance abuse generally).

When such problems are identified, attempts should be made to modify them. In many settings, the intervention options are limited to physician or nurse counseling of the pregnant woman; in others, more formal programs are available on a referral basis. Selected intervention programs are reviewed later in this chapter. Here, the point is simply that practitioners should talk with their patients to determine the existence and degree of these health-compromising risks and bring to bear the best interventions available.

6. Prenatal Education There is widespread support for more and better health education for women who are pregnant or contemplating pregnancy.[7] [8] Nonetheless, education and counseling services often are inadequate, particularly for high-risk populations. Some settings, such as health maintenance organizations, try to emphasize such care, but many do not. A variety of approaches to education and counseling have been used: one-to-one counseling, group discussions, audiovisual and written materials, and "exit interviews" with a nurse who clarifies and reinforces medical recommendations made during a health care visit.[9] [10]

Topics relevant to prevention of low birthweight that should be stressed in the prenatal period include:

- behavioral risks in pregnancy, noted above;
- early signs and symptoms of pregnancy complications, including signs of preterm labor, vaginal infection, and other medical problems, and the importance of their early detection; and
- the role that prenatal care plays in improving the outcome of pregnancy and the importance of keeping prenatal care appointments.

These topics should be included in prenatal education along with the more common ones of preparation for labor and delivery, the immediate postpartum period, infant feeding, family planning, locating a pediatrician and selecting a delivery site. Chapter 5 includes additional discussion of health education topics, though from the perspective of the interval before pregnancy.

Problems that interfere with effective education of pregnant women include the short time typically scheduled for each prenatal visit, third-party reimbursement policies that pay for diagnostic and therapeutic procedures but ignore provider costs related to patient education; and lack of patient-education interest and skills on the part of many physicians.[11] This last reason suggests that nurses and related personnel may be more appropriate than physicians as providers of prenatal education.[7]

Childbirth education classes possibly could play an important role in efforts to reduce low birthweight through prenatal education. Such classes are rapidly becoming an accepted part of prenatal care in the United States. Figures from some communities suggest that between 30 and 50 percent of mothers attend some form of prenatal class.[12] To contribute more to prevention of low birthweight, however, such classes (and indeed, patient education generally) should begin earlier in pregnancy, particularly to overcome behavioral risks. Currently, these classes usually do not begin until the third trimester of pregnancy. Also, the curriculum should place greater emphasis on the prenatal period, expanding beyond the usual focus on labor and birth to include the topics noted above.[13]

Another limitation of these classes is that they do not reach all portions of society equally. Numerous studies have shown that participants in childbirth education courses tend to be married women who are older, better educated, of a higher socioeconomic group, more likely to hold good jobs, and more positive about their pregnancies than are the women who do not participate.[14] Accordingly, efforts should be made to enroll in these classes more pregnant women from those groups that often fail to take advantage of them, particularly because many such women are at high risk of low birthweight on the basis of social, economic, and behavioral factors.

The effect of childbirth classes on pregnancy outcome has been difficult to measure. Controlled studies have found that the classes are effective in reducing the need for analgesia and anesthesia during labor, even among a group of very low-income women.[15, 16] However, neither of two controlled studies that looked for an association between the classes and low birthweight found any effect.[16] [17] This may reflect in part the emphasis on labor and delivery in these classes. Preventing low birthweight is rarely addressed.

7. Health Care System Factors Chapter 7 presented several health system characteristics that can lead to increased access to prenatal care. Several of these also could be regarded as content-of-care issues, and thus they are repeated here in the context of improving prenatal care for all women:

- the importance of communication between patients and informed staff to answer patients' questions about prenatal problems and to encourage patients to report relevant signs, symptoms, and problems;
- the intangible but essential role of a caring atmosphere in which providers pay close attention to patient attitudes, feelings, responses and complaints, and are sensitive to language and cultural barriers; and
- the importance of transportation and child care services.

Also, prenatal care providers need to organize their services so that a wider variety of patient problems and risk factors can be managed, either directly or through well-organized referrals, e.g., for nutrition-related care, psychosocial counseling, and help in modifying smoking and other health compromising behaviors. Team approaches can help to provide multiple services, although the risk of fragmentation and too many care providers remains a potential problem.[18]

Care for Women at Risk of Preterm Delivery

The information presented in Chapter 2 on the etiology of prematurity and the risk factors associated with it have led several groups to organize innovative programs aimed at preventing preterm delivery; three such programs are outlined in Appendix C. The committee has reviewed preliminary data from these and related programs. The committee concluded that expanding prenatal care in several specific ways is likely to reduce the chances of preterm delivery in women judged through risk assessment to be at elevated risk of such an outcome. These additional activities build on the seven areas of emphasis described above.

1. Risk Assessment A woman who is at higher than average risk of preterm labor requires repeated risk assessment as her pregnancy proceeds. In particular, women who have been defined as high risk because of a previous preterm birth or mid-pregnancy loss may require additional cervical assessments in the second half of pregnancy to check for early signs of dilatation or effacement. The committee is aware that the value and risks of repeated pelvic examinations in later pregnancy have not been clearly assessed.

2. Patient Education Women at elevated risk of preterm delivery should be offered special education about the factors associated with prematurity; the importance of early detection of the symptoms of preterm labor, such as bleeding and periodic contractions; how to detect mild uterine contractions and how to differentiate normal contractions that often occur throughout pregnancy from those signaling early labor; and what to do when the signs and symptoms of preterm labor appear, including how to contact an obstetric care provider or facility for consultation and help. Efforts to arrest preterm labor can hinge on its early detection and prompt management.

High-risk women also should be taught to identify and lessen events in their daily lives, such as physical stress and strenuous exercise, that can trigger uterine contractions, which in turn might lead to preterm labor. The research data supporting such advice are still tentative, but common sense and clinical judgment support such caution.

3. Provider Education Patient education should be supplemented by education of prenatal care providers about the topics mentioned above and others, including: (1) the importance of being receptive to patient problems and complaints that may be early signs of preterm labor; (2) the need for prompt identification of preterm labor, and the uses of hospitalization for observation and possible treatment; and (3) the various approaches available for arresting true preterm labor.

Clinicians also need to learn how to revise their practice patterns to accommodate the increased time and attention that such high-risk women often require. Educating patients about the risks, signs, and symptoms of preterm labor is of limited value if health care providers are not organized to be responsive to such factors. In particular, encouraging a woman to call if she believes preterm labor is under way requires that procedures be in place for admitting the woman into the hospital rapidly for observation and/or treatment if necessary. Several hours delay can decrease the likelihood of arresting preterm labor.

Finally, it is important for providers to recognize clearly the risk of iatrogenic prematurity and to ensure fetal lung maturity and a gestational age of at least 37 weeks before elective induction of labor or performance of a nonemergency cesarean section.

4. Tocolysis An important approach to reducing the incidence of prematurity has been the use of agents to inhibit preterm labor. Agents known to inhibit labor include alcohol and prostaglandin synthetase inhibitors, but these are accompanied by side-effects for mother and neonate that diminish their usefulness. Magnesium sulfate also inhibits uterine contractions. Another class of labor inhibitors are the various betamimetic drugs, several of which have been developed and marketed for many years in other countries. These include isoxsuprine hydrochloride, salbutamol, terbutaline, ritodrine hydrochloride, and hexaprenaline. Only ritodrine has been licensed as a betamimetic for use in the United States for inhibition of premature labor. It was licensed in 1980, following initiation of clinical trials in 1972.[19, 20]

Such agents, to be useful, must inhibit labor for a significant period of time and prolong pregnancy until the duration of gestation is consistent with a reduction in perinatal mortality due to preterm birth. The development of research protocols to identify and test such drugs, often called "tocolytic agents," is difficult. Uterine contractions frequently occur during the latter part of pregnancy, and thus it is often difficult to differentiate between normal Braxton Hicks' contractions and true preterm labor leading to cervical dilatation. Uterine contractions may be painful or painless and may be accompanied or unaccompanied by cervical effacement and dilatation. Contractions may cease spontaneously or with bedrest, and they may or may not be stopped by hydration or mild sedation. If tocolytic agents are withheld until cervical effacement and/or dilatation are detected to confirm the diagnosis of true labor, inhibition of labor may fail; but if cervical changes are not confirmed, it is difficult to know whether contractions would have stopped spontaneously or if only false labor was present.

Patients with ruptured membranes, significant cervical effacement, or dilatation greater than 4 or 5 centimeters usually progress to delivery despite tocolytic agents. Many patients with preterm labor have medical or obstetric complications that contraindicate the use of tocolytic agents, and in cases of vaginal bleeding, chorioamnionitis, severe preeclampsia, and other obstetric complications, delivery may be in the best interests of mother and fetus. Side-effects produced by tocolytic agents include decreased peripheral resistance, decreased blood pressure, tachycardia, and frequently, palpitation and chest pain; rarely, pulmonary edema may be life threatening or even fatal.[19 20]

Current experience with tocolysis, which is now extensive, suggests several conclusions. First, in individual cases of threatened preterm labor, tocolytic therapy can often be effective, though not always. It is nonetheless true that on a population basis, tocolysis has had little impact, as evidenced by the relatively minimal decline in the incidence of prematurity since the licensing and widespread use of ritodrine. This apparent paradox is probably explained in part by the failure to use tocolytic drugs in all suitable cases; the failure to use such agents until labor is well established, which decreases their efficacy significantly; and the number of contraindications and side-effects that limit the pool of pregnant women who could benefit from tocolysis.

The indications for and proper use of tocolytic agents need further definition and more widespread dissemination. In particular, the vital importance of early diagnosis of preterm labor must be stressed. It is likely that if both patients and providers were better informed about the early signs and symptoms of preterm labor and about the uses of tocolytic therapy, the number of cases in which tocolytic intervention could be used effectively would increase. Huszar and Naftolin report that at present, only about one-third of pregnant patients who arrive at the hospital in preterm labor are suitable candidates for tocolytic therapy, although they do not describe the reasons why the other two thirds are not; presumably, some have contraindications and many are in advanced stages of labor.[21] It is also apparent that because of the various contraindications for use of tocolytic agents and because of their side-effects, noted above, the current generation of tocolytic drugs cannot be viewed as the long-term solution to the problem of prematurity.

Care for Women at Risk of Intrauterine Growth Retardation

Many of the risk factors associated with preterm labor also are associated with intrauterine growth retardation (IUGR). Thus, the emphases in prenatal care appropriate for prevention of preterm labor often overlap with those for prevention of IUGR. For example, careful risk assessment is as important for IUGR detection and treatment as for prematurity. Nonetheless, three points specific to IUGR can be emphasized:

1. Behavioral Risks Behavioral risks are a significant factor in fetal growth retardation. Women identified as being at elevated risk of IUGR should be encouraged to pay vigorous attention particularly to smoking reduction and to avoidance of heavy or moderate alcohol use.

2. Nutrition Maternal preconception weight and weight gain during pregnancy are major determinants of birthweight (Chapter 2). The rate of weight gain during the third trimester is a particularly important determinant of birthweight.[22] Thus, monitoring adequate weight gain and offering nutritional surveillance and counseling, while central to prenatal care generally, are particularly important for women judged to be at elevated risk of IUGR. Both the content and organization of nutrition services in prenatal care have been defined,[23] and they should be major components of high quality prenatal care, especially for high-risk women.

3. Assessment of Gestational Age and of Fetal Growth and Maturity Although important for prenatal care generally, accurate assessment of gestational age and of fetal growth and maturity is critical to the early diagnosis and effective management of intrauterine growth retardation. As noted earlier, ultrasonography can help to establish gestational age when uterine size-date discrepancies are noted.

Programs Complementary to Prenatal Care

Because many of the risks associated with low birthweight have a behavioral basis, the committee examined selected interventions intended to reduce behavioral risks, including smoking reduction programs for pregnant women and nutrition intervention programs such as the Special Supplemental Food Program for Women, Infants and Children (WIC). The committee also inquired into stress and fatigue abatement approaches. Even though the data demonstrating a role for such risk factors in low birthweight are controversial (Chapter 2), their potential importance is great. Special efforts were made to determine whether interventions in all three areas could be linked to improvements in birthweight.

The interventions reviewed are not, strictly speaking, components of prenatal care, but they should be adjuncts to more routine prenatal services. Research questions in each area are numerous. But it is the committee's judgment that while research proceeds, common sense and a growing body of data suggest that elements of these programs are useful and should be linked to prenatal care, either directly or through referral.

Smoking Reduction Programs

Several types of programs have been developed in various settings to help pregnant women stop or reduce their smoking habit. Most are based on the finding that pregnancy alone provides a strong incentive to stop smoking. About 20 to 25 percent of women who smoke at the beginning of pregnancy quit on their own at some time during the 9 months. Controlled studies suggest that aggressive intervention programs can encourage up to 30 percent more (beyond those who quit spontaneously) to stop. Unfortunately, about 80 percent of women who quit during pregnancy begin smoking again after delivery.[24]

Most studies to evaluate smoking cessation programs focus on one or more of the three most common forms of intervention: one-to-one counseling by a physician or other health professional; group counseling; and provision of self-help materials. One of the earliest studies in this area examined the effect of physician advice. In a randomized controlled study performed in Britain in 1977, 280 pregnant smokers who received smoking cessation advice were compared with 308 who did not. Twenty-seven percent of the study group stopped smoking compared with 4 percent of the controls; however, half of the advised women who quit resumed smoking later in pregnancy. Interviews with women receiving advice indicated that health education and physician advice raised their motivation to quit but did not offer enough "practical help." This study also suggested the need for repetition of advice during pregnancy.[25]

A recent 3-year study by Sexton et al. demonstrated an association between a smoking cessation program and improved birthweight. Over 900 pregnant smokers from a population shown to be at relatively high risk of poor pregnancy outcome were randomly allocated to an intervention or a control group. The intervention group received special assistance and encouragement to stop smoking in the form of information, support, practical guidance, and behavior modification methods. The control group received the usual prenatal advice from their obstetricians. Forty-three percent of the intervention group stopped smoking, but only 20 percent of the control group did. In addition, treatment group infants (single live births) were 92 grams heavier and 0.6 centimeters longer than control group infants. The lesser weight and length related to smoking could not be fully explained by gestational age. These findings suggest that some fetal growth retardation can be overcome by the provision of antismoking assistance to pregnant women.[26]

Group techniques, as distinguished from one-to-one physician advice, often have been advocated in health promotion because they appear to be more efficient. In a study of the Kaiser-Permanente Medical Care Program in Portland, Oreg., Loeb et al. found that groups were not a cost-effective intervention in the area of smoking and pregnancy. They urge, instead, that resources be available for individual counseling at the time of the prenatal care visit. Groups may be effective, however, as reinforcement and support for individual counseling.[27]

The "self-care" approach to smoking in pregnancy was studied by Ershoff et al. at the Maxicare HMO in Hawthorne, Calif. The project evaluated a home correspondence smoking cessation program in which the intervention group received printed materials on a weekly basis and called in three times a week to listen to tape-recorded reinforcing messages. More women in the experimental group (49 percent) quit smoking than in the control group (37.5 percent). Ershoff et al. estimated that up to a third of pregnant smokers tend to quit on their own, and another third can be reached through intervention. The major limitations of the study were the lack of randomization and the small sample size (N = 129).[28]

Several observations made by Ershoff et al. have implications for future programs. They concluded that it appears worthwhile to provide some form of maintenance effort for women who stop smoking at pregnancy onset. For some women, abstinence in the early stages of pregnancy may be precipitated solely by the experience of nausea, and once the symptoms abate, the temptation to return to smoking may be quite strong. For others, concerns about the health consequences of smoking during pregnancy may provide the impetus for attempting to quit initially, but may not be sufficiently strong to maintain cessation over the entire course of pregnancy.

Another type of intervention program recognizes the importance of involving the woman's partner in smoking cessation programs.[29] Based on the understanding that it is more difficult for a woman to stop smoking if other members of the household smoke, Wilner et al. developed a special intervention approach, "Quitting for Two," that includes materials directed at partners. The program features written guides that can be used either in small group sessions or distributed by clinicians as a self-care program. The authors suggest, for example, that materials be distributed in pediatrician's offices--a good opportunity to reach families in the childbearing years. The materials can also be made available through childbirth preparation classes; such classes offer a special opportunity for reaching beyond the pregnant woman because spouses/partners usually attend. An important component of this program is that it encourages women planning or considering pregnancy to join. Results of the program are not yet available.

Several themes emerge from these and other programs. First, some studies suggest that social support is a critical factor in changing smoking behavior. Spouses, partners, and other family members need to be involved in intervention efforts.

Second, prenatal care providers should be reasonable in their expectation that a pregnant woman will give up an addictive habit. The effectiveness of antismoking advice and intervention may be negated if too much is attempted. A pregnant woman is often asked to alter her eating habits, avoid alcohol, perhaps to reduce her overall stress, attend prenatal classes, and avoid drugs. These recommended changes are superimposed on fatigue, shifts in body image, and other sexual and social changes associated with pregnancy and planning for a new baby. Prenatal care providers need to consider whether it is advisable to ask that many behaviors be changed simultaneously; they may need to choose those of highest priority, of which smoking is undoubtedly one.

Third, counseling by the physician or other primary clinician appears to be among the most effective intervention strategies for the pregnant smoker, particularly given the regular schedule of prenatal visits. Last year, the American Lung Associaton published a special kit for obstetricians on how to counsel their pregnant patients who smoke. Such efforts need to be reinforced by both patient and provider education.

Fourth, use of the mass media continues to play a motivating and reinforcing role, but probably is insufficient as a single intervention (Chapter 9). Attractive marketing strategies, public service announcements, and posters should be supplemented by cigarette labels that explicitly warn of the hazards of smoking during pregnancy.

Fifth, a host of research issues can be identified. For example, we need a much better understanding of the components of effective intervention strategies. It is unlikely that one intervention will be appropriate for all pregnant smokers; we need to know specifically which types of women respond best to individual counseling, groups, and self-care approaches. In particular, we need to learn more about how to structure interventions directed at pregnant adolescents who smoke and smokers who also drink, and about strategies for multiparous versus primiparous smokers, because these two groups appear to differ in their smoking practices. Research is also needed on the motivations of women who do stop successfully during pregnancy. Some women have reported stopping due to nausea, others out of concern for the baby, and others because of physician advice. Studies should probe the origins of these motivations and how they can be used to strengthen intervention approaches. Further, maintenance strategies must be given additional attention. This holds not only for continued cessation through the pregnancy, but for postpartum behavior as well. Single-episode interventions probably will be ineffective in the long term. The role of social supports such as the spouse needs to be further evaluated, particularly as a component of maintenance.

In sum, there is no question that smoking reduction or cessation is possible in pregnancy and that it has the potential to play a major role in any overall strategy to reduce low birthweight. Accordingly:

The committee urges that helping women stop or reduce smoking in pregnancy become a major concern of obstetric care providers. Research to define how best to address the smoking problem should receive high priority; simultaneously, antismoking advice should be offered routinely by physicians and other maternity care providers and supplemented, where possible, by educational materials, media-based messages, and related strategies.

Prenatal Nutrition Intervention: WIC

The nutrition data reviewed in Chapter 2 support the view that nutritional assessment and services should be major components of high-quality prenatal care, especially for women at elevated risk of IUGR. Accordingly, the committee examined the value of the Special Supplemental Food Program for Women, Infants and Children (WIC), which provides one of the principal data sets demonstrating the importance of nutrition to birthweight and represents a major public investment in the nutritional well-being of women and children. WIC is directed at high-risk pregnant and lactating women, infants, and children up to age 5 who meet certain income and nutritional-risk eligibility standards. For pregnant women, WIC provides vouchers to purchase nutritious foods, education about nutrition, and close referral ties to prenatal services. About 500,000 women receive WIC services each year, representing about 15 percent of total U.S. births. Once these high-risk women enter the WIC program, more than 90 percent participate fully until they give birth.[30]

Evaluation studies show that prenatal participation in the WIC program is associated with improved pregnancy outcomes.[30-33] While all of the studies have some methodologic problems--WIC evaluations are particularly hindered by difficulties in obtaining an appropriate comparison population and in securing a representative WIC sample--the similarity of their results supports the overall conclusion that the WIC program provides positive benefits to nutritionally and financially high-risk pregnant women.

Of particular relevance to this report is the decrease in low birthweight incidence associated with WIC participation. Kennedy et al. reported a 33 percent decrease in low birthweight status among the babies of participating women in comparison to a control group;[32] Kotelchuck et al., a 21 percent decrease;[30] and Kotelchuck and Anderka, a 22 percent decrease.[34] Metcoff et al.[33] and Kotelchuck and Anderka also reported significant decreases in the incidence of small for gestational age babies born to women who were WIC participants.[34]

Although a recent report by the U.S. General Accounting Office (GAO) notes that the quality of the evidence regarding WIC program effects is uneven, the report also states that the evidence of program benefit is strongest for increases in mean birthweight and decreases in the percentage of low birthweight infants. "Six of the WIC studies containing information about infant birthweights are of high or medium quality. They give some support, but not conclusive evidence, for the claims that WIC increases infant birthweights. In these studies, about 7.9 percent of the mothers in WIC had infants who were less than 2,500 grams at birth, compared to about 9.5 percent of the mothers who were not in WIC. This translated into the positive finding that, in the six studies, the proportion of infants who are 'at risk' at birth because of low weight decreased as much as 20 percent. Average birthweights were between 30 and 50 grams greater for WIC participants."[35]

In another comprehensive review of WIC evaluation studies, Rush et al. concluded: "The best estimates are that participation in the WIC program does lead to increased mean birthweight, probably in the range of 20 to 60 grams, with greatest effects among those at highest risk of nutritional causes of low birthweight (women with low weight at conception, blacks, smokers, etc.). Rates of birthweight under 2500 grams appear to be lowered by about one percent, and possibly as much as two percent, from base rates of around six percent of white births, and 11 or 12 percent of black births. There is reasonably consistent evidence that much of this difference is mediated by increased duration of gestation, and not just accelerated fetal growth. (Towards term, there is about a 25 gram increase in birthweight with each day's prolonged gestation.) These levels of benefit are consistent with past experience with nutritional supplementation in pregnancy. Higher estimates generally arose from studies with suspect design and analysis."[36]

The results of WIC evaluation studies also seem to indicate that early and consistent participation in the program during pregnancy is related to magnitude of benefit. Edozien et al.,[31] Kotelchuck et al.,[30] and Schram[37] all showed that the benefits of WIC accrue principally to prenatal participants of 7 or more months duration. In particular, large reductions in low birthweight incidence are noted for women participating in WIC more than two trimesters, even after controlling for possible confounding of gestational age and duration of participation. The GAO report cited earlier concludes that there is some evidence to suggest that participating in WIC for more than 6 months is associated with larger increases in birthweight and decreases in the proportion of low birthweight infants than shorter participation periods.

A recent report has also suggested that continuing to receive WIC supplementation during the interpregnancy period can help to increase birthweight in subsequent pregnancies. Caan compared the birth outcomes of a group of women who participated in WIC during a first pregnancy, continued to receive WIC in the interpregnancy period, and remained in the program during a second pregnancy, to a group of women who also participated in WIC during both pregnancies but received very little supplementation in the interpregnancy period. The difference in mean birthweight adjusted for gestational age between the two groups was 160 grams.[38]

WIC is not the only prenatal nutrition intervention program that has been associated with improvement in low birthweight status. Results from other countries are consistent with the WIC results,[39,40] although the applicability of the programs evaluated to the United

States is unclear. Prenatal participation in the U.S. Commodity Supplemental Food Program also has been associated with a decrease in the low birthweight rate among participating women.[41] In sum, supplemental food programs seem to be associated with significant reductions in low birthweight.

It is also important to note again that WIC is not simply a nutrition supplementation program. It is a three-part intervention program involving supplemental food, nutritional counseling, and close ties to prenatal care. Each component is believed to contribute to the improved pregnancy outcome. The value of WIC as a tool for recruiting high-risk women into prenatal care is discussed in Chapter 7. Research has not isolated the differential effects of the three WIC components.

> The committee urges that nutrition supplementation programs such as WIC be a part of comprehensive strategies to reduce the incidence of low birthweight among high-risk women. Such programs should be closely linked to prenatal services.

Stress and Fatigue Alleviation

Even though the evidence associating stress with low birthweight is of uneven quality, several programs have tried to reduce the levels of stress experienced by pregnant women in an effort to improve pregnancy outcome. Some are concerned primarily with physical stress and fatigue, others more with psychosocial and emotional stress. Although the committee makes no recommendation in this report for a major commitment to stress reduction during pregnancy, it highlights this as potentially an important area. Several approaches to stress reduction are described below to give an indication of current work in this area.

Efforts to reduce physical stress to improve pregnancy outcome include the study reported in 1974 by Jeffrey et al. on the effect of bed rest in twin pregnancy. The study concluded that bed rest appeared to reduce perinatal mortality rates; however, when gestations of less than 30 weeks were excluded, bed rest did not significantly alter the perinatal mortality rate or the length of gestation. However, the incidence of small-for-gestational-age infants at all ages over 30 weeks was decreased--thus the conclusion that bed rest encourages intrauterine growth, at least in twin pregnancies.[42]

Reduction of physical stress is also part of Papiernik's low-birthweight prevention program in France (Appendix C). In that program, women with several risk factors (especially a history of preterm delivery, incompetent cervix, and/or a particularly strenuous lifestyle) are advised to reduce stress, especially physical stress, by taking a leave of absence from their jobs or by getting additional help at home from a friend, family member, or paid helper.

Approaches to reduce psychosocial and emotional stress include programs that encourage the use of social support networks. For example, Nuckolls et al. found that utilization of social support systems can reduce pregnancy complications among women exposed to multiple life crises during pregnancy.[43]

Some programs address psychosocial and physical stress simultaneously. An example is the March of Dimes continuing education program for nurses developed by Herron and Dulock, which is used in the University of California at San Francisco prematurity prevention program described in Appendix C. Nurses interview pregnant women regarding lifestyle factors that can cause excessive fatigue and that may trigger uterine contractions, such as strenuous work or activities, climbing more than three flights of stairs on a routine basis to reach living quarters, and commuting more that 1-1/2 hours daily. In addition, the nurses are instructed to determine whether pregnant women have experienced any event or series of events precipitating unusual anxiety, such as the death of a family member or close friend, loss of employment by either the pregnant woman or her partner, or separation of the pregnant woman from her partner by a dissolved relationship or divorce. Once stresses are identified, the nurses work actively to help the women toward resolution of problems. The nurses also are taught to encourage patients to seek and use the assistance of supportive individuals in their own environments and to refer patients to a social worker or psychiatrist as appropriate.[44] High-risk patients in the San Francisco program also receive psychological support during pregnancy from a member of the "Preterm Labor Support Group," consisting of nonpregnant women who have experienced preterm labor, and are encouraged to develop close relationships with the nurse practitioners who manage their prenatal care.[45]

Another potentially important stress reducing intervention is maternity leave. In a review of maternity policies in the United States, Kamerman et al. detail the inadequacies of protections for working pregnant women who wish to take leave from work before and/or after childbirth.[46] The patchwork arrangements in this country of sick leave, disability leave, leave without pay, and other leave categories provide seriously inadequate income and job security for pregnant women and new mothers who participate in the labor force. Inadequate maternity policies also make it exceedingly difficult for women to stop working in later pregnancy to reduce stress-related risk factors, such as employment requiring long periods of standing. Adequate maternity leave before childbirth may be both helpful and hard to arrange.

The committee recognizes that revising maternity policies touches complicated issues concerning women's participation in the labor force. It is reasonable to suggest, nonetheless, that more adequate maternity leave, particularly for certain high-risk women, could contribute to the reduction of low birthweight. Labor unions, women's groups, and health professionals at a minimum should direct attention to this major issue.

Encouraging Change in Prenatal Services

To encourage the provision of improved, more flexible prenatal services, particularly for women at elevated risk of low birthweight, the committee recommends four specific strategies. First, the committee recommends that:

> The suggestions made here for strengthening the capacity of prenatal care to reduce the incidence of low birthweight should be reviewed carefully by the professional societies of the major maternity care providers and by others concerned with prenatal care, to determine whether their general guidelines for clinical practice should be revised or enriched accordingly. These organizations include the American College of Obstetricans and Gynecologists, the American College of Nurse-Midwives, the American Academy of Family Practice, the Nurses Association of the American College of Obstetricians and Gynecologists, the various state level Perinatal Associations, and the American Public Health Association (particularly its Public Health Nursing section).

Second, there is a role for federal leadership in enhancing the capacity of prenatal care to reduce low birthweight. By contributing public funds to Medicaid, health departments, community and migrant health centers, and other health services, the federal government is able to influence strongly the content of care it purchases or provides directly. This influence can be used not only to improve prenatal care supported by public funds, but also to improve prenatal care in the private sector by providing a worthy example. Accordingly, the committee urges that:

> The Division of Maternal and Child Health (DMCH), in concert both with consumers and the major professional societies concerned with maternity care, should define a model of services to be used in publicly financed facilities providing prenatal care. Such standards should be flexible enough to accommodate the needs of high-risk women; deal not only with clinical/medical issues but also with behavioral issues such as smoking; include formalized risk assessment and adequate health education; and address the major barriers that decrease access to prenatal care. DMCH and appropriate state agencies should be provided with sufficient funds to monitor the adoption of the model in public facilities.

A federal statement describing model prenatal care would contribute to a uniform understanding of what the content of prenatal care should be and would help providers tailor care to specific health goals, including prevention of IUGR and preterm labor. It is important that such a statement be updated and revised frequently to incorporate new knowledge and experience and that it be used in a way that does not discourage research on improved approaches to prenatal care.

Third, the committee recommends that:

The professional societies of the major maternity care providers should undertake educational efforts for their memberships based on the prenatal care elements emphasized in this report.

The committee recognizes that the issue of how best to structure education for health care providers is complex. The following are suggested as additions to the existing system of continuing education for clinicians:

- Summary articles and reviews on ways to reduce the incidence of low birthweight should appear more frequently in professional newsletters and journals. For example, the "technical bulletin series" of the American College of Obstetricians and Gynecologists (ACOG) is believed by ACOG to be read widely by obstetricians and gyncologists and other maternity care providers. Accordingly, ACOG could use this communication source to emphasize to providers the prenatal care issues outlined in this report. Similar communications could be used by other organizations.
- Individual education/tutorials could be modeled, for example, on the Bowman Gray School of Medicine's Prevention of Prematurity Program. This program, which involves meetings between specially trained health professionals based in medical schools and community clinicians, demonstrates the leadership role that medical schools can play in reducing the incidence of low birthweight.[47]
- County medical society gatherings and meetings of national professional organizations are important sources of information for their members. At the scientific meetings of such groups, the topic of how to strengthen the capacity of prenatal care to reduce low birthweight should be given increased emphasis.
- Public information campaigns can be structured to help focus the attention of health care providers (not just the general public) on important risks such as nutritional inadequacies (Chapter 9).

Fourth and finally, it is widely recognized that reimbursement policies and practices exert enormous influence over the content of medical care. Services that are paid for adequately are provided more often than services that are covered inadequately or not at all. Many of the clinical emphases advocated in this report require services for which third party reimbursement is problematic, such as counseling and education to reduce behavioral risks; intensive prenatal services for high-risk women (which may exceed the number of visits covered in set packages of care or include more technologically intensive services); education about pregnancy risks generally, and signs and symptoms of preterm labor specifically; hospitalization for suspected preterm labor or for rest therapy; and ancillary services such as transportation to health care facilities.

There is no single, simple solution to the problem of ensuring adequate reimbursement for such services. Providers such as health maintenance organizations often support them, but most third-party payers do not. It is reasonable to argue that progress would be made, however, if at least the following were to occur:

• Both the professional societies of the major maternity care providers and the federal government stress forcefully that adequate prenatal care includes counseling and related support services and that reimbursement should be provided for them. Stipulating such services in a federal definition of comprehensive prenatal care would provide tangible evidence of such a view.

• Labor unions, businesses, and other organizations negotiate health insurance benefits that cover more comprehensive prenatal services (suggestions for revising Medicaid reimbursement policies related to prenatal care are in Chapter 7).

• Governmental agencies increase their support of research to define selected classes of services more adequately--both their content and effectiveness. Some reluctance to reimburse for services such as smoking cessation programs is undoubtedly based on understandable confusion on the part of third-party payers as to what the service actually is, who provides it, and what the level of cost-effectiveness and utilization are likely to be. Where such unanswered questions are the clear cause of reluctance to reimburse, research should be pursued to resolve the issues.

Research Needs

The field of prenatal care is filled with unanswered research questions. In Chapter 6, the evidence that prenatal care decreases the incidence of low birthweight is presented. As noted in that section, however, "prenatal care" is not carefully defined or uniformly practiced. In particular, it is not well understood which components of prenatal care lead to improved pregnancy outcome. Some practice settings offer a package of prenatal care services that is quite extensive--rich in education, screening and diagnostic services, and counseling, and closely linked to other services; other settings offer a less complete set of services. Differences in content may explain a significant part of the variation in the effects of prenatal care reported across studies.

The committee has concluded that research on the content of prenatal care should be a high funding priority for foundations, public agencies, and institutions concerned with improving maternal and child health. Research of three kinds is needed:

1. description and analysis of the <u>current</u> composition of prenatal care;
2. assessment of the efficacy and safety of numerous <u>individual components</u> of prenatal care, some of which already are widely employed and others of which are only emerging; and

3. evaluation of certain well-defined <u>combinations</u> of specific prenatal interventions designed to meet the widely varied needs and risks among pregnant women.

Making major progress in reducing low birthweight, as contrasted to the small but steady improvements in recent years, requires a far more sophisticated understanding of prenatal care content than we have at present. Over the longer term, the full promise of prenatal care lies in vigorous research to develop ways that can make it even more effective.

Describing the Current Content

Little is known about what now is included in prenatal care provided in a variety of settings, although there are stated standards of what prenatal care should include. For example, ACOG periodically publishes Standards for Obstetric-Gynecologic Services, which outlines both the recommended content and scheduling of prenatal care.[1] These standards are a codification of current understanding of important prenatal problems and their management, as are the Guidelines for Perinatal Care developed jointly by ACOG and the American Academy of Pediatrics.[2]

Adequate data do not exist, however, on the extent to which these standards are followed in various practice settings. Information is available regarding the brief amount of time obstetricians typically spend with patients in routine prenatal visits[4,8] and about the schedule of prenatal visits followed by some groups of women.[4,9] However, the extent to which prenatal care providers follow specific ACOG suggestions regarding formalized risk assessment, nutritional status assessment, prenatal education, efforts to reduce smoking in pregnant patients, and related interventions is unknown. The documented brevity of most prenatal visits suggests that many recommended activities are omitted. Accordingly, the committee recommends that:

> The Assistant Secretary for Health should take the lead in organizing activities to increase our knowledge of current prenatal care practices. Existing surveys conducted by the National Center for Health Statistics could include a special emphasis on prenatal care content.* Consumer

---

*For example, the National Survey of Family Growth and the Health Interview Survey could provide information on prenatal care from the recipient's point of view; and the National Ambulatory Medical Care Survey (NAMCS) could provide information from the provider side. However, because NAMCS surveys only office-based private practice, it will be important to develop ways to survey the content of prenatal care in other settings, such as health departments, hospital outpatient departments, nurse-midwifery services, and various public programs.

experience with prenatal care should be analyzed and the professional societies of the major maternity care providers should be consulted about ways to survey their members regarding various content issues. In some instances, it may prove necessary to undertake direct studies of provider practices.

Baseline data assembled from these sources will play a major role in the longer-term effort to better define and improve the content of prenatal care.

Research on Individual Care Components

Over the course of the study, the committee compiled a long list of research topics centered on specific interventions in prenatal care; noted below are topics judged particularly important. Some pertain to IUGR and others to preterm delivery. For the sake of simplicity, no distinction is made.

Clinical Topics

- improving various risk assessment techniques (such as risk scoring systems and assessment of cervical changes) to better identify high-risk patients;
- evaluating tocolytic drug therapy in well-defined subpopulations, including studies to compare the effectiveness of hydration, rest, and stress reduction with and without tocolysis;
- understanding the long-term effects on mother and infant of ultrasonography and of tocolytic drugs; and, similarly, studying the efficacy and long-term effects of prophylactic tocolysis in high-risk women;
- continuing to refine and evaluate the use of ultrasound imaging to diagnose pregnancy problems;
- assessing the effects of altered schedules of visits for prenatal care (in particular, could low-risk women have fewer prenatal visits than is currently recommended? Do high-risk women need more visits?);
- evaluating the efficacy and safety of various prenatal progestational agents; and
- assessing the effect on pregnancy outcome of treating a range of genitourinary tract infections and organisms.

Behavioral and Environmental Topics

- determining the best techniques of educating pregnant women (particularly high-risk women) about self-detection of the early symptoms of preterm labor, and what to do if such symptoms are detected; and evaluating the effects of such education on pregnancy outcome;

• developing and evaluating improved techniques, usable in a variety of settings, to help pregnant women reduce or quit smoking;

• developing and evaluating more effective approaches to reducing alcohol and other substance abuse in pregnant women;

• evaluating the effects of stress reducing activities such as bed rest on specific clinical conditions and the outcome of pregnancy generally, including low birthweight; in such studies, it will be important to disentangle physical stress and fatigue, psychosocial and emotional stress, and general social policies that may create stress--designing and evaluating intervention programs in this area will also require greater specificity in both measures and concepts of stress;

• developing and evaluating techniques to assess and improve the nutritional status of pregnant women, particularly those with nutritional deficiences; and

• expanding and refining the content of childbirth education classes and determining the effects of such instruction on pregnancy outcome.

Research on Combinations of Interventions

Of equal importance to studying individual components of prenatal care is research to determine the effects of various combinations of interventions. The great variation in risk status among pregnant women suggests that prenatal care should vary significantly in its content for individual women and across populations of women. For example, it is probably the case that the schedule and content of visits for poor, adolescent girls with numerous risk factors such as smoking and poor nutritional status should be quite different from the care offered middle class, low-risk women. Certainly variations in care already exist, but research to probe the results of carefully constructed combinations of interventions is rare. The prematurity prevention program at the University of California at Los Angeles and the March of Dimes multicenter prevention program described in Appendix C are important steps in this direction.

Several other innovative programs are under way or soon to start that attempt to study prenatal care content and effects more carefully. Some are quite clinical in their orientation, involving small populations and designed to evaluate a few well-defined interventions. Others are more accurately described as "community based," often involving larger numbers of women and addressing issues of access, financing, and linkages among care providers, as well as prenatal care content. Such projects include, for example, the Better Babies project in Washington, D.C.; the Florida and North Carolina prematurity prevention activities; the efforts in South Carolina directed at low birthweight prevention; and the program being planned by the Department of Obstetrics and Gynecology of the Albert Einstein College of Medicine in New York.

Such programs, if carefully designed to relate specific prenatal interventions to well-defined pregnancy outcomes, should contribute over time to improving the capacity of prenatal care to reduce low birthweight. Accordingly, the committee urges that:

Both public and private institutions should support studies to assess the effectiveness of well-defined combinations of prenatal interventions in reducing low birthweight and improving pregnancy outcomes generally. The prenatal care analyzed in such studies should reflect the highly varied needs of individual women and groups. In particular, such studies should assess the merits of different combinations of prenatal interventions for women at elevated risk of prematurity or IUGR.

In short, defining and improving the content of prenatal care requires sustained, high-quality research and a commitment of resources adequate to the task. Too often, discussion and research on prenatal care has been oriented to the broad question of whether it improves pregnancy outcome. The appropriate question now is to identify the components and combinations of prenatal care services that are effective in reducing specified risks for well-defined groups of women.

Summary

Prenatal care as currently offered in the United States has demonstrated its capacity to reduce low birthweight, but emphasizing certain elements of its content could make its contribution even greater. More weight should be placed on careful risk assessment and appropriate intervention to reduce identified risks; on early identification and management of threatened preterm labor and IUGR; and on comprehensive patient and provider education. Both the federal government and the major maternity care providers have specific roles to play in encouraging these new emphases in prenatal care.

A variety of research programs should be developed in both the public and private sectors to increase the ability of prenatal care to reduce low birthweight. Research efforts should focus on three areas: analyses of current prenatal care practices in multiple settings; assessments of the efficacy of individual components of prenatal care; and evaluations of combinations of prenatal interventions specifically designed to meet the widely varying needs of pregnant women.

References and Notes

1. American College of Obstetricians and Gynecologists: Standards for Obstetric-Gynecologic Services, Fifth Edition. Washington, D.C., 1982.
2. American Academy of Pediatrics and American College of Obstetricians and Gynecologists: Guidelines for Perinatal Care. Washington, D.C., 1984.
3. Committee to Study the Prevention of Low Birthweight: Risk assessment of low birthweight and preterm birth for the individual.

Unpublished paper prepared by B Selwyn. Washington, D.C.: Institute of Medicine, 1984.

4. Hall MH, Chng PK, and MacGillvray I: Is routine antenatal care worthwhile? Lancet II:78-80, 1980.
5. Read MS, Catz C, Grave G, McNellis D, and Warshaw JB: Intrauterine growth retardation--identification of research needs and goals. Seminar Perinatol. 8:2-4, 1984.
6. National Institutes of Health: Diagnostic Ultrasound Imaging in Pregnancy. Report of a Consensus Development Conference. NIH No. (PHS) 84-667. Public Health Service. Washington, D.C.: U.S. Government Printing Office, 1984.
7. U.S. General Accounting Office: Better Management and More Resources Needed to Strengthen Federal Efforts to Improve Pregnancy Outcome. Report to the Congress of the United States. GAO No. HRD-80-20. Washington, D.C.: U.S. Government Printing Office, January 21, 1980.
8. Select Panel for the Promotion of Child Health: Better Health for Our Children: A National Strategy. Vol. I. DHHS No. (PHS) 79-55071. Washington, D.C.: U.S. Government Printing Office, 1981
9. American Hospital Association: Health Education: Role and Responsibility of Health Care Institutions. Chicago: American Hospital Association, 1975.
10. Select Panel for the Promotion of Child Health: Behavioral aspects of maternal and child health: Natural influences and educational intervention. Prepared by PD Mullen. In Better Health for Our Children: A National Strategy. Vol. IV, pp. 127-188. DHHS No. (PHS) 79-55071. Public Health Service. Washington, D.C.: U.S. Government Printing Office, 1981.
11. Select Panel for the Promotion of Child Health: A child's beginning. Prepared by SS Kessel, JP Rooks, and IM Cushner. In Better Health for Our Children: A National Strategy. Vol. IV, pp. 199-242. DHHS No. (PHS) 79-55071. Public Health Service. Washington, D.C.: U.S. Government Printing Office, 1981.
12. Cogan R: Effects of childbirth preparation. Clin. Obstet. Gynecol. 23:1-14, 1980. See also Perkins ER: The pattern of women's attendance at antenatal classes: Is this good enough? Health Educ. J. 39:3-9, 1980.
13. Davis CD and Marrone FA: An objective evaluation of a prepared childbirth program. Am. J. Obstet. Gynecol. 84:1196-1206, 1962.
14. Nurses Association of the American College of Obstetricians and Gynecologists (NAACOG): Guidelines for Childbirth Education. Washington, D.C.: NAACOG, 1981. See also: International Childbirth Education Association (ICEA): Position Paper on Planning Comprehensive Maternal and Newborn Services for the Childbearing Years. Minneapolis: ICEA, 1979.
15. Enkin M: Antenatal classes. In Effectiveness and Satisfaction in Antenatal Care, edited by M Enkin and I Chalmers, pp. 151-162. Philadelphia: Spastics International Medical Publications, 1982.
16. Timm M: Prenatal education evaluation. Nurs. Res. 28:338-342, 1979.

17. Robitaille Y: The effect of prenatal courses on maternal health behavior and neonatal outcome. Doctoral Dissertation, Department of Epidemiology and Health, McGill University. Montreal, Canada, 1983.

18. Sokol RJ, Woolf RB, Rosen MG, and Weingarden K: Risk, antepartum care, and outcome: Impact of a maternity and infant care project. Obstet. Gynecol. 56:150-156, 1980.

19. Barden TP, Peter JB, and Merkatz IR: Ritodrine hydrocholoride: A betamimetic agent for use in preterm labor. I. Pharmacology, clinical history, administration, side effects, and safety. Obstet. Gynecol. 56:1-6, 1980.

20. Merkatz IR, Peter JB, and Barden TP: Ritodrine hydrochloride: A betamimetic agent for use in preterm labor. II. Evidence of efficacy. Obstet. Gynecol. 56:7-12, 1980.

21. Huszar G and Naftolin F: The myometrium and uterine cervix in normal and preterm labor. N. Engl. J. Med. 311:571-581, 1984.

22. Stein ZA and Susser MW: The Dutch famine, 1944/45 and the reproductive process. 1. Effects on six indices at birth. Pediatr. Res. 9:70-76, 1975.

23. Committee on Nutrition of the Mother and Preschool Child: Nutrition Services in Perinatal Care. Food and Nutrition Board, National Research Council. Washington, D.C.: National Academy Press, 1981.

24. Committee to Study the Prevention of Low Birthweight: Efforts to change smoking and drinking behavior in pregnant women. Unpublished paper by S Wilner. Washington, D.C.: Institute of Medicine, 1984.

25. Donovan JW: Randomized controlled trial of anti-smoking advice in pregnancy. Br. J. Prev. Social Med. 31:6-12, 1977.

26. Sexton M and Hebel JR: A clinical trial of change in maternal smoking and its effect on birth weight. JAMA 251:911-915, 1984.

27. Bailey JW, Loeb BK, and Waage G: A randomized trial of smoking intervention during pregnancy. Paper presented at the 111th Annual Meeting, American Public Health Association, Dallas, Tex., 1983.

28. Ershoff DH, Aaronson NK, Danaher BG, and Wasserman FW: Behavioral, health and cost outcomes of an HMO-based prenatal health education program. Public Health Rep. 98:536-547, 1983.

29. Wilner S, Schoenbaum SC, Palmer RH, and Fountain R: Approaches to intervention programs for pregnant women who smoke. In Proceedings of the Fifth World Conference on Smoking and Health, Winnipeg, Canada, July 1983.

30. Kotelchuck M, Schwartz JB, Anderka MT, and Finison KS: WIC participation and pregnancy outcomes: Massachusetts statewide evaluation project. Am. J. Public Health 74:1086-1092, 1984.

31. Edozien JC, Switzer BR, and Bryan RB: Medical evaluation of the Special Supplemental Food Program for Women, Infants and Children. Am. J. Clin. Nutr. 32:677-692, 1972.

32. Kennedy ET, Gershoff S, Reed R, and Austin JE: Evaluation of the effect of WIC supplemental feeding on birthweight. J. Am. Dietetic Assoc. 80:220-227, 1982.

33. Metcoff J, Costiloe P, Crosby W, Sandstead H, Bodwell CE, and Kennedy E: Nutrition in Pregnancy. Final report submitted to the Food and Nutrition Service, U.S. Department of Agriculture, Washington, D.C., 1982.
34. Kotelchuck M and Anderka MT: Massachusetts Special Supplemental Program for Women, Infants and Children (WIC) Follow-up Study. Final report submitted to U.S. Department of Agriculture, Washington, D.C., 1982.
35. U.S. General Accounting Office: WIC Evaluations Provide Some Favorable But No Conclusive Evidence on the Effects Expected for the Special Supplemental Program for Women, Infants and Children, pp. ii-iv. Report to the Committee on Agriculture, Nutrition, and Forestry, United States Senate. GAO No. PEMD-84-4. Washington, D.C., January 30, 1984.
36. Rush D, Alvir JM, Garbowski GC, Leighton J, and Loan NL: National Evaluation of the Special Supplemental Food Program for Women, Infants and Children (WIC): Review of past studies of health effects of the Special Supplemental Food Program for Women, Infants and Children (WIC), p. 103. Submitted to the Office of Analysis and Evaluation, Food and Nutrition Service, Department of Agriculture. June 30, 1984.
37. Schram WF: An Analysis of the Effects of WIC. Jefferson City, Mo.: Missouri Department of Public Health, 1983.
38. Caan B: An evaluation of the effect of supplemental feeding during the interpregnancy interval on birth outcomes. November 1984. Unpublished paper cited with permission of the author. Contact Caan at the California State Department of Health Services, Berkeley, Calif.
39. Mora JO, de Pardes B, Wagner M, de Navarro L, Suescun J, Christiansen N, and Herrera MG: Nutritional supplementation and the outcome of pregnancy. I. Birthweight. Am. J. Clin. Nutr. 32:455-462, 1979.
40. Habicht JP, Yarborough C, Lechtig A, and Klein RE: Relation of maternal supplementary feeding during pregnancy to birthweight and other sociobiological factors. In Proceedings of the Symposium on Nutrition and Fetal Development, edited by M Winick, pp. 127-145. New York: John Wiley & Sons, 1973.
41. Monrad DM and Pelavin SH: Evaluation of the Commodity Supplemental Food Program. Durham, N.C.: NTS Corporation, 1982.
42. Jeffrey RL, Bowes WA Jr, and Delaney JJ: Role of bed rest in twin gestation. Obstet. Gynecol. 43:822-826, 1974.
43. Nuckolls KB, Cassel JC, and Kaplan BH: Psychosocial assets, life crisis and prognosis of pregnancy. Am. J. Epidemiology 95:431-441, 1972.
44. Herron MA and Dulock HL: Preterm Labor: A Staff Development Program in Perinatal Nursing Care. White Plains, N.Y.: March of Dimes Birth Defects Foundation, 1982.
45. Herron MA, Katz M, and Creasy RK: Evaluation of a preterm birth prevention program: Preliminary report. Obstet. Gynecol. 59:452-456, 1982.

46. Kamerman SB, Kahn AJ, and Kingston PW: Maternity Policy and Working Women. New York: Columbia University Press, 1983.
47. Mary Lou Moore, Bowman Gray School of Medicine, Winston-Salem, N.C. Personal communication, 1984.
48. National Center for Health Statistics: Office Visits by Women: The National Ambulatory Medical Care Survey. Prepared by BK Cypress. Vital and Health Statistics, Series 13, No. 45. DHHS No. (PHS) 80-1976. Public Health Service. Washington, D.C.: U.S. Government Printing Office, March 1980.
49. Kessel SS and Kleinman J. Preliminary data from the 1980 National Natality and Fetal Mortality Follow Back Surveys. National Center for Health Statistics (Kleinman). Personal communication, 1984.

CHAPTER 9

A Public Information Program

The federal government has long sponsored public information efforts directed to pregnant women. A basic premise of these campaigns has been that more informed mothers would take better care of themselves and thereby increase their chances of delivering healthy babies. In recent years, the materials and media messages that constitute these public information efforts have increased in number and sophistication.

The committee believes that public information programs can contribute to the prevention of low birthweight. Such campaigns can help create a climate in which change and progress are possible, in addition to conveying specific types of information. This chapter describes several elements that characterize successful campaigns and sketches the outlines of a public information program directed specifically at low birthweight prevention. The chapter concludes with a discussion of the Healthy Mothers, Healthy Babies Coalition.

Conditions For Success

A growing body of research suggests that public information programs can help achieve change in health-related behaviors, but their success depends on a variety of interrelated conditions.

Social Support

Perhaps most important, a public information program must enjoy wide social, political, and scientific support.[1] Also, it should be part of a spectrum of related activities throughout society, not an isolated effort.

Two public health issues--smoking and childhood immunization--illustrate these fundamentals. The intense public information program on smoking and health that began after the first report to the Surgeon General in 1964, although contributing greatly to the success of this nation's effort to curtail cigarette use, was only one part of a broader strategy that included scientific research, legislation and regulation, and public debate.[2] The decrease in American smoking prevalence since then is attributable in some part to all of these interrelated efforts, and probably cannot be credited solely to the public information campaign.

Similarly, the effective childhood immunization initiative of the 1970s included a widespread public information program aimed at parents and children, but it also was built on solid scientific agreement that childhood immunization was effective and free of substantial risk, on state laws requiring proof of immunization in order to attend school, and on the easy availability of vaccines and services.[3]

Scientific consensus must form the basis of public information programs designed to change behavior in health. Public disagreement among experts leads to confusion and less inclination to change behavior. For example, in 1980, the American Cancer Society, reacting to the Canadian Walton Commission Report on how frequently Pap smears should be obtained, recommended that after two negative smears, a woman could space future Pap tests 3 years apart. The American College of Obstetricians and Gynecologists reacted with a scientific opinion that disputed this stand and called for yearly Pap tests. The public was left confused.[4]

The success of an information program also depends on the availability of necessary services and resources to back up the campaign message. It is futile to urge immunization or prenatal care in the absence of easily accessible facilities to provide such services.

Consistency of Effort

Public information programs designed to change people's behavior must operate over an extended period with a fairly consistent and reinforcing set of messages.[2 5] There is little likelihood, except in rare circumstances, that changes will be swift or dramatic; thus, small changes over time must be recognized as signs of success.

Private advertising builds product acceptance through consistent reinforcement over time of product identity, which is intended to lead to increased use of the advertised item.[6] Millions of dollars are spent in long-term advertising campaigns to achieve small, incremental changes. For example, low tar cigarettes, which had a negligible share of the market in 1967, are the market leaders today.[7] In the field of health, as in the commercial world, incremental changes in behavior signal progress, particularly if sustained over several years.[2]

Use of Multiple Mass Media

Long-range strategies to influence behavior change should take advantage of multiple media. Communicating a health message by means of only one medium limits the size of the audience. Thus, radio music shows may be the best way to capture the attention of teenagers, while television soap operas may be the preferred channel to reach housewives.[1]

The importance of using multiple media, each of which reinforces the messages of others, is emphasized in the literature about marketing family planning programs. In many of these programs, promotion to consumers typically includes advertising through the mass media, point of purchase promotion, face-to-face salesmanship, and special events or other techniques to attract media coverage and improve public acceptance. For example, in the 1970s, a successful marketing campaign in Sri Lanka helped increase use of a brand of condoms named "Preethi," or "happiness." The sale of the condoms was supported through a mass media campaign including newspapers and radio ads, films, and a booklet entitled "How to Have Children by Plan and Not by Chance." Point of purchase displays were provided to the distributors. As a result of the entire campaign, Preethi sales rose from 300,000 a month in July 1974 to an average of 500,000 a month by 1977.[8]

Audience Definition and Message Development

Public information campaigns should begin with an explicit definition of audience. Sometimes, nearly the entire population is the target audience, as in many seatbelt campaigns. More often, a subgroup is the campaign focus--teenagers, smokers, the elderly, and so forth. Campaign messages must fit the defined audience. Messages designed to attract attention and motivate behavior change in particular target groups must be developed carefully and market tested to ensure their appeal to those groups.

For example, through careful market research, the Healthy Mothers, Healthy Babies Coalition developed a series of posters and matching cards for distribution through clinics, WIC programs, and other places where high-risk groups receive prenatal care and information. The posters featured fantasy themes with beautiful women and healthy children in dreamlike settings. Because the presentations were deliberately outside the target women's day-to-day experiences, the posters and cards were subjected to pretests at clinics in several locations to see if they would be acceptable. These tests showed that the materials appealed to the test groups; almost 100 percent liked something about the posters, and 90 percent indicated that the posters were "eye catching." Few respondents reacted negatively to the fantasy concept or felt that the posters were for someone unlike themselves. The recall and understanding of the messages were high.[9] The posters and cards, used by more than 8,000 clinics, achieved widespread acceptance by clinic populations, even where the clinic staff and professionals had doubts about their acceptability.

The public service announcements (PSAs) developed by the Office on Smoking and Health during the past 5 years have employed different messages for specific subsets of the general audience. A set of PSAs featuring "Star Wars" robots was aimed at children to reinforce the message that smoking is an unhealthy practice. For the teenage target audience, announcements featuring a rock group and an antismoking song were developed for use on rock programs to convey the message that smoking is not "in." Other PSAs, featuring a conversation with the U.S. Surgeon General, were directed at the general adult audience to reinforce the message that smoking increases the risk of cancer, heart disease, and other health problems. Each message was aimed at a well-defined audience and tailored to attract the attention of that group.

Messages also may get attention by surprising or shocking the audience.[5] In the 1970s, the British Health Education Council developed a poster featuring the profile of a nude and obviously pregnant woman who was smoking. The poster achieved instant attention and notoriety. Its message was simply, "Is It Fair to Force Your Baby to Smoke?" The poster and additional text triggered a greater than expected drop-off in smoking among pregnant women, a much higher message recall than normal, and a significant change in behavior that carried over after pregnancy.[10]

Quality of Materials

One element that unfortunately receives limited attention in many health information programs is the quality of the materials and messages. Too often this lack of attention is the result of limited budgets for entire programs, of which the public information element is often only a small part. It is especially important that material developed to change health attitudes and behavior be of high, professional quality. Without this quality, some of the credibility of the message may be lost on the target group.[11]

A Public Information Program on Low Birthweight Prevention

With these principles in mind, the committee considered the merits of a public information program in the United States directed at low birthweight prevention. It concluded that such a program would be useful and would complement the other strategies outlined in this report. In the sections below, some elements of such a program are outlined.

Program Objectives and Audience

A public information initiative directed at low birthweight prevention should be built around at least two objectives. The first is to call the problem of low birthweight to the public's attention and to reinforce its importance with the nation's leaders.

This objective is partially achieved through the release periodically of major reports by various public and private organizations. Reports such as _Healthy People_, the _Report of the Select Panel for the Promotion of Child Health_, the _Surgeon General's Workshop on Maternal and Infant Health_, the annual report by the Public Health Service, _Health: United States_, and reports from advocacy groups such as the Children's Defense Fund, all have called attention to the national significance of low birthweight. These reports, aimed at the nation's opinion leaders, are major resource documents for administrators, planners, and legislators. Media represenatives, too, find such reports useful in developing general interest stories that give high visibility to the problem of low birthweight. Reports compiled and disseminated by the federal government often receive particularly widespread attention and therefore are excellent vehicles in which to define the problem and suggest preventive strategies.

> The committee recommends that the Office of the Assistant Secretary for Health develop and publicize a report every 3 years on the nation's progress in reducing low birthweight. The report should explore relevant data, trends, and research that could contribute to easing the problem, and should describe successful programs completed or under way to reduce the incidence of low birthweight. The development, presentation, and dissemination of the report should be managed to reach as many concerned groups and individuals as possible. Additionally, the statistical profile of the nation's health developed by the National Center for Health Statistics, <u>Health: United States</u>, periodically should include a special supplement or profile on low birthweight and its prevention.

The second objective of a national public information campaign should be to help reduce low birthweight by conveying a set of ideas to the public generally, with specific messages tailored to high-risk groups. The balance of this chapter is addressed to this second objective.

The committee considered carefully whether a public information program should focus on only a few target groups and again reviewed the risk factor and epidemiologic literature in this regard. Because many of the risk factors for low birthweight are widely distributed throughout the population, and because a substantial amount of low birthweight occurs among women judged to be at low risk, the committee concluded that the program should embrace a broad audience. At the same time, a subset of messages should be developed to reach several well-defined groups known to be at high risk of low birthweight--pregnant smokers, young teenagers, and poor, socially disadvantaged women. The latter two groups in particular often live in environments in which health information is scant, health matters are of low priority, and motivation to plan for a healthy pregnancy is lacking.

Any public information campaign designed to reduce the incidence of low birthweight should focus on the partners, spouses, boyfriends, and families of women, as well as the women themselves. Such individuals can play an important part in providing the support necessary to help women plan for pregnancy and undertake difficult behavior changes, such as reducing smoking or altering eating habits.[5]

Messages

A public information initiative directed at the prevention of low birthweight should have two themes, (1) planning for pregnancy and (2) adopting good health practices in the childbearing years, especially during pregnancy. Messages based on these themes should be supplemented by others that call attention generally to the implications of low birthweight. Some message topics are noted below; actual wording would require careful development and market testing:

• the problem of low birthweight--even in a society devoted to thinness, it is important that babies be born of adequate weight;
• the many benefits of planning for pregnancy and related family planning concepts;
• the risks of smoking in pregnancy;
• the benefits of good nutritional practices before and during pregnancy;
• the risks of both moderate and heavy alcohol use in pregnancy (and substance abuse generally); and
• the importance of obtaining prenatal care and beginning such care early in pregnancy.

Information Channels

According to the market research performed for the Healthy Mothers, Healthy Babies Coalition, the channels for relaying these messages that offer the best chances of reaching two of the groups meriting special attention--teenagers and poor, socioeconomically disadvantaged women--are: (1) clinics where women from these groups often go for prenatal care, (2) WIC program offices, (3) schools, and (4) selected media.[12] Family planning clinics are an additional locus for presenting these messages.

Prenatal care and family planning clinics provide a captive audience that visits frequently, typically for a substantial amount of time. Suitable films, videotapes, posters, and publications should be made available in the clinics themselves to capitalize on this opportunity. Similarly, clinic staff should build the recommended messages into their health education and counseling activities.

WIC program workers, who are often reported to have good relationships with their clients, appear to be in a good position to influence behavior. Most women who have direct contact with WIC have high regard for its staff services. This favorable environment should be exploited for relaying campaign messages.

Schools are a natural setting for communicating important health education and information themes to all young people. In Chapter 5, this topic is discussed in greater depth.

Undoubtedly, the mass media offer tremendous opportunities for reaching pregnant women. Television, in particular, has come to dominate our lives. Ninety-eight percent of all households in the United States have at least one television set. The average TV household views an estimated 6 hours and 26 minutes a day, with Sunday night as the most popular viewing time and situation comedies as the most popular type of program during prime time.[13]

Mindful of the pervasiveness of television, many groups have tried to use this medium as part of public information efforts. Because paid advertising is beyond the financial capability of most public information campaigns, and because of certain legal restrictions, most campaigns rely on PSAs, the traditional way to present public interest health messages on television. Unfortunately, the cost of production, the competition for air time, and the small likelihood of good placement and repeated airings often make this approach impractical and unattractive as the prime effort in a health promotion campaign.

Integrating health-related messages into the story lines of certain television shows, such as soap operas, also has been proposed as a way to influence behavior. The committee finds this intuitively appealing and urges that its merits be explored, particularly given the fact that many high-risk women belong to groups that are known to watch daytime television. If the cooperation and commitment of network programming executives could be obtained, it might be possible to launch an effort to alert target groups to the set of messages outlined earlier.

Related to this concept is the finding in one survey that the ABC-TV program "F.Y.I." was mentioned most often by socially disadvantaged women respondents as a believable source of health information.[12] It was aired at regularly scheduled times during breaks in afternoon soap operas. ABC-TV has since canceled the program, but has said that it might begin airing it again.

Radio is another medium that should be used to communicate the campaign messages. Some 456.2 million radio sets were in use in 1980,[13] and surveys have shown that radio listening is especially prevalent in poor, socially disadvantaged groups.[14] One of the attractions of using radio is that it is less costly than television.

The print mass media, newspapers and magazines, also could be useful. Selected newspapers or magazines can be used to transmit messages to specific groups because of their specialized readerships. For example, <u>Jet</u> magazine is read widely by black women; so is the Sunday newspaper, especially the magazine sections. Similarly, comic books, photo stories, and simplified illustrated booklets and similar materials should be developed for use in a range of settings. All such materials require careful testing to make sure that they are effective in communicating campaign messages.

Leadership and Organizational Structure

The comprehensive public information program advocated by the committee clearly needs an organizational home and a stable leadership structure. It must be well funded and should embrace a wide variety of groups and institutions to increase the number of ways in which the campaign messages can be disseminated. The committee suggests that the Healthy Mothers, Healthy Babies Coalition fulfill this leadership role. As an established organization, it has many attributes that make it a logical leader for a public information program directed at low birthweight prevention. Indeed, many of the Coalition's efforts to date are highly relevant to the prevention of low birthweight, even though directed at more general issues of maternal and infant health.

The Coalition grew out of the recommendations of the Surgeon General's 1980 Workshop on Maternal and Infant Health, which called for the Surgeon General to use the influence of his office to develop a program of public information and education to enhance the health of pregnant women and infants.[15] In response to this recommendation, the Public Health Service and five other organizations set up a loose coalition of 36 voluntary, professional, and governmental groups to find ways of improving public education aimed at the nation's high-risk women, with a special focus on improving the outcome of pregnancy. The Coalition has now grown to more than 60 national organizations with networks in 25 states and is perhaps the largest attempt thus far to concentrate the activities of so many groups on the common objective of improving infant and maternal health. Coalition activities have included development of materials for clinics, including posters and information cards, as well as booklets, newspaper columns, and radio programs. The Coalition also has conducted market research on how women, especially low-income women, receive their prenatal information.[16]

The Coalition has no permanent source of funding, however. Funds have been raised only for specific projects, not to build a stable institution capable of sustaining a long-term, high-quality public information program. The poster project, for example, was supported by a consortium of six organizations, each of which donated $25,000. This money covered design, production, and distribution of the posters, as well as a promotional campaign to let prenatal clinics know they were available. Although such project-specific funding is useful, it does not ensure the survival of such campaigns over time.

The committee has concluded that the Coalition has the potential for playing a larger, more permanent role in improving maternal and child health and in reducing the incidence of low birthweight. Accordingly:

> The committee urges that the Healthy Mothers, Healthy Babies Coalition lead a comprehensive public information program directed at low birthweight prevention. The program should be aimed at the general public, but also include messages specially designed to reach low-income women, teenagers, and pregnant smokers. It should follow the themes of planning for pregnancy and of adopting good health practices in the childbearing years, especially during pregnancy. The Coalition should establish a formal executive secretariat to provide stability and permanence. Both public and private funds should be provided the Coalition in amounts adequate to its task. Activities should include the production and distribution of high quality, well-tested public information materials, and special efforts should be made by the Coalition to urge that television programming include the campaign themes. Similarly, the radio and print media should be enlisted in this long-term, national effort.

In urging a public information program directed at low birthweight prevention, the committee emphasizes again that this should be but one element in a more comprehensive program, that it must be sustained over time, and that it must be integrated with complementary activities in the health care sector in particular. For example, public messages pointing out the importance of prenatal care must coincide with a commitment to making prenatal care accessible; and messages to decrease smoking in pregnancy must be reinforced and elaborated in individual clinic and office settings. Finally, such a campaign must pay careful attention to audience definition, message development, and use of multiple media to channel information. The Healthy Mothers/Healthy Babies Coalition, if more adequately funded, is a logical leader for the program.

References

1. Hamburg DA: Changing behavior for health. Am. J. Cardiol. 47:736-740, 1981.
2. Warner KE and Murt HA: Impact of the antismoking campaign on smoking prevalence: A cohort analysis. J. Public Health Policy 3:374-390, 1982.
3. Hinman AR, Brandling-Bennett AD, and Nieburg PI: The opportunity and obligation to eliminate measles from the United States. JAMA 242:1157-1162, 1979.
4. Pap smear controversy pits cancer society vs. ob-gyns. Hosp. Pract. 16:16-29, February 1981.
5. Flay BR, DiTecco D, and Schlegel RP: Mass media in health promotion: An analysis using an extended information processing model. Health Educ. Q. 7:127-147, 1980.
6. Siano JJ: Consistency is key in building brand identity. Advertising Age, M 46-48, February 20, 1984.
7. Hutchings R: A review of the nature and extent of cigarette advertising in the United States. In National Conference on Smoking and Health: Developing a Blueprint for Action, Proceedings, pp. 249-263. New York: American Cancer Society, November 1981.
8. Social Marketing: Does it Work? Population Reports, Series J, No. 21. Baltimore, Md.: Johns Hopkins University, January 1980.
9. Test Results of the Healthy Mothers Posters, Health Message Testing Service, Public Health Service, Bethesda, Md., February 1982.
10. Morton Lebow: Administrator for Public Affairs, American College of Obstetricians and Gynecologists, Washington, D.C., personal communication.
11. Atkin CK: Research evidence on mass mediated health communication campaigns. In Communication Yearbook 3, edited by D Nimmo, pp. 655-668. New Brunswick, N.J.: Transaction--International Communication Association, 1979.

12. Juarez and Associates, Inc: Healthy Mothers Market Research: How to Reach Black and Mexican American Women. Final report submitted to the Office of Public Affairs, Public Health Service, DHHS Contract No. 282-81-0082. Washington, D.C., September 14, 1982.
13. Profile: Broadcasting. Washington, D.C: National Association of Broadcasters, 1981.
14. Green D: Exposure to Print and Electronic Media: Women Age 18-34. Report submitted to the Public Health Service by Chilton Research Services. Radnor, Pa., January 1982.
15. U.S. Department of Health and Human Services: The Surgeon General's Workshop on Maternal and Infant Health. DHHS No. (PHS) 81-50161. Public Health Service. Washington, D.C.: U.S. Government Printing Office, January 1981.
16. Bratic E: Healthy Mothers, Healthy Babies Coalition--A joint private-public initiative. Public Health Rep. 97:503-509, 1982.

CHAPTER 10

Prenatal Care and Low Birthweight: Effects on Health Care Expenditures

Public policy decisions about health promotion strategies should incorporate an understanding of their costs as well as their benefits. Ideally, for each strategy summarized in Chapter 4, policymakers would be able to determine the net public and private costs per case of low birthweight averted. Equipped with data on the most cost-effective means to reduce low birthweight, policymakers would then weigh the additional costs of intervention against the public and private benefits from reducing the low birthweight rate. Unfortunately, lack of adequate data on the costs of these strategies, alone or in combination, placed such a goal beyond the committee's reach.

In general, estimates of the costs of measures that should be implemented in the period before pregnancy to reduce the risks associated with low birthweight are not available. Information does exist on the costs of family planning, but it does not include calculations of the economic impact of projected changes in the low birthweight rate resulting from family planning practices, and the committee did not undertake such an analysis. Lack of adequate data also prevented the committee from estimating the additional public expenditures that would be required to finance the recommended public information program and research efforts.

With regard to extending the availability of prenatal care, however, the committee found that a straightforward, common sense analysis could be performed regarding some of the financial implications involved in the provision of prenatal services to pregnant women. Formal cost-benefit and cost-effectiveness analyses, including estimates of the present value of low birthweight infants, were not feasible, however, because of problems in the quality and uniformity of available cost data, uncertainties about the life expectancy of low birthweight infants with significant morbidity, difficulties in delineating the services received, and uncertainties about target populations.

Within the domain of prenatal care costs, the committee elected to undertake a narrow set of tasks. First, a target population of high-risk pregnant women was identified. Second, within the target population, the additional public fiscal outlays required to provide these women with more complete prenatal care services than they now obtain were estimated. Third, the direct medical care expenditures resulting from a low-weight birth were assessed for a single year. Finally, the additional public fiscal outlays for adequate prenatal care of the target group mothers were compared with the potential savings in single-year medical care costs that might result from reduction in the low birthweight rate, resulting from increased receipt of prenatal care. The estimated costs of extending more complete prenatal services to the target group would represent potential expenditures of new dollars; the reductions in the costs of caring for low birthweight infants, by virtue of reducing the low birthweight rate in the target group, would be a return on these new dollars.

Even the narrow agenda of this chapter is fraught with uncertainties. For example, the committee focused on high-risk women receiving public assistance; it did not analyze outcomes for other women at high risk. To assess the costs of prenatal care, the committee relied on data from current obstetrical practice; it did not speculate on the costs of changes in the content of care, such as those outlined in Chapter 8, that might be appropriate for high-risk mothers.

Although prescription of a particular set of prenatal services to produce a defined reduction in low birthweight is not possible at this time, the estimates of a reduced rate of low birthweight used in this analysis appear achievable. This judgment is based in part on studies reviewed in Chapter 6 that, despite qualifications, demonstrate reductions in low birthweight associated with adequate prenatal care, and in part on the multivariate analysis presented in Chapter 3, which indicates that a significant reduction in low birthweight rates could result from changes in the timing and frequency of prenatal visits. The analysis presented in this chapter supports the widely shared view that, with adherence to current standards for timing and frequency of prenatal visits, the Surgeon General's national goal of a 5 percent rate of low birthweight overall and a maximum rate of 9 percent in high-risk subpopulations,* can be met through provision of such prenatal services.[1]

The committee's focus on mothers receiving public assistance permits a calculation of the direct budgetary consequences of subsidizing prenatal care. In most instances, both the predelivery services consumed by these high-risk mothers and the postdelivery care of their low-weight infants would be paid by governmental programs. If the postdelivery cost savings outweigh the additional predelivery expenditures, then a net reduction in public expenditures will be obtained. It must be emphasized, however, that net savings in governmental budgets is a limited criterion. A society concerned with the health and productivity of all its citizens might choose to reduce low-weight births even if the budgetary outlays were to exceed savings.

---

*The Surgeon General's objective states, "By 1990, low birth weight babies . . . should constitute no more than 5 percent of all live births . . . (and) no county and no racial or ethnic group of the population (e.g. black, Hispanic, American Indian) should have a rate of low birth weight infants . . . that exceeds 9 percent of all live births."[1]

In the following analysis, the cost of prenatal care comprises the expenditures required for routine prenatal services as currently provided by most qualified physicians and nurse-midwives. The costs of a more comprehensive package of care, including psychological and social counseling, behavioral modification, nutritional planning, and special diagnostic studies, are excluded. The cost of low birthweight reflects initial expenditures on intensive care; rehospitalization costs of survivors during the first year and a single-year estimate of the annual long-term medical expenses of those who survive the first year of life and do not require institutionalization. The cumulative direct long-term medical expenses of both institutionalized and noninstitutionalized survivors are excluded, as are the indirect costs of lost productivity from infants who survive with handicaps and from the family members who care for them.

Overview of the Analysis

In the sections below, the major components of the committee's computation are defined and discussed. Later in the chapter, the specific figures used for the cost elements are presented.

Target Population

The target population was identified as the total national cohort of women aged 15 to 39 years who receive public assistance and who have less than 12 years' education.

To assess the number of low-weight births in this group, the committee proceeded in three stages. First, it estimated the total size of the target population for 1980 from a 1/1,000 sample of the 1980 U.S. Census.[2] In that year, an estimated 2,981,000 black and white women aged 15 to 39 years received public assistance. Among such women, an estimated total of 1,399,000 had completed less than a high school education (Population P_0 in Figure 10.1).

Second, to estimate the total number of live births among the target group, the population was further disaggregated by age (15 to 17, 18 to 19, 20 to 24, 25 to 29, 30 to 34, and 35 to 39 years) and race (black and white only). Age- and race-specific national fertility rates for 1979 were then applied to each subgroup.[3] Among the target population, a total of 110,600 live births were estimated for 1980 (Population P_1 in Figure 10.1).

Third, for each age/race subgroup of the target population, the committee estimated the total number of low-weight births from age- and race-specific low birthweight rates in 1980.[4] (The 1980 data are used here instead of the 1981 data presented in Table 3.6 of Chapter 3 to be consistent with the census data.) Among the 110,600 live births in the target cohort, 12,719 (11.5 percent) were estimated to be low-weight babies (Population P_2 in Figure 10.1).

The population of less educated women on public assistance was, in the committee's view, the most easily identifiable population for

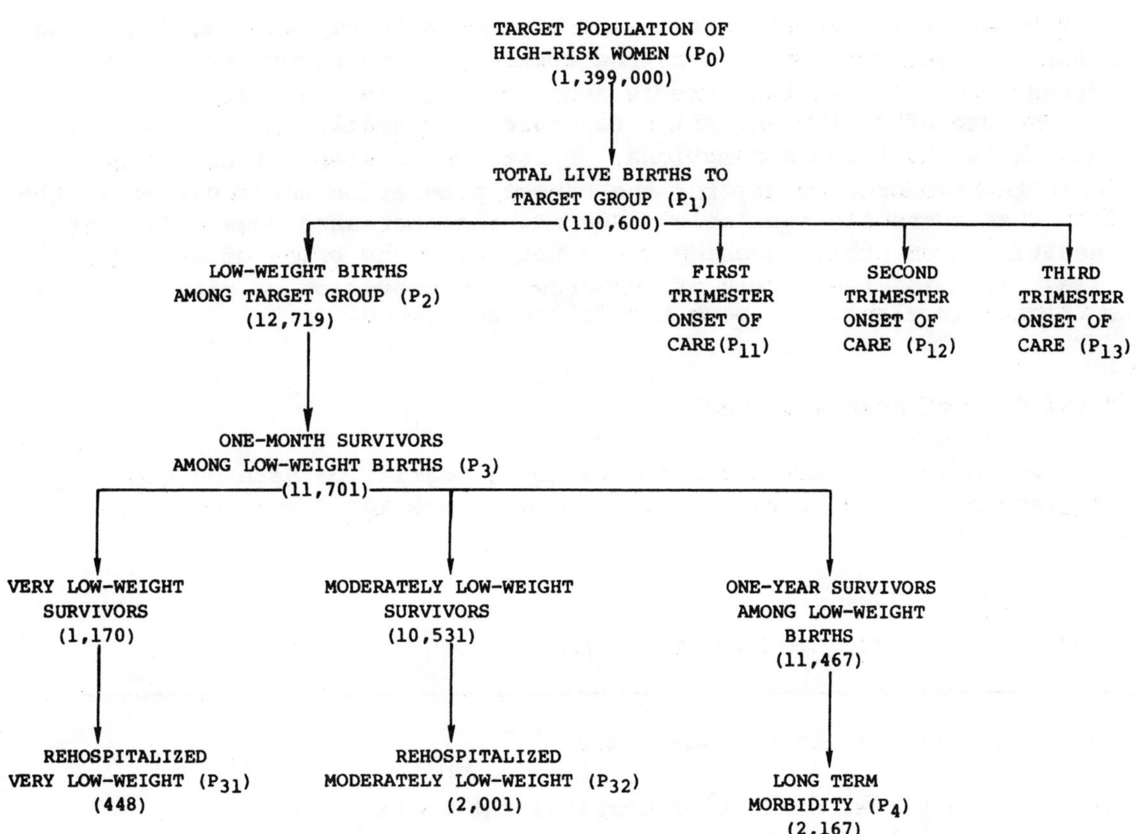

FIGURE 10.1 Population calculations for cost analysis.

analysis. Though many women with at least a high school education also could be classified as high risk on the basis of other factors, the important relationship between education and low birthweight risk (chapters 2 and 3) motivated the committee's choice. Moreover, because women receiving public assistance also are likely to receive public subsidy for medical care, both the outlays for additional prenatal care and the savings from a reduced incidence of low birthweight involve governmental funds.

In computing the number of births among the target group, the committee used age- and race-specific, but not education-specific, natality rates. Accordingly, the total number of births in the target population (and thus the total number of low-weight births) may be underestimated. Low-weight birth rates, however, were specific for infants whose mothers had less than a high school education.

Unit Cost of Prenatal Care

The committee assumed that the additional cost of providing prenatal care to a mother with no prior care was equal to the current average charge for routine care in the United States. The average charge was ascertained by reviewing a wide range of sources, including a small survey commissioned by the committee, described below. The current cost of prenatal care is denoted by C_1 in Table 10.1.

The use of an average price for currently available, routine care entails two critical assumptions. First, the content of care (and hence the resource costs) for the target population would differ little from that currently available. Second, the increased demand for care resulting from public subsidy would not cause the price of care to rise. That is, the supply of resources for provision of care would be sufficiently elastic to meet the increased demand.

Total Cost of Prenatal Care

The committee examined national vital statistics data on the timing of prenatal care in relation to race and educational status.[5] For a

TABLE 10.1 Total Cost Computations

C_1	=	unit cost of prenatal care	
C_2	=	unit cost of initial hospitalization of low-weight infant	
C_3	=	unit rehospitalization cost of surviving low-weight infant	
C_4	=	unit long-term, single year morbidity cost of surviving low-weight infant	
TC_1	=	total additional cost of prenatal care	$= C_1 \times (P_{13} + 0.5P_{12})$
TC_2	=	total cost of initial hospitalization	$= C_2 \times P_2$
TC_3	=	total cost of rehospitalization	$= C_3 \times (P_{31} + P_{32})$
TC_4	=	total long-term morbidity cost	$= C_4 \times P_4$
TC_5	=	total cost of low-weight births in target group	$= C_2 + C_3 + C_4$
r	=	low birthweight rate per 100 in target population after introduction of prenatal care	
TC_6	=	total reduction in cost of care of low-weight births	$= (1 - r/11.5) \times TC_5$

population of pregnant women with the same racial and educational distribution as the target group, the committee estimated the following distribution of timing of care: 57 percent initiate care in the first trimester, 32 percent in the second trimester, and 11 percent initiate care in the third trimester or receive no care (see groups P_{11}, P_{12}, and P_{13} in Figure 10.1). Given the total size of the target population, the estimated cost of care, and the estimated current distribution of care, the committee computed the estimated total additional cost of providing first-trimester care to the entire high-risk cohort (see Table 10.1).

Costs of Care of Low-Weight Births

The committee's analysis includes a single-year estimate of the costs of care per low-weight birth. The figure used has three components: initial hospitalization costs; the costs of repeat hospitalizations during the year following birth among those infants who were initially discharged alive; and an estimate of annual noninstitutional, nonhospital morbidity costs incurred by those infants surviving the first year of life.

Each component of the cost of care for low-weight infants was taken from the literature reviewed below. Total costs for initial hospitalization equaled the average cost per infant (C_2) multiplied by the total population of 12,719 low-weight births in the target groups (P_2 in Figure 10.1). Total costs for repeat hospitalization were computed separately for moderately low-weight and very low-weight births.[5] Thus, among the 12,719 low-weight births in the target group, 11,701 were expected to survive the neonatal period (P_3), comprising about 1,170 very low-weight and 10,531 moderately low-weight infants. These separate population totals were in turn multiplied by the estimated probabilities of rehospitalization. This procedure yielded 448 very low-weight and 2,001 moderately low-weight rehospitalized infants (populations P_{31} and P_{32}). The latter population figures were multiplied by the estimated unit cost of rehospitalization (C_3) to calculate the total costs. Finally, among the 11,719 infants who survived the neonatal period (P_3), a total of 11,467 were estimated to survive the first year, of whom 2,167 were expected to suffer long-term morbidity (P_4). The annual morbidity costs for noninstitutionalized, nonhospitalized survivors were derived by multiplying the estimated unit cost of morbidity (C_4) by the latter population total. The population subtotals used in each stage of the analysis are diagrammed in Figure 10.1. The total cost computations are summarized in Table 10.1.

In the estimate of the initial hospitalization costs, the committee included an unknown number of infants (probably of moderately low birthweight) who would not have required or received intensive care in Level II or III neonatal intensive care units. This may appear to result in an overstatement of these costs. However, when the large cohort of moderately low birthweight infants is excluded from the initial hospitalization figures, the committee's conclusions remain unchanged. Further, the low base charge used to determine the initial hospitalization costs probably does not adequately reflect all of the current hospital and professional charges for the care of low birthweight infants. It is not possible to determine the degree to which these adjustments offset each other.

The dollar figure used for the per diem charge for rehospitalization of infants would tend to produce an underestimation of costs, because it does not include any professional charges or reflect the higher than average hospital resource utilization by infants admitted to general pediatric wards or to intensive care units.

The annual morbidity costs also are underestimated because they do not include charges for institutionalization or the discounted present value of expenditures over the lifetime of the low birthweight infant. This estimate of the ambulatory medical care costs of low birthweight infants must be interpreted cautiously, however, because it assumes that their chronic care is similar in its pattern of resource utilization to that of other children with chronic disabilities. This has not been established.

Computation of single-year expenditures attributable to the care of low-weight infants does not by itself gauge the incremental costs incurred by delivery of a low-weight neonate. For example, if all live births were shifted to the normal weight category, there would still be some expected costs due to hospitalization, rehospitalization, and long-term morbidity.[6] Alternatively, no adjustment has been made for cost savings in infant care associated with the improved health of normal birthweight infants born to pregnant women who have received improved prenatal management. These factors have not been incorporated, because the committee believes they would not affect the outcome of the analysis significantly.

More importantly, confining the cost estimates for the care of low birthweight infants used in this analysis to a single year underestimates the actual costs over the long term. Thus the committee's estimates of this variable must be viewed as conservative.

Estimated Cost Savings

If the current low birthweight rate of 11.5 percent among the target population were reduced only to 10 percent, then the total number of low-weight neonates would decline from 12,719 (population P_2 in Figure 10.1) to 11,060. If the subsequent survival probabilities, rehospitalization probabilities, and long-term morbidity probabilities remained unchanged, then the total costs associated with low-weight births would be reduced by a factor of 10/11.5 = 0.87. Similarly, if the low birthweight rate were reduced to 9 percent, with all other probabilities unchanged, the population P_2 would be only 9,954, and total costs would be reduced by a factor of 9/11.5 = 0.78.

To assess the potential cost savings from reduced low-weight births in the target group, the committee computed the total costs for low birthweight rates of 11.5 percent, 10 percent, and 9 percent, respectively. Such a procedure assumes that the reduction in low-weight rates does not affect subsequent probabilities of initial hospitalization, rehospitalization, or long-term morbidity.

In the results below, all cost magnitudes are stated in constant 1984 dollars. Adjustments for changes in the general price level were based on the medical care component of the consumer price index.

Additional Assumptions and Comments

Many assumptions had to be made to perform this analysis, and they must be taken into consideration when interpreting the committee's conclusions. First, the dollar figures used as a basis for the cost calculations represent what the committee considered to be reasonable estimates of the current charges for the particular medical services discussed. No attempt was made to analyze the current sources of reimbursement by patients, public agencies, insurance companies, or other third parties for prenatal services or for the subsequent care of low birthweight infants. Similarly, no attempt was made to analyze the effect of reimbursement of less than charges on potential cost shifting by providers or on access to care.

Second, the estimates used for health care charges (both for prenatal services and for services used by infants) do not generally include all of the medical services provided and thus underestimate the costs per patient, especially in the cost of care of the hospitalized low birthweight child. For example, charges for the medically indicated use of ultrasound to evaluate the fetus generally would not be included in routine prenatal care costs. Similarly, charges for the appropriate use of CT and ultrasound head scanning of low birthweight neonates for detection of intracranial hemorrhages and any related surgical procedures might not be included in estimates of initial hospitalization costs.

Third, women at high risk of bearing a low birthweight infant who were not on public assistance because they did not apply or qualify, or who were not represented in the census data used in this analysis, are not included in the target group of pregnant women at high risk. The total costs both of prenatal care and the care of low birthweight children would be increased by including these additional groups, but the increases might have a different pattern than that projected for the cohort presented.

Fourth, the estimate of prenatal care costs may be understated to a degree that cannot be adequately quantified because of a greater use of these services by women at greater risk, and because changes in the content of prenatal care services may be implemented and add more to the expense. However, even if additional prenatal care costs were substantially greater, the committee's conclusions would still be valid.

Fifth, this analysis does not take into consideration the possible costs of appropriate medical interventions during the prenatal period that might not have occurred without the increased provision of prenatal services to these high-risk pregnant women. For example, early identification of preterm labor might lead to the use of tocolytic agents and hospitalization before admission for delivery, which would increase medical costs. Alternatively, early identification of toxemia might lead to diet counseling and bed rest, which could decrease the need for hospitalization or shorten the length of stay and thus reduce medical costs.

Finally, no adjustment has been made for fetal wastage, which might reduce prenatal care costs and low birthweight child care costs. Alternatively, higher fertility rates than those utilized might be appropriate for this high-risk cohort of pregnant women, and this would increase both the costs of prenatal services and of low birthweight infant care.

Description of Costs

This section summarizes the costs reported in the literature for the provision of prenatal and delivery services to pregnant women, of neonatal intensive care to low birthweight infants, of subsequent postneonatal hospitalization to surviving infants, and of long-term medical care to survivors. It also presents and justifies the estimates used by the committee for each cost component in the analysis. All costs and charges have been adjusted for inflation to March 1984 dollars.

Prenatal and Delivery Costs

The range of costs and charges for prenatal care reported in the literature is substantial.[7] This variability is due in large part to differences in the content of the prenatal services, to differences in the reimbursable costs or charges allowed by third party payors, and to variations in the methods of partitioning the total costs of maternity care into prenatal, delivery, and postpartum components. For example, the cost of the prenatal care services may be defined as the "reimbursable cost" provided by Medicaid, or as the professional "charges" that are paid fully or in part by private insurance companies or individuals. Further, it is customary for payment to physicians for prenatal services to be included as part of the comprehensive fee for delivery.

Published data on the separate cost of prenatal services is limited. Therefore, an independent survey of prenatal care charges in the United States was undertaken.[8] One hundred perinatal health care professionals from 38 of the 50 states were queried and responses were obtained from 34 of these individuals. The average physician fee for prenatal care was $365; obviously this figure could be affected significantly by the experiences of the nonresponders. This survey also indicated the following averages for physician comprehensive fees for a cluster of services including prenatal care, delivery, and postpartum in-hospital care: $804 for a vaginal delivery and $1,179 for a cesarean delivery.

The Health Insurance Association of America (HIAA), in a publication entitled "The Cost of Having a Baby," reports that the average charge for a physician's obstetrical services in the United States, including prenatal and delivery services, is $730 for a vaginal delivery and $941 for a cesarean delivery. HIAA data also indicate that the average national hospital charge for a delivery, based on a hospital per diem, is $1,648 for a vaginal and $2,853 for a cesarean delivery. Total charges for professional services (obstetric, anesthesia, pediatric) and the hospital maternity stay for the United States average $2,620.[9]

The committee also reviewed other data on prenatal charges. For example, in a report submitted to the state legislature, the Michigan Department of Public Health proposed a reimbursement sum of $350 per patient for providing an estimated 12 prenatal visits and a postpartum visit, nutritional and psychosocial assessment, laboratory services, prescriptions, and parent education for Medicaid patients through local health departments.[10] Malitz, analyzing the cost implications of extending Medicaid in Texas to low-income pregnant women, estimated that "birth-related" services to a majority of Medicaid recipients for prenatal care averaged $266 per woman.[11] There is no description of the services provided to these Medicaid recipients. The Colorado Department of Health reported that prenatal services cost an average of $461 per woman,[12] and the Ohio Department of Health estimated that the cost of providing prenatal services in public health clinics was $365 per patient.[13] McManus reports, in an analysis of Medicaid's impact on prenatal care to low-income women, that in 1982, obstetricians were reimbursed an average of $398 and "specialists" $417 for prenatal, delivery, and postpartum care. There is no description, however, of the services rendered and no indication of the proportion of the total reimbursement that could be allocated to prenatal care alone.[14]

The Oakland, Calif., "OB Access Project" reported $870 as the average fee-for-service payment financing a rich array of obstetrical services including prenatal and delivery care to a group of Medi-Cal patients.[15] This contrasted with an average physician fee reimbursement of $620 for routine prenatal, intrapartum, and postpartum care under the regular Medi-Cal program. The $250 differential financed a more comprehensive set of prenatal services that went beyond routine care to include psychosocial and nutritional assessments,[16] childbirth education, and other care components described in Chapter 6.

Based on the available literature and the survey, the committee estimates the cost for professional services associated with prenatal care, excluding delivery and postpartum charges, to be approximately $400. The cost comparison analysis in this chapter uses this figure for the additional cost of prenatal care in determining the expense of providing prenatal services (as currently practiced) beginning in the first trimester to women on public assistance who are at high risk of delivering a low birthweight infant.

Initial Hospitalization Costs

Reported costs and charges for the initial hospitalization of low birthweight infants in intensive care units vary enormously, from only several thousand dollars to as high as $134,173.[10 17-28] A few of the studies are summarized below. The costs attributable to the use of standard newborn nurseries for the care of low birthweight babies are not described in this report.

In an analysis of the cost of providing health services to low birthweight infants and low-income pregnant women, the Michigan Department of Health reported that the average approximate cost of neonatal intensive care was $20,000, with an average length of stay of 17 to 27 days; it was not indicated whether these were reimbursed costs or charges.[10] Pomerance et al. reported an average cost of $62,730 for the hospital component of neonatal intensive care provided to low birthweight infants born at less than 35 weeks of gestation.[17] Bragonier, Cushner, and Hobel estimated the average charges for initial hospitalization (including neonatal intensive care), intrapartum care, and all professional services for low birthweight infants at $90,880.[18] Their analysis used the findings of Phibbs et al. that 16 percent of the total medical care expense for a low birthweight infant's neonatal intensive care stay can be attributed to professional fee charges, and the remainder to hospital and ancillary service charges.[19]

In a paper describing the hospital costs of caring for infants weighing 1,000 grams or less, Pomerance et al. analyzed the hospital charges, excluding physician fees and bad debt, for caring for 75 infants.[21] The average charge per infant admitted (regardless of survival) was $61,196. The survival rate for the 75 infants in the sample was 40 percent, with an average total charge of $99,993 per survivor. The average length of stay for survivors was 89 days, with a range of 51 to 194 days.

Rajagopalan et al. analyzed the cost of neonatal intensive care for 492 infants admitted to Babies Hospital, Columbia Presbyterian Medical Center, New York.[26] Seventeen percent of these infants had one or more operations and incurred an average cost of $35,834. These infants were responsible for 37 percent of the aggregate cost of care for the study population. The infants weighing less than 1,500 grams incurred an average cost of $37,392. Fifty percent of the sample had total expenses of less than $9,000. The average total neonatal intensive care expense for hospitalization and professional fees was $16,826.

The lower the newborn infant's birthweight, the greater the resource consumption and cost of services.[27] Smaller infants require more extensive medical support for longer periods of time. Survivors consume more services than infants who die. Diagnosis also has a major impact on resource consumption and medical costs.

Budetti estimated that the average sum of physician and hospital charges for a newborn infant's initial hospitalization in a Level II or III neonatal intensive care unit is $13,616 (adjusted to 1984 dollars).[28] This figure is used in the committee's cost comparison analysis. Although it probably represents a low estimate, the quality of the data on which it is based makes it the most appropriate information available for the committee's purposes. In Budetti's study, the average length of stay in neonatal intensive care units for low birthweight infants was 8 to 18 days, with a mean of 13 days.

Rehospitalization Costs

An estimate of the costs of rehospitalization during the first year of life of low birthweight infants who survive the neonatal period is important in determining the financial consequences of a reduction in the incidence of low birthweight births, because it has been established that surviving infants are at high risk for later serious morbidity and mortality. As in the preceding section, a few studies that have estimated rehospitalization costs are summarized below.

Rajagopalan et al. reported that a total of 77 of 492 surviving low birthweight infants (16 percent) were readmitted to the hospital within the first year of life.[26] Thirty-seven were readmitted for a mean of 19 days with an average charge of $10,821 for direct complications of their neonatal illnesses. Forty infants were hospitalized for a mean of 11 days at an average charge of $6,457 for problems not directly related to their neonatal illnesses.

The Virginia Perinatal Association estimated the average Medicaid-reimbursed cost for rehospitalization of low birthweight infants by various birthweights based on studies by McCormick.[29] They estimated that 19 percent of the moderately low birthweight infants (1,501-2,500 grams) and 38.3 percent of the very low birthweight infants (1,500 grams or less) were rehospitalized, with an average length of stay of 12.5 and 16.2 days, respectively. Hack et al. reported in a Cleveland study that 90 very low birthweight infants discharged after an average length of stay of 62 days experienced 51 separate admissions during the first year of life.[30] These admissions represented 30 (33 percent) of the 90 discharged newborn infants. The reasons for readmission were primarily for management of chronic conditions related to the initial neonatal hospitalization and for respiratory tract and other infections.

The American Hospital Association reported $372 as the average cost of an inpatient hospital day.[31] This figure is used in our cost comparison analysis. It underestimates the true cost of caring for rehospitalized low birthweight infants because their care on general pediatric wards requires the utilization of substantially more personnel services and other expensive resources than that of the average patient, and because many of these infants are admitted to intensive care units. This figure also does not include charges for professional services.

National data on the proportion of low birthweight infants who survive their initial intensive care hospitalization are not available, although some informal estimates have been made.[32] In a population-based study of the impact of the regionalization of perinatal care on infant mortality in Alabama, Goldenberg et al. estimate that 8 percent of low birthweight infants do not survive their initial hospitalization.[33] This percentage is used in the committee's cost comparison analysis to identify the population of infants at risk for rehospitalization.

Long-Term Morbidity Costs

Estimates of long-term morbidity costs vary significantly. For example, Butler et al. estimate that the average annual hospital expenditure for children with chronic disabilities who require periodic hospitalization is $3,268;[34] 36 percent of the total hospital days used by children are attributed to chronically ill children with 11 major chronic conditions. Chronically ill children utilize more health services than children with acute illnesses--the average length of hospital stay for children with chronic disabilities is 9 days, compared with 4.8 days for children without limitations of activity.

McManus reports that the estimated cost of institutional care for developmentally disabled children is $359,124 per child, the present value of 20 years of care discounted at 10 percent per year.[14] Smyth-Staruch et al. reported in a study of chronically ill or disabled children in Cleveland that the chronically ill/disabled child consumed, on the average, 10 times the amount of health care services consumed by the normal child ($5,447 versus $511).[35]

Breslau and Salkever estimate that the average annual direct medical cost of caring for noninstitutionalized low birthweight infants surviving into childhood with activity limitations because of chronic disease is $1,405 per child.[36] [37] Additional costs of long-term care include many nonmedical expenses of chronic illness born by the child and family, such as work loss by parents. Salkever states that mothers of children with cystic fibrosis experience a 50 percent work loss following the diagnosis.[37]

Breslau estimates that 18.9 percent of low birthweight infants who survive the first year of life will have activity limitations.[36] She also reports that low-income, nonwhite, two-parent families have the largest loss of work income because of the additional care these children require from their parents.[38] Single-parent families must work and often cannot respond to the increased time requirements associated with raising a chronically ill or disabled child; the impact of this phenomenon on the development of these children is unknown.

Data suggest that 1.5 to 2 percent of low birthweight infants who survive the neonatal period will not survive beyond the first year of life.[29] [33] The 2 percent estimate is used in projecting the costs of long-term morbidity of the surviving low birthweight infants.

Results of the Cost Comparison

In this section, the committee presents the results of its cost comparison. The cost of providing additional prenatal care to the target population is compared with the potential reduction in single-year medical care costs of low birthweight infants that would result from a decrease in the low birthweight rate (following the increased use of prenatal care). Savings in the cost of caring for low birth-weight children are presented, broken down into initial hospitalization cost savings; rehospitalization cost savings during the first year of life; and long-term, single-year morbidity cost savings. Finally, overall cost savings are estimated.

As detailed earlier, for the 2,981,000 black and white (only) women on public assistance, ages 15 to 39, a total of 255,149 births were projected on the basis of birth rates by race and age (Table 10.2).[3] From this, it was projected that a total of 23,766 low birthweight infants would be born to the population of women on public assistance (Table 10.2). The average national fertility rates that were used probably underestimate the number of births, especially low birthweight births, for this population of women on public assistance with less than 12 years of education.

Within the total population of women of childbearing age on public assistance, 1,399,000 women between 15 and 39 years of age who had completed less than a high school education were considered to be at

TABLE 10.2 Total Live Births and Low Birthweight (LBW) Births to Women on Public Assistance by Age and Race, 1979

	15-17	18-19	20-24	25-29	30-34	35-39	Total
Live Births[a]							
Black	7,189	13,790	43,043	28,893	12,730	3,709	109,354
White	3,441	9,478	51,778	51,570	23,777	5,751	145,795
Total	10,630	23,268	94,821	80,463	36,507	9,460	255,149
LBW Births[b]							
Black	1,046	1,849	5,628	3,730	1,658	501	14,412
White	273	661	3,375	3,222	1,428	395	9,354
Total	1,319	2,510	9,003	6,952	3,086	896	23,766

[a]Data from analysis of 1980 Census Public Use, Microdata Sample, provided by Northern Ohio Data and Information Service. Cleveland, Ohio, Spring 1984. (Income data in the 1980 census microdata sample reports income received in 1979 by source.) Natality data from National Center for Health Statistics: Advance Report of Final Natality Statistics, 1979, Vol. 30, No. 6 (supplement 2). Table 3: Birth rates by age of mother, live birth order and race of child: United States, 1979. DHHS No. (PHS) 81-1120. Public Health Service. Washington, D.C.: U.S. Government Printing Office, September 29, 1981.

[b]Age- and race-specific rates of low birthweight from National Center for Health Statistics: Advance Report of Final Natality Statistics, 1980, Vol. 31, No. 8 (supplement). Table 13: Number and percent low birthweight and live births by birthweight, by age of mother and race of child: United States, 1980. DHHS No. (PHS) 83-1120. Public Health Service. Washington, D.C.: U.S. Government Printing Office, November 30, 1982.

high risk of delivering low birthweight infants if they became pregnant (Figure 10.1). These women were projected to have 110,601 pregnancies at risk for low birthweight, of which 12,719 would result in a low birthweight infant, given a low birthweight rate for this high-risk population of 11.5 percent (Table 10.3).

TABLE 10.3 Total Live Births and Low Birthweight (LBW) Births to Women on Public Assistance Who Completed Less Than 12 Years of School by Age and Race

	15-17	18-19	20-24	25-29	30-34	35-39	Total
Live Births[a]							
Black	6,416	6,935	17,308	12,677	5,866	2,221	51,423
White	2,176	4,954	20,953	19,138	9,136	2,821	59,178
Total	8,592	11,889	38,261	31,815	15,002	5,042	110,601
LBW Births[b]							
Black	955	1,026	2,797	1,882	871	329	7,860
White	244	415	1,739	1,534	682	245	4,859
Total	1,199	1,441	4,536	3,416	1,553	574	12,719

[a]Data from analysis of 1980 Census Public Use, Microdata Sample, provided by Northern Ohio Data and Information Service. Cleveland, Ohio, Spring 1984. (Income data in the 1980 census microdata sample reports income received in 1979 by source.) Natality data from National Center for Health Statistics: Advance Report of Final Natality Statistics, 1979, Vol. 30, No. 6 (supplement 2). Table 3: Birth rates by age of mother, live birth order and race of child: United States, 1979. DHHS No. (PHS) 81-1120. Public Health Service. Washington, D.C.: U.S. Government Printing Office, September 29, 1981.

[b]Rates of low birthweight from National Center for Health Statistics: Advance Report of Final Natality Statistics, 1980, Vol. 31, No. 8 (supplement). Table 13: Number and percent low birthweight and live births by birthweight, by age of mother and race of child: United States, 1980. DHHS No. (PHS) 83-1120. Public Health Service. Washington, D.C.: U.S. Government Printing Office, November 30, 1982.

TABLE 10.4 Total Additional Cost of Providing Prenatal Care Beginning in the First Trimester to the Full Target Population

Onset of Prenatal Care (trimester)	Distribution of Onset of Prenatal Care[a] (percent)	Incremental Prenatal Costs (dollars)	Number of High-Risk Pregnant Women to Receive Prenatal Care	Cost of Prenatal Care (dollars)
First	56.5	0	62,517	--
Second	32.2	200	35,632	7,126,400
Third or None	11.3	400	12,452	4,980,800
Total	100.0		110,601	12,107,200

[a]National Center for Health Statistics: Vital Statistics of the United States, 1981, Vol. 1, Natality. Table 1.45: Percent distribution of live births by month of pregnancy prenatal care began, by years of school completed by mother and race of child. Public Health Service. Washington, D.C.: U.S. Government Printing Office, in press.

New Prenatal Care Expenditures

The committee judged that $400 per pregnant woman was a reasonable estimate of the unit cost of providing prenatal care to the specified population of pregnant women. To calculate the total incremental cost of providing prenatal care to the target population, the unit cost was adjusted to reflect the different levels of care already received (Table 10.4).[5] The committee concluded that an additional $12,107,200 would be required to provide all of these high-risk women with prenatal care beginning in the first trimester of pregnancy.

A potential weakness of this computation is that the pattern of initiation of prenatal care services for women receiving public assistance may be different from the national pattern that has been assumed, because a greater proportion may be receiving late or no prenatal care or "nonadequate" care, as discussed in chapters 3 and 7. In addition, this cost estimate does not take into consideration the number of women at high risk of delivering a low birthweight infant who may enter prenatal care early. Further, the improved content of the prenatal care outlined by the committee in Chapter 8 probably would be more expensive to provide than that based on current practices, the cost of which was estimated and used in the analysis. These circumstances would increase the costs of prenatal care services, but the magnitude of the increase cannot be determined at this time. However, the following cost comparison shows that even if the fiscal outlays to provide prenatal services to this population of women were arbitrarily increased by 100 percent over the estimate of average current practice costs used here, there would still be a net cost savings in attaining the Surgeon General's goal.[1]

Savings in the Cost of Caring for Low Birthweight Children

A decrease in the number of low birthweight infants would lead directly to decreases in neonatal mortality and morbidity and in the volume of medical services used to care for these children, especially in terms of days of hospitalization in neonatal intensive care units and rehospitalization during the first year of life.

To determine the reduction in costs that might result from the provision of prenatal care to the target population, the committee examined incremental reductions in the low birthweight rate from 11.5 percent to 10 percent to 9 percent. These decrements would represent a 13 percent and a 22 percent reduction in the low birthweight rate, which is within the range of changes that may be anticipated (chapters 3 and 6). The committee estimated only the resulting annual expenditures for direct medical care during the initial hospitalization, for rehospitalization of neonatal survivors during the first year, and for medical services provided for noninstitutionalized, long-term survivors during 1 year.

Initial Hospitalization Cost Savings The 12,719 low birthweight infants (P_2 in Figure 10.1) born to the target population are assumed to require Level II or III neonatal intensive care during the period of initial hospitalization. Using Budetti's charges of $13,616 ($C_2$ unit costs in Table 10.1) for Level II and III neonatal intensive care, the total initial hospitalization cost (TC_2 in Table 10.1) for these low birthweight infants would be $173,181,904. A projected reduction in the low birthweight rate to 9 percent would reduce the number of low birthweight infants to 9,954. Initial hospitalization costs at this 9 percent rate would be $135,533,664--a cost savings of $37,648,240. If only a 10 percent low birthweight rate were achieved by the provision of prenatal care to these high-risk pregnant women, the total initial hospitalization costs would be $150,592,960--a cost savings of $22,588,944 (Table 10.5).[39]

The application to the initial hospitalization of all low birthweight infants of Budetti's estimated charges for hospitalization in Level II and III intensive care units tends to overestimate these expenses. For example, some infants, generally a subpopulation within the 2,250- to 2,500-gram weight group, may be cared for in Level I nurseries and some will have a pattern of care similar to normal birthweight infants. To evaluate the fiscal impact of these adjustments on the cost comparison, the committee estimated the effect of excluding the initial hospitalization and subsequent care costs attributable to all infants weighing 2,250 to 2,500 grams, which should eliminate the costs related to almost all of the moderately low birthweight infants not receiving intensive care, as well as the costs of many other infants who would have received intensive care (and,

TABLE 10.5 The Cost of Initial Hospitalization of Low Birthweight (LBW) Infants and Savings at Different LBW Rates

LBW Rate (percent)	Total Cost[a] (dollars)	Cost Savings[b] (dollars)
11.5	173,181,904	
10	150,592,960	22,588,944
9	135,533,664	37,648,240

[a]Based on an average neonatal intensive care charge (professional and hospital) of $13,616 (1984 dollars).
[b]The cost savings are the reduced expenditures for initial hospitalization of fewer low birthweight infants at the 10 percent and 9 percent low birthweight rates, respectively.

thus, whose costs should be included). In 1981, this cohort represented 43 percent of all low birthweight infants. The effect of this percentage reduction on the total low birthweight infant costs at each low birthweight rate (Table 10.9) does not invalidate the committee's conclusions, although it reduces the magnitude of the net cost savings.[40 41]

Budetti's original estimate did not include all charges for Level II and III care of infants.[28] In addition, the adjustment to 1984 dollars does not take into account the growing use of increasingly expensive resources in caring for low birthweight infants, resulting from changes in medical diagnosis, treatment, and technology since Budetti gathered his data. These considerations may explain, in part, why many of the cost estimates for neonatal intensive care found in more recent studies are higher than those of Budetti. Finally, the trend toward a reduction in the number of term low birthweight infants (Chapter 3) will raise the proportion of very low birthweight and preterm moderately low birthweight infants, which in turn could result in increasing expenditures for the initial hospitalization of low birthweight infants. On balance, in the judgment of the committee, the costs of the initial hospitalization of low birthweight infants used in this analysis have not been overestimated.

Rehospitalization Cost Savings During the First Year The costs of rehospitalization of low birthweight infants who survive the neonatal period were calculated utilizing data reported by McCormick and the Virginia Perinatal Association.[29] The rehospitalization rate was 38.3 percent for very low birthweight infants (1,500 grams or less) and 19 percent for moderately low birthweight infants (1,501 to 2,500 grams). The average lengths of stay were 16.2 days and 12.5 days, respectively. An average hospital charge of $372 per day is used as

TABLE 10.6 Rehospitalization Costs During Initial Year for Very Low Birthweight (VLBW) and Moderately Low Birthweight (MLBW) Infants at Different Low Birthweight (LBW) Rates

LBW Rate (percent)	Number of Infants	Number of Infants Rehospitalized	Total Days of Care	Total Hospital Costs (dollars)
VLBW				
11.5	1,170	448	7,258	2,699,976
10	1,017	390	6,318	2,350,296
9	915	351	5,687	2,115,564
MLBW				
11.5	10,531	2,001	25,013	9,304,836
10	9,158	1,740	21,750	8,091,000
9	8,243	1,567	19,588	7,286,736

the unit cost (C_3 in Table 10.1).[31] The limitations of this estimate are described above.

An 8 percent mortality rate was used to estimate the number of low birthweight infants who would not survive the neonatal period.[33 42] Estimated total costs (TC_3 in Table 10.1) for rehospitalization of the 2,449 low birthweight infants (at a low birthweight rate of 11.5 percent) who would survive the neonatal period and require rehospitalization are $12,004,812 (Table 10.6). At a 10 percent low birthweight rate, rehospitalization cost savings are projected to be $1,563,516 (Table 10.7); at a 9 percent rate, these savings are projected to be $2,602,512.

Long-Term, Single-Year Morbidity Cost Savings Breslau estimates that 18.9 percent of low birthweight infants surviving the first year of life will have long-term morbidity.[36] Salkever estimates the annual unit medical costs (C_4 in Table 10.1) for noninstitutionalized children with limitations of activities due to chronic disease to be more than $1,405 per child.[37] The committee projected that there would be an additional 2 percent mortality among the low birthweight infants during the first year of life, leaving 11,467 surviving infants, of whom 2,167 (P_4 in Figure 10.1) would suffer long-term morbidity.[32] The long-term morbidity costs for these infants would be $3,044,635 per year. This figure does not include the costs of care

TABLE 10.7 Rehospitalization Cost Savings

LBW Rate (percent)	VLBW Costs (dollars)	MLBW Costs (dollars)	Total Rehospital-ization Costs (dollars)	Cost Savings[a] (dollars)
10	2,350,296	8,091,000	10,441,296	1,563,516
9	2,115,564	7,286,736	9,402,300	2,602,512

[a]The cost savings are the reduced expenditures for rehospitalization of fewer low birthweight infants at the 10 percent and 9 percent low birthweight rates, respectively.

for infants with disabilities severe enough to require institutionalization, because adequate data to make such an estimate were not available. Annual long-term morbidity cost savings from a reduction of the low birthweight rate to 10 percent would be $396,210; at 9 percent, the savings would be $661,755 (Table 10.8). Obviously, in order to estimate the cumulative savings in long-term morbidity costs, these annual calculations would need to be multiplied by the average life expectancy of low birthweight infants and take into consideration the discounted present value of such long-term expeditures. Adequate data on the life expectancy of these infants are not available, but there is little reason to suspect that the longevity of infants surviving the first year would be markedly reduced. Thus, in using an estimated cost saving for only 1 year, the committee has substantially understated the cost savings for noninstitutional ambulatory direct medical care of low birthweight children in the calculation of net cost savings.[39 40]

These estimates assume that low birthweight infants with long-term morbidity are comparable in their resource utilization to other groups of chronically ill children. Although there are some data suggesting that the proportion of very low birthweight infants with disabilities decreases with age, and expenditures for institutionalization may be changing because of deinstitutionalization policies, adequate information is not available to make a more discriminating analysis at this time. Long-term follow-up studies of low birthweight infants are needed to explore these and many other issues.

Overall Cost Savings

Table 10.9 summarizes the costs of caring for low birthweight infants in the target population (Figure 10.1). Table 10.10 presents the reductions in the direct medical costs of care for low birthweight infants that might occur if the rates of such births were reduced to 10 percent and 9 percent, respectively. It also includes a calculation of the net reduction in fiscal outlays for medical care that might occur

TABLE 10.8 Long-Term, Single-Year Morbidity Costs at Different Low Birthweight (LBW) Rates

LBW Rate (percent)	Number of Infants with Long-Term Morbidity	Annual Direct Medical Expenses (dollars)	Cost Savings[a] (dollars)
11.5	2,167	3,044,635	
10	1,885	2,648,425	396,210
9	1,696	2,382,880	661,755

NOTE: This assumes a 2 percent mortality rate after rehospitalization during the first year of life, resulting in 11,466 low birthweight infants at risk of long-term morbidity.

[a]The cost savings are the annual reduced expenditures for long-term morbidity of fewer low birthweight infants at the low birthweight rates of 10 percent and 9 percent, respectively. If these infants have a life expectancy of 60 years, for example, the cost savings might be 60-fold greater discounted by the present value of such long-term expenditures.

as a consequence of increasing expenditures for prenatal care services to pregnant women in the target population. Within the limits of the assumptions of the committee's analysis, the provision of more adequate prenatal care services to a cohort of women who are at high risk of delivering a low birthweight infant could reduce total expenditures for direct medical care of their low birthweight infants by $3.38 for each additional $1.00 spent on their prenatal care. This would occur if increasing the amount of prenatal care obtained by these women decreased their rate of low birthweight from its present level of 11.5 percent to the 9 percent level, which is the Surgeon General's goal for a maximum low birthweight rate in high-risk groups in the United States. At a low birthweight rate of 10.76 percent, the savings in low birthweight infant care costs would equal the additional costs of prenatal care services.

Finally, although the committee's calculations and examples focus only on governmental fiscal outlays for a selected group of women receiving public assistance, there are, of course, many more women at high risk of bearing a low birthweight infant. Low birthweight infants born to these women incur costs that are met by private insurance or out-of-pocket expenditures, or are unmet and result in hospital bad debts. The provision of more adequate prenatal care to these women, too, is likely to reduce such fiscal outlays.

TABLE 10.9 Summary of Medical Costs of Low Birthweight (LBW) Child Care at Different Low Birthweight Rates

LBW Rate (percent)	Number of LBW Infants	Initial Hospitalization Costs (dollars)	Rehospitalization Costs (dollars)	Long-Term Morbidity Costs (dollars)	Total LBW Infant Costs[a] (dollars)
11.5	12,719	173,181,904	12,004,812	3,044,635	188,231,351
10	11,060	150,592,960	10,441,296	2,648,425	163,682,681
9	9,954	135,533,664	9,402,300	2,382,880	147,318,844

[a]These are calculations of the total cost of care (TC_5) based on the formulas given in Table 10.1.

Summary

The birth of infants weighing less than 2,500 grams, and particularly those of 1,500 grams or less, imposes a large economic burden on our nation by contributing substantially to neonatal mortality, to disability among surviving infants, and to the cost of health care.

The provision of adequate prenatal services, as currently practiced, to all pregnant women who receive public assistance and who have attained less than a high school education would require increased expenditures, but would decrease the overall fiscal outlays of governmental agencies for the care of the low birthweight infants born to these high-risk women. Savings in the cost of care of low birthweight children would probably more than offset the additional cost for the prenatal services. Similarly, further net savings in overall fiscal outlays for the care of low birthweight children would be likely to result from the provision of appropriate prenatal services to other groups of women who are at high risk of delivering low birthweight infants.

TABLE 10.10 Cost Savings at Different Low Birthweight (LBW) Rates

LBW Rate (percent)	Total LBW Infant Costs (TC_5) (dollars)	Reduction in Cost of LBW Infant Care (TC_6) (dollars)	Outlays for Additional Prenatal Care (TC_1) (dollars)	Net Gost Savings (TC_6-TC_1) (dollars)
11.5	188,231,351	--	--	--
10	163,682,681	24,548,670	12,107,200	12,439,470
9	147,318,844	40,912,507	12,107,200	28,805,307

NOTE: See Table 10.1 for definitions and formulas.

References and Notes

1. Public Health Service: Promoting Health/Preventing Disease: Objectives for the Nation. Washington, D.C.: U.S. Government Printing Office, Fall 1980.
2. Analysis of 1980 Census Public Use, Microdata Sample, provided by Northern Ohio Data and Information Service. Cleveland, Ohio, Spring 1984.
3. National Center for Health Statistics: Advance Report of Final Natality Statistics, 1979, Vol. 30, No. 6 (supplement 2). Table 3: Birth rates by age of mother, live birth order and race of child: United States, 1979. DHHS No. (PHS) 81-1120. Public Health Service. Washington, D.C.: U.S. Government Printing Office, September 29, 1981.
4. National Center for Health Statistics: Advance Report of Final Natality Statistics, 1980, Vol. 31, No. 8 (supplement). Table 13: Number and percent low birthweight and live births by birthweight, by age of mother and race of child: United States, 1980. DHHS No. (PHS) 83-1120. Public Health Service. Washington, D.C.: U.S. Government Printing Office, November 30, 1982.
5. National Center for Health Statistics: Vital Statistics of the United States, 1981, Vol. 1, Natality. Table 1.45: Percent distribution of live births by month of pregnancy prenatal care began, by years of school completed by mother and race of child. Public Health Service. U.S. Government Printing Office. In press.
6. Shapiro S, McCormick MC, Starfield BH, Krischer JP, and Bross D: Relevance of correlates of infant deaths for significant morbidity at one year of age. Am. J. Obstet. Gynecol. 136:363-373, 1980. See also McCormick MC, Shapiro S, and Starfield BH: Injury and its correlates among 1-year-old children: Study of children with both normal and low birthweights. Am. J. Dis. Child. 135:159-163, 1981. See also Shapiro S, McCormick MC, Starfield BH, and Crawley B: Changes in morbidity associated with decreases in neonatal mortality. Pediatrics 72:408-415, 1983.
7. Committee to Study the Prevention of Low Birthweight: Prenatal care and low birthweight: Effects on health care expenditures. Unpublished paper prepared by S Smookler and RE Berhman. Washington, D.C.: Institute of Medicine, 1984.
8. Committee to Study the Prevention of Low Birthweight: A rapid survey of prenatal care charges in the United States. Unpublished paper prepared by C Korenbrot. Washington, D.C.: Institute of Medicine, May 1984.
9. Health Insurance Association of America: The Cost of Having a Baby. Washington, D.C., 1983.
10. Michigan Department of Public Health: Prenatal Care: A Healthy Beginning for Michigan's Children. Report of the Director's Special Task Force. Lansing, Mich., 1984.
11. Malitz D: Cost benefit analysis of extending Texas Medicaid coverage to provide prenatal care to pregnant women. Submitted to the Texas Department of Human Resources, May 1983.

12. Colorado Department of Health: Cost Benefit Analysis of Excess Prematurity Versus Prenatal Care. Denver, Colo., 1977.
13. Lazarus W: Right from the Start: Improving Health Care for Ohio's Pregnant Women and Their Children. Columbus, Ohio: Children's Defense Fund-Ohio, 1983.
14. Committee to Study the Prevention of Low Birthweight: The role of Medicaid in delivering prenatal care to low income women. Unpublished paper prepared by MA McManus. Washington, D.C.: Institute of Medicine, November 1983.
15. Korenbrot C: Risk reduction in pregnancies of low income women, Mobius 4:34-43, July 1984.
16. In an HMO setting, the costs of providing prenatal nutrition counseling and a smoking cessation program were estimated to be $118.00 per patient. Ershoff D, Aaronson N, Danaher B, and Wasserman FW: Behavioral, health and cost outcomes of an HMO-based prenatal health education program. Public Health Rep. 98:536-547, 1983.
17. Pomerance JJ, Schifrin BS, and Meredith JL: Womb rent. Am. J. Obstet. Gynecol. 137:486-490, 1980.
18. Bragonier JR, Cushner IM, and Hobel CJ: Social and personal factors in the etiology of preterm birth. In Preterm Birth: Causes, Prevention and Management, edited by F Fuchs and PG Stubblefield, pp. 64-85. New York: Macmillan, 1984.
19. Phibbs CS, Williams RL, and Phibbs RH: Newborn risk factors and costs of neonatal intensive care. Pediatrics 68:313-321, 1981.
20. Korenbrot C, Aalto C, and Laros R: The cost-effectiveness of stopping preterm labor with beta-adrenergic treatment. N. Engl. J. Med. 310:691-696, 1984.
21. Pomerance JJ, Ukrainski CT, Ukra T, Henderson H, Nash AH, and Meridith JL: Cost of living for infants weighing 1,000 grams or less at birth. Pediatrics 61:908-910, 1978.
22. McCarthy JT, Koops BL, Honeyfield PR, and Butterfield LJ: Who pays the bill for neonatal intensive care? J. Pediatr. 95:755-761, 1979.
23. Kaufman SL and Shepard SS: Costs of neonatal intensive care by length of stay. Inquiry 19:167-178, 1982.
24. Weitz J: Improvements for Maternity and Infant Care. Washington, D.C.: Children's Defense Fund, July 11, 1983.
25. Boyle MH, Torrance GW, Sinclair J, and Horwood SP: Economic evaluation of neonatal intensive care of very-low-birth-weight infants. N. Engl. J. Med. 308:1330-1337, 1983.
26. Rajagopalan R, Stickle G, Kairam R, and Driscoll J: Some clinical determinants of the cost of neonatal intensive care. Unpublished paper, 1984.
27. Walker DB, Feldman A, Vohr BR, and Oh W: Cost-benefit analysis of neonatal intensive care for infants weighing less than 1,000 grams at birth. Pediatrics 74:20-25, 1984.
28. Office of Technology Assessment, U.S. Congress: The Implications of Cost-Effectiveness Analysis of Medical Technology, Background Paper No. 2: Case studies of medical technologies. Case Study No. 10: The costs and effectiveness of neonatal intensive care.

Prepared by P Budetti, MA McManus, N Barrand, and LA Heinen. GPO Stock No. 052-003-00845-9. Washington, D.C.: U.S. Government Printing Office, 1981.

29. McCormick MC, Shapiro S, and Starfield BH: Rehospitalization in the first year of life for high-risk survivors. Pediatrics 66:991-999, 1980. Also see Virginia Perinatal Association, Inc.: Cost/Benefit Analysis of Virginia Senate Bill 200 (Expanding Medicaid Eligibility to Include First Time Pregnant Women). This cost-benefit analysis is based on a 1984 Medicaid cost-saving formula devised by the Children's Defense Fund, Washington, D.C. The 1983 Virginia Statewide Perinatal Services Plan is a major compendium of the perinatal health statistics used in this analysis.
30. Hack M, DeMonterice D, Merkatz IR, Jones P, and Fanaroff A: Rehospitalization of the very low birthweight infant--a continuum of perinatal and environmental morbidity. Am. J. Dis. Child. 135:263-266, 1981.
31. Freeland MS and Schendler CE: Health spending in the 1980s: Integration of clinical practice patterns with management. Health Care Financ. Rev. 5:1-68, 1984.
32. National Association of Children's Hospitals and Related Institutions, Inc.: Survey for Surgeon General's Conference on Handicapped Children and Their Families, 1982. The survey reports data from 11 children's hospitals.
33. Goldenberg R, Koski J, Ferguson C, Wayne J, Hale C, and Nelson K: Infant mortality: The relationship between neonatal and post-neonatal mortality during a period of increasing perinatal center utilization. J. Pediatr., in press.
34. Butler J, Budetti P, McManus P, Stenmark S, and Newacheck P: Health care expenditures for children with chronic disabilities. Center for the Study of Families and Children, Institute for Public Policy Studies, Vanderbilt University. Paper prepared for Public Policies Affecting Chronically Ill Children and Their Families, September, 1982.
35. Smyth-Staruch K, Breslau N, Weitzman M, and Gortmaker S: Use of health services by chronically ill and disabled children. Med. Care 22:310-328, 1984.
36. Committee to Study the Prevention of Low Birthweight: Medical care costs of prematurity. Unpublished paper prepared by N Breslau. Washington, D.C.: Institute of Medicine, 1984.
37. Salkever D: Parental opportunity costs and other economic costs of children's disabling conditions. In Chronically Ill Children, A Stacked Deck, edited by NJ Hobbs and J Perrin. San Francisco: Jossey-Bass Inc., 1984.
38. Breslau N, Salkever D, and Smyth-Staruch K: Women's labor force activity and responsibilities for disabled dependents: A study of families with disabled children, J. Health Soc. Behav. 23:169-183, 1982.
39. The cost savings are the reduced expenditures for initial hospitalization of fewer low birthweight infants at the 10 percent and 9 percent low birthweight rates, respectively.

40. The net cost savings are the differences in total low birthweight infant costs at low birthweight rates of 10 percent and 9 percent, respectively, compared to the total low birthweight costs at 11.5 percent, less the $12,107,200 expenditure for additional prenatal services.
41. In an alternative approach to this problem, it could be assumed that all infants weighing 1,500 grams or less would require intensive care during initial hospitalization at a unit cost of $40,000 per infant and that 40 percent of infants weighing 1,501 to 2,500 grams would require intensive care at a unit cost of $20,000 per infant. If 1,800 infants born to women in the target population were in the former group and 10,900 in the latter group, the total cost of intensive care during initial hospitalization would be $159,200,000 ([$40,000 x 1,800] + [$8,000 x 10,900]). This would not affect the validity of the committee's basic conclusion that there would be a net cost saving from additional prenatal care services if the low birthweight rate were reduced to 9 percent.
42. This calculation assumes an 8 percent mortality rate during initial hospitalization (per Goldenberg et al.[33]), resulting in 11,597 low birthweight survivors and rehospitalization rates of 38.3 percent for very low birthweight infants (1,500 grams or less) and 19 percent for moderately low birthweight infants (1,501 to 2,500 grams). Average lengths of stay are assumed to be 16.2 days for very low birthweight infants and 12.5 days for moderately low birthweight infants. A hospital charge of $372 per day is used in this calculation. The ratio of very low birthweight to moderately low birthweight infants is assumed to be .10, based on data from the Robert Wood Johnson Foundation's regionalization of perinatal care project.

APPENDIXES

APPENDIX A

Risk Factors Associated with Low Birthweight

The following chart lists the major risk factors for low birthweight and notes (with an "x") whether an individual factor has been associated with intrauterine growth retardation (IUGR), preterm delivery (PTD) or both; or whether it has been linked only to low birthweight, not further specified (LBW). In some instances, a factor has been linked to all three outcome measures; in others, the association is with only one or two.

For some of these factors, the committee was able to locate relative and attributable risk values;* these appear on the chart under the headings RR and AR, respectively. In general, relative risk values were recorded only if at least one value of 1.8 or greater was found in the articles reviewed, although several values less than 1.8 that are drawn from Chapter 3 are noted on the chart. Attributable risks were recorded whenever a number was located. The control variables used by various studies in computing the relative and attributable risks are not listed; nor, in most instances, are the characteristics of the populations from which the data were gathered.

Documentation justifying the presence of a given factor on the chart is drawn either from the articles providing the RR or AR values, or from the data presented in Chapters 2 and 3. For those factors that have no RR or AR values on the chart and that are not discussed in Chapters 2 or 3, a reference is provided. Reference numbers appear in parentheses, corresponding to the citations following the chart.

Following the references and notes to the appendix is a list of several additional articles that discuss the risk factors associated with preterm delivery, IUGR, or both.

---

*Chapter 1 contains a definition of relative risk and attributable risk.

APPENDIX A

Risk Factors Associated With Low Birthweight

Risk Factors	Intrauterine Growth Retardation			Preterm Delivery			Low Birthweight (unspecified)			Comments
	Risk	RR	AR	Risk	RR	AR	Risk	RR	AR	
I. Demographic										
A. Age (generally <17 or >34)	x			x	2.6(1)		x			RR value for white, <15
					1.8(1)					RR value for white, ≥40
		1.5(2)								RR value for <17
								1.84 (3)		RR value for white, <15
								1.3 (3)		RR value for black, <15
								1.3 (3)		RR value for white, ≥40
								1.1 (3)		RR value for black, ≥40
B. Unmarried	x	1.8(2)		x			x			
								1.8 (3)		RR value for white, <15 and ≥35
								1.6 (3)		RR value for white, ages ages 15 to 34
								1.3 (3)		RR value for black, <15 and ≥35
								1.15 (3)		RR value for black, ages 15 to 34
C. Black	x	2.4(2) 2.3(7)		x			x	1.39 (4)		
D. Low socioeconomic status	x		5.2(8)							"manual" social class
				x		40-60(5) (6)	x			
E. Poor level of education				x			x	1.47(3)		RR for white, ≤11 years education
								1.18(3)		RR for black, ≤11 years education
II. Risks/Conditions Pre-Existing Current Pregnancy										
A. Low maternal prepregnant weight	x	3.6 (2)		x	2.1 (2)		x			≤100 lb
		1.84(8)	13.8(8)							RR range 1.22-2.8; AR range 6.6-20.5
		2.4(7)								
	x			x						≤50.8 kg (24)(25)
								2.2(9)		≤110 lb, compared to wt. of ≥130 lb, white term births

B. Small stature	x	2.03(8)	15.8(8)							white, exact height not specified. RR range 1.3-3.1, AR range 9.0-22.0
		2.3 (10)		x			x			<1.5 m
		1.7 (2)								<52 in.
		1.5 (7)								<62 in.
C. Genital anomalies	x	1.1 (1)		x	3.1(5) (1)	<0.5(5)				
		0.8 (1)		x	1.9(1)	0.5(5)				uterine myomas
						16-18(5)				general uterine
					2.1(2)					general uterine/ cervical
		1.9 (2)								clinically small pelvis
D. Maternal diseases/ disorders, not pregnancy-related.										
1. general							x		7.7(12)	white
									20.0(12)	white
									3.8(12)	nonwhite
				x		4.0-9.0(5)				
						3.8-19.8(5)				
						9.0(6)				"maternal illness"
	x			x						"chronic medical diseases"
2. diabetes mellitus	x			x	5.5(2)					
3. liver disease	x	2.0(1)		x	4.1(5) (1)	0.5(5)				
4. nephritis	x	1.7(2) 1.0(1)		x	4.8(5) (1)	<.5(5)				
5. absent kidney	x	1.1(1)		x	2.1(1)					
6. chronic hypertension	x	1.8(2) (1)		x	1.9(1)					
7. viral pneumonia	x	1.6(1)		x	2.0(1)					
8. heart/cardiovascular disease	x	1.3(1)		x	1.8(1)	<.5(5)				
E. Obstetric history										
1. previous antepartum bleeding/hemmorhage	x	2.0(2)		x	1.7(2)					
2. previous "LBW baby"	x	1.7(7)		x	2.3(2)					
3. previous IUGR baby	x	2.9(10)					x	5.2(11)[a]	20.0(11)[a]	
		7.98(8)	56(8)							RR range 4.7-13.5; AR range 46.9-63.5
		3.4(11)	27.7(11)							

[a]For additional values referring to previous pregnancy outcomes, see referenced article.

Risk Factors	Intrauterine Growth Retardation			Preterm Delivery			Low Birthweight (unspecified)			Comments
	Risk	RR	AR	Risk	RR	AR	Risk	RR	AR	
4. previous PTD	x	2.4(1)		x	3.7(5)(1)					2 previous
		3.3(1)			4.9(1)					3 previous
						18(5)[a] (6)				1 or more, incl. fetal deaths
					2.2(1)					1 previous
					4.4(11)	12.5(2)				1 previous
5. previous abortions	x	1.3(1)		x	1.7(1)		x			2 previous abortions
		1.1(1)			2.2(1)					3 or more; spontaneous vs induced not stated
					1.4(2)					"abortion"
					4.4(2)					"habitual abortion"
						18(5)[b]			18(6)[b]	
6. previous fetal/ neonatal deaths	x	1.2(1)		x	1.7(2)		x	1.1-1.2(3)		1 fetal death
					1.9(1)	18(5)[b]		2.63(4)		
		1.9(1)			3.8(1)					2 or more
					2.1(2)					fetal anomaly
	x				2.5(2)					1 neonatal death
		1.4(1)			2.2(1)					
		1.1(1)			3.7(1)					2 or more
7. incompetent cervix/ previous cone biopsy				x			x		2.6(12)	white
									1.5(12)	non white
8. previous abruptio placentae	x	1.5(1)		x	2.6(1)					
9. previous placenta previa(1)	x			x						
10. previous isoimmunization	x	1.1(1)		x	4.8(1)					
F. DES exposure(18)				x						
G. Selected maternal genetic factors(19)(27)	x						x			
III. Medical Risks, Current Pregnancy										
A. Parity 0,1	x	1.1(1)		x	1.5(2)		x	1.0 (3)		
		1.5-2.0(2)								
		3.0(10)								over age 35
		1.3(10)								all ages

B. High parity(20)	x		x			x			
C. Short pregnancy interval						x	1.63(3) 1.46(3)		white[c] black[c]
D. Multiple pregnancy	x		x	5.5(5)	10.0(12) 10.0(5) (6)	x		14.5(12)	white
				2.0(2)					twins
		5.3(1)		5.5(1)					
E. Polyhydraminos/ oligohydraminos	x	1.4(1)	x	2.6(1)	}				
F. Hyperemesis	x	1.9(1)	x	4.1(1)	} 2.4(5)				
G. Isoimmunization	x	1.1(1)	x	4.3(1)	}				
H. 1st or 2nd trimester bleeding/hemmorhage	x		x	2.1(2)	}				
I. Infections									
1. chorioamionitis			x			x			
2. pyelonephritis			x			x		1.00(5)	
3. other maternal febrile states			x			x			genital/vaginal infection
4. Rubella	x								
5. Cytomegalovirus	x								
6. urinary tract	x		x			x			
7. retained IUD			x		4x as much (5)				
8. appendicitis	x	0.8(1)	x	2.8(1)	<.5(5)				
9. sexually transmitted diseases	x	1.8(2)	x						gonorrhea
J. Anemia/"abnormal hemoglobin"	x	0.8(1)	x	4.2(1)					Hg <7g
		1.0(1)		3.3(1)					Hg 7-7.9g
		1.2(1)		2.1(1)					Hg 8-8.9g
		1.5(1)		3.3(1)	.7(5)				
						x		1.1(12) 1.4(12)	nonwhite, Hg <9 white, Hg <11
K. Fetal anomaly	x	1.7(1)	x	2.4(1)	6(6)(5)	x		1.5(12)	white

[a]For additional values referring to previous pregnancy outcomes, see referenced article.
[b]AR values refer to two or more miscarriages or ≥ 1 previous preterm delivery.
[c]interval <6 months, where prior pregnancy resulted in single, live birth.

Risk Factors	Intrauterine Growth Retardation Risk	RR	AR	Preterm Delivery Risk	RR	AR	Low Birthweight (unspecified) Risk	RR	AR	Comments
L. Abruptio placentae	x	2.0(1)		x	8.0(5) (1)					
							x		6.5(12) 4.9(12)	white nonwhite
						10.0 (5)(6)				
M. Placenta previa	x	1.4(1)		x	6.0(5) (1)					
							x		2.8(12) 1.7(12)	white nonwhite
N. Low systolic BP	x			x	2.5(2)					≤100
		1.4(2)								≤120
O. Low diastolic BP (≤60)	x	1.5(2)		x	3.1(2)					
P. High systolic BP (≤160)	x	2.5(2) 2.84(8)	1.3(7) 18.4(8)	x	2.0(2)					hypertension without preeclampsia. RR range 1.9-4.2; AR range 12.5-24.0
		1.6(7)								
Q. Preeclampsia/toxemia	x	2.3(10) 15.8(8)	9.8(8)							RR range 6.2-40.4; AR range 6.4-13.1
		1.8(1)								
				x		6.4(12) 1.4(1)				white
							x		.68(12) 14.0(12) .75(12)	toxemia; white toxemia; white toxemia; nonwhite
R. Eclampsia	x	2.4(1)		x	5.8(5) (1)					
S. Spontaneous PROM[a]	x	1.4(1)		x	2.0(1)	26(5)				

Risk factor										
IV. Behavioral/Environmental Risks in Current Pregnancy										
A. Smoking	x	3.04(8)	39.7(8)	x			x			IUGR RR range 2.2-4.2, AR range 32.9-45.8
		1.4(2)				11.0(12)		1.5(13)		
						4-14(5)		1.56(14)		
						(6)				
									30.0(12)	white
									21-39(15)	
		1.6(7)								>1 pack/day
B. Nutritional deprivation/ poor weight gain	x	1.78(8)	10.2(8)	x						RR range 1.1-2.8, AR range 3.3-16.6
		1.9(2)								wt. gain <.5 lb/wk
							x		65.0(12)	white
									57.0(12)	nonwhite (of term births)
								2.3(9)		compared to wt. gain of ≥21 lb, white term births
C. Heavy alcohol use	x	1.49(23)		x			x			1-2 drinks/week
		1.86(23)								3-5 drinks/week
		2.19(23)								≥6 drinks/week
								1.1(16)		
D. High altitude(21)	x						x			
E. Marijuana/substance abuse	x	3.0(2)		x	3.4(2)		x			non-narcotic abuse
		2.8(2)			2.3(2)					narcotic abuse
		2.1(7)								
V. Health Care Risk Factors										
A. Iatrogenic prematurity induction of labor/ cesarean section				x	3.0(5)					
					(6)					
B. Absent or inadequate prenatal care	x	2.0(1)		x	3.1(1)		x			none
								1.41(17)		native born white
								1.78(17)		native born black
								1.56(3)		white, 7th mo. start or none
								1.35(3)		black, 7th mo. start or none
								1.2-2.33(17)[a]		inadequate, white
								1.76-1.94(17)[b]		inadequate, black
								2.88(3)		white, none
								2.21(3)		black, none

[a]PROM = spontaneous premature rupture of the membranes.

Risk Factors	Intrauterine Growth Retardation			Preterm Delivery			Low Birthweight (unspecified)			Comments
	Risk	RR	AR	Risk	RR	AR	Risk	RR	AR	
VI. Evolving Concepts of Risk										
A. Stress (physical and psychosocial/emotional)	x			x	3.0(2)					psychosocial problems
B. Uterine irritability				x						
C. Events triggering premature uterine contractions, such as hard physical work, sexual intercourse/orgasm, and general physical stress				x						
D. Selected cervical changes detected before onset of labor				x						
E. Progesterone deficiency				x						
F. Selected environmental toxins/occupational exposure (i.e, air pollution, pesticides, ionizing radiation, lead, anesthetic gasses)(22)(26)	x			x			x			
G. Inadequate plasma volume expansion	x			x			x			
H. Selected genitourinary infections	x			x			x			

[a]1.2 for private hospital service patients, 2.33 for general maternity service patients.
[b]1.76 for patients with no adverse pregnancy conditions, 1.94 for patients with adverse pregnancy conditions.

References and Notes

1. Kaltreider DF and Kohl S: Epidemiology of preterm delivery. Clin. Obstet. Gynecol. 23:27-31, 1980.
2. Rosen MG: The biological vulnerability of the low birthweight infant. In Infants at Risk for Developmental Dysfunction. Institute of Medicine, Pub. No. 82-001, Washington, D.C., 1982.
3. See Chapter 3, Tables 3.6-3.8 and 3.10-3.12.
4. Linn S, Schoenbaum SC, Monson RR, Rosner R, Stubblefield PG, and Ryan KJ: The association of marijuana use with the outcome of pregnancy. Am. J. Public Health 73:1161-1164, 1983.
5. Johnson JWC and Dubin NH. Prevention of preterm labor. Clin. Obstet. Gynecol. 23:51-73, 1980.
6. Mahan CS: New strategies for preventing an old problem: Low birthweight. J. Fla. Med. Assoc. 70:722-727, 1983.
7. Sokol RJ: Clinical risks and laboratory evaluations of intrauterine growth retardation. National Institute of Child Health and Human Development Workshop on Intrauterine Growth Retardation, July 17-20, 1983. National Institutes of Health, Bethesda, Md.
8. Scott A, Moar V, and Ounsted M: The relative contribution of different maternal factors in small-for-gestational-age pregnancies. Eur. J. Obstet. Gynecol. Reprod. Biol. 12:157-265, 1981.
9. Taffel SM and Keppel KG: Implications of mother's weight gain on the outcome of pregnancy. Paper presented at the American Statistical Association meeting, Philadelphia, Pa., August 13-16, 1984. Forthcoming in Proceedings of the American Statistical Association, Winter, 1984-1985.
10. Butler N: Risk factors in human intrauterine growth retardation. In Size at Birth, Ciba Foundation Symposium 27, pp. 379-382. Amsterdam: Associated Science Publishers, 1974.
11. Bakketeig LS, Hoffman HJ, and Harley EE: The tendency to repeat gestational age and birthweight in successive births. Am. J. Obstet. Gynecol. 135:1086-1103, 1979.
12. Hemminki E and Starfield B: Prevention of low birthweight and pre-term birth. Milbank Mem. Fund Q. 56:339-361, 1978.
13. Breart G, Goujard J, Blondel B, Maillard F, Chavigny C, Sureau C, and Rumeau-Rouquette C: A comparison of two policies of ante-natal supervision for the prevention of prematurity. Intern. J. Epidemiol. 10:241-244, 1981.
14. Longo LD: Maternal blood volume and cardiac output during pregnancy: A hypothesis of endocrinologic control. Am. J. Physiol. 245:R720-R729, 1983.
15. Guyer B, Wallach LA, and Rosen SL: Birth-weight-standardized neonatal mortality rates and the prevention of low birth weight: How does Massachusetts compare with Sweden? N. Engl. J. Med. 306:1230-1233, 1982.

16. Marbury MC, Linn S, Monson R, Schoenbaum S, Stubblefield PG, and Ryan KJ: The association of alcohol consumption with outcome of pregnancy. Am. J. Public Health 73:1165-1168, 1983.
17. Gortmaker SL: The effects of prenatal care upon the health of the newborn. Am. J. Public Health 69:653-660, 1979.
18. Herbst AL, Hubby MM, Azizi F, and Makii MM: Reproductive and gynecologic surgical experience in diethylstilbestrol-exposed daughters. Am. J. Obstet. Gynecol. 141:1019-1028, 1981.
19. Committee to Study the Prevention of Low Birthweight: Genetic factors in low birthweight infancy. Unpublished paper by JL Simpson. Washington, D.C.: Institute of Medicine, 1984.
20. National Center for Health Statistics: Factors Associated with Low Birthweight: United States, 1976. Prepared by S Taffel. Vital and Health Statistics, Series 21, No. 36. DHEW No. (PHS) 80-1915. Public Health Service. Washington, D.C.: U.S. Government Printing Office, April 1980.
21. Moore LG, Rounds SS, Jahnigen D, Grover RF, and Reeves JT: Infant birthweight is related to maternal arterial oxygenation at high attitude. J. Appl. Physiol. 52:695-699, 1982.
22. Committee to Study the Prevention of Low Birthweight: Prevention of low birthweight: Environmental and occupational factors. Unpublished paper by V Hunt. Washington, D.C.: Institute of Medicine, 1984.
23. Mills JL, Graubard BI, Harley EE, Rhoads GG, and Berendes HW: Maternal alcohol consumption and birthweight: How much drinking during pregnancy is safe? JAMA 252:1875-1879, 1984.
24. Fedrick J and Anderson ABM: Factors associated with spontaneous preterm birth. Br. J. Obstet. Gynaecol. 83:342-350, 1976.
25. Galbraith RS, Karchmar EJ, Piercy WN, and Low JA: The clinical prediction of intrauterine growth retardation. Am. J. Obstet. Gynecol. 133:281-286, 1979.
26. Vianna NJ and Polan AK: Incidence of low birth weight among Love Canal residents. Science 226:1217-1219, December 7, 1984.
27. Hackman E, Emanuel I, van Belle G, and Daling J: Maternal birthweight and subsequent pregnancy outcome. JAMA 250:2016-2019, 1983.

Additional Reading on Risks Associated With Low Birthweight

Bragonier JR, Cushner IM, and Hobel CJ: Social and personal factors in the etiology of preterm birth. In Preterm Birth: Causes, Prevention and Management, edited by F Fuchs and PG Stubblefield. New York: MacMillan, 1983.

Fedrick J and Adelstein P: Factors associated with low birthweight of infants delivered at term. Br. J. Obstet. Gynaecol. 85:1-7, 1978.

Huddleston JF: Preterm labor. Clin. Obstet. Gynecol. 25:123-136, 1982.

Stickle G and Ma P: Some social and medical correlates of pregnancy outcome. Am. J. Obstet. Gynecol. 127:162-166, 1977.

Thomasson JE and Giles HR: Identification and management of intrauterine growth retardation. In Controversy in Obstetrics and Gynecology III, edited by FP Zuspan and CD Christian, pp. 247-252. Philadelphia: W.B. Saunders, 1983.

Widness JA and Oh W: Intrauterine growth retardation: The current approach to perinatal diagnosis and management. In Controversy in Obstetrics and Gynecology III, edited by FP Zuspan and CD Christian, pp. 265-271, Philadelphia: W.B. Saunders, 1983.

APPENDIX B

Data on Selected Low Birthweight Trends

(Supplement to Chapter 3)

The following tables supplement those contained in Chapter 3. They include data for the United States as a whole and for five states: California, Massachuetts, Michigan, North Carolina, and Oregon.

For assistance in compiling the tables included in this appendix and in Chapter 3, the committee gratefully acknowledges contributions of the following individuals: Selma Taffel, Joel Kleinman, Jacob Feldman, and Paul Placek at the U.S. National Center for Health Statistics; Gary B. Pohl and Jeffrey Taylor at the Office of Vital and Health Statistics, Michigan Department of Public Health; David Hopkins and Nancy Clarke at the Center for Health Statistics, Oregon Department of Human Resources, Health Division; Peter M. Chen, Elizabeth J. Clingman, and Ronald L. Williams at the Community and Organization Research Institute, University of California, Santa Barbara; Charles G. Rothwell and Michael Patetta at the State Center for Health Statistics, North Carolina Division of Health Services; and Charlene Zion, Irene Klangos, and Sharon Rosen at the Division of Health Statistics, Massachusetts Department of Public Health.

TABLE B.1 Percentage of Live Births by Low Birthweight and Race in the United States, 1971-1981

	All Races			White			Black		
	2,500 g or Less	1,500 g or Less	1,501-2,500 g	2,500 g or Less	1,500 g or Less	1,501-2,500 g	2,500 g or Less	1,500 g or Less	1,501-2,500 g
1971	7.64	1.14	6.50	6.55	0.92	5.63	13.31	2.28	11.03
1972	7.65	0.87	6.78	6.47	0.94	5.53	13.54	2.37	11.17
1973	7.53	1.16	6.37	6.39	0.94	5.45	13.21	2.28	10.93
1974	7.40	1.13	6.27	6.28	0.91	5.37	13.09	2.26	10.83
1975	7.37	1.15	6.22	6.24	0.92	5.32	13.05	2.37	10.68
1976	7.24	1.15	6.09	6.11	0.91	5.20	12.93	2.40	10.53
1977	7.07	1.13	5.94	5.92	0.86	5.02	12.77	2.37	10.40
1978	7.10	1.16	5.94	5.90	0.91	4.99	12.90	2.43	10.47
1979	6.90	1.15	5.75	5.74	0.90	4.84	12.50	2.35	10.15
1980	6.82	1.15	5.67	5.68	0.90	4.78	12.47	2.43	10.04
1981	6.80	1.16	5.64	5.66	0.90	4.76	12.50	2.47	10.03
Percent Decrease									
Absolute									
1971-1976	0.40	(0.01)[a]	0.41	0.44	0.01	0.43	0.38	(0.12)	0.50
1976-1981	0.44	(0.01)	0.45	0.45	0.01	0.44	0.43	0.07	0.50
1971-1981	0.84	(0.02)	0.86	0.89	0.02	0.87	0.81	(0.19)	1.00
Relative									
1971-1976	5.23	(0.88)	6.31	6.72	1.09	7.64	2.86	(5.26)	4.53
1976-1981	6.08	(0.87)	7.39	7.36	1.10	8.46	3.33	2.92	4.75
1971-1981	10.99	(1.75)	13.23	13.59	2.17	15.45	6.09	(8.33)	9.07

[a]Parentheses indicate increase.

TABLE B.2 Low-Weight Births (Less Than 2,500 Grams) per 1,000 Live Births in Five States, 1968-1982

	Calif.[a]	Mass.[b]	Mich.[c]	N.C.[d]	Oreg.[e]
1968	73			97	
1969	71	76		91	
1970	69	74	78	92	
1971	66	71	77	87	57
1972	65	70	78	88	58
1973	65	71	77	87	59
1974	63	67	74	87	56
1975	63	68	74	87	57
1976	62	66	75	83	54
1977	61	64	72	80	52
1978	62	64	72	81	51
1979	60	61	71	79	52
1980	59	61	69	80	50
1981	58	59	69	79	50
1982			69	80	
Average Annual Percent Decline[f]	1.6 (0.1)	2.0 (0.1)	1.2 (0.1)	1.3 (0.1)	1.7 (0.2)

NOTE: All data include both singleton and multiple births. Births with unknown birthweights are excluded.

[a]Based on tabulations provided by the Community and Organization Research Institute, University of California, Santa Barbara.

[b]Computed from vital records data provided by the Division of Health Statistics, Massachusetts Department of Public Health.

[c]Based on tabulations provided by Michigan Department of Public Health, Office of Vital and Health Statistics.

[d]Computed from vital records data provided by the Division of Health Services, North Carolina State Center for Health Statistics.

[e]Based on tabulations provided by the Center for Health Statistics, Oregon Department of Human Resources, Health Division.

[f]Estimated from ordinary least squares regression of the natural logarithm of the low-weight rate against time. Standard errors in parentheses.

TABLE B.3 Low-Weight Births and Late Fetal Deaths per 1,000 Live Births and Late Fetal Deaths in Four States, 1968-1982

	Calif.[a]	Mich.[b]	N.C.[b]	Oreg.[b]
1968	78		102	
1969	76		96	
1970	74		97	
1971	71		93	60
1972	70	81	93	61
1973	69	81	93	63
1974	68	77	91	59
1975	66	77	91	60
1976	66	77	87	57
1977	64	74	83	54
1978	66	74	84	53
1979	63	73	85	54
1980	62	72	83	52
1981	61	72	82	51
1982		72	83	
Average Annual Percent Decline[c]	1.8 (0.1)	1.3 (0.1)	1.5 (0.1)	2.0 (0.3)

[a]Late fetal deaths include all fetal deaths weighing 500 grams or more.
[b]Late fetal deaths include all fetal deaths of at least 28 weeks gestation.
[c]See Table B.2, note f.

SOURCES: See footnote a, c, d, and e on Table B.2.

TABLE B.4 Effect of Adding Fetal Deaths to Live Births on Changes in Low Birthweight Rates, by Race in the United States, 1973 and 1977 (Rates per 100 Live Births and Fetal Deaths)

Birthweight (grams)	White			Black		
	1973	1977	Percent Change[a]	1973	1977	Percent Change[a]
Live Births						
≤1,500	0.94	0.89	5.3	2.28	2.37	(4.3)[b]
≤2,500	6.4	5.9	7.2	13.3	12.8	3.5
Live births plus fetal deaths, ≥28 weeks gestation						
≤1,500	1.14	2.06	7.0	2.66	2.72	(2.3)
≤2,500	6.8	6.3	7.7	13.9	13.3	4.0
Live births plus fetal deaths, ≥20 weeks gestation						
≤1,500	1.40	1.29	7.8	3.27	3.24	0.1
≤2,500	7.0	6.5	8.1	14.5	13.8	4.4

[a]Percent change based on birthweight rates to 2 decimal places.
[b]Parentheses indicate increase.

TABLE B.5 Percentage Distribution of Live Births By Detailed Birthweight and Race in the United States, 1971, 1976, and 1981

Birthweight (grams)	All Races			White			Black		
	1971	1976	1981	1971	1976	1981	1971	1976	1981
Total	100.00	100.00	100.00	100.00	100.00	100.00	100.00	100.00	100.00
≤1,000	0.51	0.53	0.55	0.41	0.41	0.41	1.04	1.18	1.24
1,001-1,500	0.63	0.62	0.61	0.51	0.50	0.49	1.24	1.22	1.22
1,501-2,000	1.43	1.42	1.30	1.22	1.18	1.08	2.68	2.57	2.41
2,001-2,500	5.05	4.68	4.35	4.41	4.02	3.68	8.35	7.96	7.62
2,501-3,000	18.68	17.16	16.34	17.20	15.50	14.56	25.88	24.94	24.26
3,001-3,500	38.32	37.44	36.97	38.30	37.16	36.53	38.08	38.33	38.28
3,501-4,000	26.43	27.98	29.03	28.17	29.92	31.12	17.86	18.81	19.77
4,001-4,500	7.22	8.18	8.85	7.94	9.09	9.89	3.74	3.95	4.26
4,501-5,000	1.27	1.51	1.59	1.41	1.70	1.80	0.65	0.63	0.97
≥5,001	0.17	0.20	0.22	0.18	0.22	0.24	0.13	0.11	0.12
Not Stated	0.26	0.29	0.20	0.23	0.30	0.19	0.35	0.33	0.21

TABLE B.6 Low-Weight Births per 1,000 Live Births in Relation to Race for Five States, 1968-1982

	Calif.[a]			Mass.[b]		Mich.[b]		N.C.[b]		Oreg.[b]	
	W	B	S	W	B	W	B	W	B	W	B
1968	58	116	57					78	147		
1969	55	115	55	73	135			72	142		
1970	53	113	53	71	136	66	143	72	145		
1971	51	111	53	65	113	64	144	70	135	56	118
1972	49	113	52	66	137	63	145	69	138	57	152
1973	49	112	51	68	135	63	143	70	133	57	122
1974	48	110	48	64	111	62	135	67	135	54	129
1975	47	109	49	65	115	61	138	68	135	55	109
1976	46	108	47	63	125	61	140	64	130	52	127
1977	45	108	46	61	116	59	135	61	126	50	110
1978	46	107	48	60	123	59	137	64	124	49	109
1979	44	103	46	57	114	58	137	63	126	50	111
1980	45	103	44	56	114	57	133	62	123	48	104
1981	44	101	45	55	111	57	137	61	124	47	103
1982						56	141	61	126		
Average Annual Percent Decline[c]	1.9 (0.2)	1.0 (0.1)	1.8 (0.1)	2.2 (0.2)	1.4 (0.5)	1.3 (0.1)	0.4 (0.2)	1.6 (0.2)	1.2 (0.1)	2.0 (0.3)	2.6 (1.0)

[a]W = white births of non-Spanish surname. B = black births. S = white births inferred to be Spanish by surname. "Race" refers to race of newborn. Only singleton live births included. Births of unknown weight excluded.

[b]W = white births. B = black births. "Race" refers to race of mother. Both singleton and multiple live births included. Births of unknown weight excluded.

[c]See Table B.2, note f.

SOURCES: See footnotes a through e on Table B.2.

TABLE B.7 Percentage of Live Births By Low Birthweight, Age of Mother, and Race in the United States, 1971, 1976, and 1981

Maternal Age (years)	2,500 Grams or Less			1,501 Grams or Less			1,501-2,500 Grams		
	1971	1976	1981	1971	1976	1981	1971	1976	1981
<u>All Races</u>	7.64	7.24	6.80	1.14	1.15	1.16	6.50	6.09	5.64
Less than 15	16.65	14.69	13.96	3.70	3.51	3.14	12.96	11.18	10.82
15-19	10.14	9.88	9.43	1.72	1.69	1.72	8.42	8.19	7.71
15-17	--	--	10.62	--	--	2.06	--	--	8.56
18-19	--	--	8.77	--	--	1.60	--	--	7.17
20-24	7.08	7.11	6.94	1.01	1.11	1.13	6.07	6.00	5.81
25-29	6.63	5.96	5.81	0.92	0.91	0.97	5.71	5.05	4.84
30-34	7.16	6.46	5.80	1.05	1.00	1.01	6.11	5.46	4.98
35-39	8.79	7.91	7.06	1.25	1.18	1.25	7.54	6.73	5.81
40 or older	9.11	9.20	8.43	1.21	1.32	1.26	7.90	7.88	7.17
<u>White</u>	6.55	6.11	5.66	0.92	0.91	0.90	5.63	5.20	4.76
Less than 15	12.78	11.69	10.40	3.34	2.79	2.60	9.44	8.90	7.80
15-19	8.27	8.05	7.70	1.38	1.31	1.30	6.89	6.74	6.40
15-17	--	--	8.70	--	--	1.60	--	--	7.10
18-19	--	--	7.20	--	--	1.20	--	--	6.00
20-24	6.09	6.01	5.80	0.82	0.89	0.90	5.27	5.12	4.90
25-29	5.99	5.27	5.00	0.79	0.75	0.80	5.20	4.52	4.20
30-34	6.44	5.77	5.00	0.88	0.82	0.80	5.56	4.95	4.20
35-39	7.87	6.95	6.20	1.04	0.97	1.10	6.83	5.98	5.10
40 or older	8.23	8.36	7.40	1.11	1.16	1.00	7.12	7.20	6.40
<u>Black</u>	13.31	12.93	12.50	2.28	2.40	2.47	11.02	10.53	10.03
Less than 15	19.03	16.99	16.60	3.94	4.13	3.20	15.09	12.86	13.40
15-19	15.08	13.78	14.00	2.62	1.79	2.80	12.46	11.99	11.20
15-17	--	--	14.60	--		3.00	--	--	11.60
18-19	--	--	13.60	--		2.60	--	--	11.00
20-24	12.75	12.59	12.50	2.12	2.25	2.40	10.63	10.34	10.10
25-29	11.72	11.28	11.40	2.02	2.14	2.30	9.70	9.14	9.10
30-34	11.83	11.52	11.30	2.15	2.32	2.40	9.68	9.20	8.90
35-39	13.51	13.05	12.40	2.31	2.36	2.50	11.20	10.69	9.90
40 or older	12.89	13.02	13.33	1.70	2.11	2.32	11.19	10.91	10.98

TABLE B.8 Low-Weight Births Per 1,000 Live Births in Relation to Maternal Age in Four States, 1968-1982

	Mass.			Mich.			N.C.			Oreg.		
	<20	20-34	≥35	<20	20-34	≥35	<17	17-34	≥35	<18	18-34	≥35
1968							166	94	109			
1969	103	72	85				149	88	108			
1970	110	69	92	105	72	83	150	89	100			
1971	115	66	89	104	70	85	147	83	109	80	56	62
1972	127	66	78	106	70	83	140	85	98	76	56	79
1973	126	67	83	102	71	84	134	85	101	81	56	86
1974	125	62	81	101	67	88	139	84	95	75	55	69
1975	126	63	83	101	67	87	131	85	98	92	54	71
1976	120	63	73	104	68	84	138	81	88	91	51	73
1977	114	60	74	97	71	90	138	77	97	79	50	63
1978	113	60	67	100	66	84	129	79	90	86	49	55
1979	109	57	70	96	65	91	135	80	85	72	51	53
1980	106	57	66	97	64	76	131	77	91	87	48	56
1981	100	56	67	98	65	76	141	77	89	92	48	52
1982				99	65	73	133	79	87			
Average Annual Percent Decline[a]	1.2 (0.2)	1.9 (0.1)	2.7 (0.3)	0.7 (0.2)	0.9 (0.2)	0.8 (0.5)	1.1 (0.3)	1.2 (0.2)	1.6 (0.2)	-0.9 (0.8)	1.8 (0.2)	3.9 (1.1)

[a]See Table B.2, note f.

SOURCES: See footnotes b through e on Table B.2.

TABLE B.9 Percentage of Live Births at Low Birthweight (2,500 Grams or Less) by Age and Educational Attainment of Mother and Race, 1971, 1976, and 1981

Maternal Age and Educational Attainment	All Races			White			Black		
	1971	1976	1981	1971	1976	1981	1971	1976	1981
Total	7.7	7.4	7.0	6.6	6.2	5.7	13.5	13.1	12.6
0-8 years	10.2	9.9	9.6	8.9	8.6	8.3	14.6	14.9	14.7
9-11 years	10.3	10.2	10.2	8.7	8.4	8.4	14.9	14.7	14.9
12 years	6.9	6.8	6.6	6.1	5.8	5.5	12.4	12.0	12.0
13-15 years	5.9	5.9	5.5	5.3	5.1	4.6	10.9	11.2	10.5
16 years or more	5.3	4.9	4.6	4.9	4.5	4.2	10.0	9.4	9.0
Under Age 15									
0-8 years	16.4	15.1	14.8	11.6	12.3	10.6	19.4	17.2	17.3
9-11 years	17.9	15.1	14.6	14.2	12.2	12.0	19.6	16.5	15.7
Age 15-19									
0-8 years	12.0	11.8	11.3	10.4	10.3	9.9	16.2	16.7	16.0
9-11 years	11.2	10.8	10.6	9.2	8.7	8.7	15.8	15.3	14.7
12 years	8.6	8.5	8.1	7.0	6.8	6.4	14.2	13.2	12.7
13-15 years	7.8	9.0	8.3	6.6	6.6	6.8	11.2	12.6	11.7
Age 20-34									
0-8 years	9.3	8.7	8.4	8.3	7.6	7.5	13.3	13.6	13.2
9-11 years	9.5	9.5	9.9	8.3	8.1	8.1	13.8	13.7	14.9
12 years	6.7	6.5	6.4	6.0	5.7	5.4	11.7	11.4	11.7
13-15 years	5.7	5.8	5.4	5.3	5.1	4.5	10.2	10.8	10.3
16 years or more	5.2	5.0	4.6	4.9	4.6	4.1	10.0	9.5	9.0
Age 35 or Older									
0-8 years	8.9	12.2	9.4	8.1	10.7	7.7	10.9	16.9	12.3
9-11 years	11.2	12.2	9.2	10.1	11.4	11.7	13.7	13.7	18.8
12 years	8.7	9.0	14.0	8.0	8.2	8.6	12.5	13.7	11.4
13-15 years	7.2	6.4	9.2	6.5	6.2	6.1	16.7	12.0	14.0
16 years or more	5.9	7.0	7.5	5.9	6.3	4.6	5.7	12.3	10.5

NOTE: Includes 49 states and Washington, D.C., in 1981; 44 states and Washington, D.C.; in 1976, 38 states and Washington, D.C., in 1971.

TABLE B.10 Low-Weight Births Per 1,000 Live Births in Relation to Years of Maternal Education in Four States, 1968-1982

	Mass.			Mich.			N.C.			Oreg.		
	<12	12	≥13	<12	12	≥13	<12	12	≥13	<12	12	≥13
1968							119	85	68			
1969	98	71	67				114	80	64			
1970	99	69	65	104	72	57	114	82	64			
1971	93	69	57	106	70	55	110	78	60	80	54	44
1972	94	69	55	107	69	56	111	80	59	78	56	48
1973	97	70	55	108	69	57	110	80	61	84	56	45
1974	91	65	54	106	68	54	109	80	61	79	55	43
1975	93	67	52	105	67	57	113	79	61	76	54	48
1976	88	67	52	106	68	57	109	76	59	77	50	45
1977	89	64	50	102	66	55	106	73	56	71	53	40
1978	88	64	50	106	66	54	107	77	58	72	52	48
1979	86	61	47	100	67	53	110	78	57	72	52	40
1980	88	61	46	102	63	54	107	75	58	68	48	42
1981	87	59	46	104	66	53	110	76	55	71	48	40
1982				108	65	52	106	80	60			
Average Annual Percent Decline[a]	1.1 (0.2)	1.4 (0.2)	2.9 (0.3)	0.2 (0.2)	0.8 (0.1)	0.6 (0.1)	0.5 (0.1)	0.5 (0.2)	1.0 (0.2)	1.9 (0.4)	1.3 (0.4)	1.0 (0.7)

[a]See Table B.2, note f.

SOURCES: See footnotes b through e on Table B.2

TABLE B.11 Percentage of Live Births by Low Birthweight, Live Birth Order, and Race in the United States, 1971, 1976, and 1981

	2,500 Grams or Less			1,501 Grams or Less			1,501-1,500 Grams		
Live Birth Order	1971	1976	1981	1971	1976	1981	1971	1976	1981
All Races	7.64	7.24	6.80	1.14	1.15	1.16	6.50	6.09	5.64
First birth	7.68	7.58	7.07	1.14	1.22	1.22	6.54	6.34	5.85
Second birth	7.10	6.52	6.15	1.07	1.02	1.04	6.03	5.50	5.11
Third birth	7.46	7.06	6.60	1.09	1.06	1.08	6.37	6.00	5.52
Fourth birth	8.07	8.04	7.68	1.17	1.27	1.28	6.90	6.77	6.40
Fifth birth and over	8.96	8.44	8.32	1.34	1.30	1.40	7.62	7.14	6.92
White	6.55	6.11	5.66	0.92	0.91	0.90	5.63	5.20	4.76
First birth	6.59	6.50	6.09	0.95	1.00	0.99	5.64	5.50	5.10
Second birth	6.07	5.45	5.10	0.85	0.80	0.81	5.22	4.65	4.29
Third birth	6.44	5.93	5.30	0.86	0.81	0.78	5.58	5.12	4.52
Fourth birth	7.12	6.74	6.10	0.98	0.99	0.98	6.14	5.75	5.12
Fifth birth and over	7.64	6.95	6.29	1.09	1.01	0.98	6.55	5.94	5.31
Black	13.31	12.93	12.50	2.25	2.40	2.47	11.03	10.53	10.03
First birth	13.59	10.93	12.54	2.24	2.47	2.56	11.35	8.46	9.98
Second birth	13.42	12.72	11.94	2.46	2.34	2.36	10.96	10.38	9.58
Third birth	13.29	12.60	12.36	2.38	2.27	2.37	10.91	10.33	9.99
Fourth birth	12.66	12.16	13.22	2.10	2.39	2.33	10.56	10.77	10.89
Fifth birth and over	12.78	12.72	14.04	2.08	2.19	2.60	10.70	10.53	11.44

TABLE B.12 Low Birthweight Rate (2,500 Grams or Less) per 1,000 by Month Mother Began Prenatal Care and Race, 1971, 1976 and 1981

Prenatal Care Began (month)	All Races			White			Black		
	1971	1976	1981	1971	1976	1981	1971	1976	1981
First-second	65.9	62.6	59.2	59.8	55.2	51.4	123.6	117.3	114.6
Third	68.6	67.8	64.0	60.6	57.8	53.6	123.9	124.4	117.7
Fourth-sixth	85.7	83.5	79.9	71.5	68.8	64.7	128.9	127.8	125.8
Seventh-ninth	84.7	81.8	78.4	71.0	68.0	64.2	119.4	121.7	119.8
No prenatal care	216.8	201.9	200.4	177.7	162.8	162.9	284.7	284.1	274.7
Seventh month or later or no care	114.2	111.4	110.4	92.1	90.0	88.5	164.9	168.8	168.3
Fourth month or later or no care	92.3	89.6	86.6	75.9	73.2	69.6	138.6	137.4	136.1

NOTE: Includes total United States in 1981; 44 states and Washington, D.C., in 1976; 39 states and Washington, D.C., in 1971.

TABLE B.13 Low-Weight Births per 1,000 Live Births in Relation to Timing of First Prenatal Visit in Four States, 1968-1982

	Mass.		Mich.		N.C.		Oreg.	
	First Trim.	Other & Unknown	First Trim.	Other & Unknown	First Trim.	Other & Unknown	First Trim.	Other & Unknown
1968					85	119		
1969	70	93			78	117		
1970	62	88	69	100	82	113		
1971	64	87	69	97	79	107	53	69
1972	66	93	69	99	79	108	53	73
1973	62	101	69	99	80	107	53	74
1974	62	90	68	92	78	111	51	72
1975	63	95	67	96	79	110	50	75
1976	62	89	67	96	76	106	46	78
1977	60	85	64	93	72	104	46	68
1978	60	88	65	94	75	102	45	67
1979	57	86	64	93	75	105	47	67
1980	56	92	63	90	74	100	44	68
1981	55	90	62	95	75	97	46	62
1982			63	97	76	97		
Average Annual Percent Decline[a]	1.5 (0.2)	0.3 (0.4)	1.0 (0.1)	0.5 (0.2)	0.8 (0.2)	1.3 (0.1)	2.3 (0.3)	0.8 (0.6)

NOTES: "First Trim." = Prenatal care initiated in the first trimester of pregnancy. "Other & Unknown" = other prenatal care, no care, or unknown care.

[a]See Table B.2, note f.

SOURCES: See footnotes b through e on Table B.2.

APPENDIX C

A Summary of Three Prematurity Prevention Programs

Described below in outline form are three innovative programs designed to reduce the occurrence of preterm delivery.

I. The March of Dimes Multicenter Prevention of Preterm Delivery Program*

A. Location: This program originated at the University of California, San Francisco (UCSF). It has been expanded to include studies at the University of California, San Diego; Northwestern University, Chicago; the University of Alabama, Birmingham; Vanderbilt University, Nashville; and Ohio State University, Columbus.

B. Investigators responsible for program: Robert K. Creasy, M.D.; Richard Depp, M.D.; Stephen Entmen, M.D.; Thomas Key, M.D.; Robert Goldenberg, M.D.; and Jay Iams, M.D.

C. Funding source: The March of Dimes Birth Defects Foundation.

D. Dates of implementation:

1. Original UCSF program: July 1, 1978 to May/June, 1985.
2. Pilot Phase of multicenter program: November 1, 1982 to April 30, 1983 (baseline preprogram data collected before any intervention initiated).
3. Implementation of multicenter program began July 1, 1982.
4. Tentative concluding date: January 1, 1986.

E. Program description

1. Basic type of program: The original San Francisco program was a longitudinal demonstration project to test the effectiveness of an educational program for patients at risk of preterm labor and for providers of obstetric care. This program focused on self-detection of early signs of preterm labor to allow patients to be treated as soon as possible with tocolysis.† The program also

*Program summary prepared by committee member Calvin J. Hobel in consultation with Robert K. Creasy.

†The use of a medication to inhibit uterine activity, described more fully in Chapter 8.

included intensive in-service education for the obstetric care providers. The same basic program will be implemented in the five new areas; however, at these sites, high-risk patients will be divided randomly into a study group (basic program) and a control group.

2. Health care providers: The program utilizes both physicians and nurse practitioners to carry out risk assessment, to allocate into study/control groups, to provide primary care, and to supervise the overall program.
3. Entry into the study: All new patients who enroll for prenatal care at the designated study sites will have an opportunity to participate in this program. Informed consent will be obtained. Risk assessment will be performed using modifications by Creasy of the scoring system developed by Papiernik (Chapter 2). High-risk patients will be randomized into either the study group or the control group. High-risk patients in the study group will receive weekly pelvic exams to identify early cervical changes. At 22 to 26 weeks of pregnancy, low-risk patients will be rescreened to determine whether events warrant their transfer to the high-risk group.
4. Patient self-detection education program (for study patients only): The program emphasizes the importance of early preterm labor detection and provides instruction on self-detection of the subtle symptoms of preterm labor. Patients are trained in self-detection of painless contractions by palpation and are requested to report immediately if any one of five different symptoms develops. All study patients are reevaluated weekly by specially trained nurses.
5. Interventions: The early evaluation of patients, the self-detection education program, and the weekly exam are considered the main interventions in this program.
6. Staff training/education program: In-service training for all providers is given to ensure a prompt response to patient complaints, liberal and early hospitalization, an aggressive therapeutic approach, and awareness of certain contraindications for therapeutic measures.

F. Program effectiveness: Preliminary results indicate that during the first 2 years of the San Francisco study, early recognition of preterm labor was significantly improved. About 93 percent of high-risk patients who went into preterm labor and 79 percent of low-risk patients who went into preterm labor were candidates for tocolytic treatment, compared with less than 20 percent before introduction of the program.* In addition, a significant reduction occurred in

*Herron MA, Katz M, and Creasy RK: Evaluation of a preterm birth prevention program: Preliminary report. Obstet. Gynecol. 59:452-456, 1982.

TABLE C.1 Comparison of Preterm Births at University of California at San Francisco (UCSF) and an Affiliated Institution (AI)

	1978/79	1979/80	1980/81	1981/82	1982/83
UCSF	6.75	6.75	2.40	3.5	NA[a]
AI	6.90	6.20	7.00	NA	NA

[a]NA means not available.

the preterm delivery rate compared to the same institution in earlier years and to an affiliated institution. See Table C.1.

II. The Los Angeles Prematurity Prevention Program*

A. Location: This program is being implemented in selected health centers in the west health districts of Los Angeles. There are five study clinics and three nonstudy clinics (controls). These health centers provide prenatal care for patients who deliver at Harbor-UCLA Medical Center.

B. Investigators responsible for program: Calvin J. Hobel, M.D.; Robert Bragonier, M.D., Ph.D.; Michael Ross, M.D.; Rose Bemis, R.N.N.P.

C. Funding source: California Department of Health.

D. Dates of implementation:

1. Pilot Phase: April 15, 1983 to July 15, 1983.
2. Full Implementation: August 15, 1983 to present; anticipated completion date is June 30, 1986.

E. Program description

1. Basic type of program: This is a randomized trial to test the effectiveness of five different interventions designed to prevent preterm labor, superimposed on an intensive educational program for both patients and providers.
2. Health care providers: The program uses nurse practitioner teams to carry out risk assessment; allocation of intervention; primary care; and supervision of the program components, including education, social service, nutrition, home visits, and the audit of outcome.
3. Entry into the study: All new patients less than 31 weeks pregnant receive an orientation and a welcome pamphlet. If the patient elects to participate, she signs an informed consent form. All patients complete a psychological questionnaire, whether or not they choose to participate. Data for risk assessment is collected using

*Program summary prepared by committee member Calvin Hobel.

the Problem Oriented Perinatal Risk Assessment System (POPRAS) perinatal record. A complete history is taken, followed by a physical exam with pelvic assessment. All data are entered into a computer system and the patient is designated as high or low risk based on a scoring system derived for this population of patients.* If low-risk, the patient is assigned randomly to either a standard visit schedule or an abbreviated visit schedule. If the low-risk patient is in one of the study clinics, she also receives the education program--thus, within the low-risk population, this study will evaluate the impact of clinic visits and education in preventing a low-risk pregnancy from becoming high-risk. All low-risk patients are reassessed at 28 weeks. If high-risk, the patient is assigned randomly to one of four intervention groups or a control group.

4. Education program: Education is provided for both the health care providers (clinic and hospital) and the patients within the designated health districts.
   a. The education program for the provider concentrates on the concept of the prevention program, the importance of program design, methods of risk assessment, justification for the interventions, description of the patients' education program, reasons for hospitalization for early preterm labor, importance of continuity of care, and benefits of a successful program.
   b. The education program for patients is based on three special preterm labor classes that cover the following: a general overview of the prevention program, the detection of signs and symptoms of preterm labor and several other problems that may develop, and information about going to the hospital if preterm labor is suspected and what to expect. Information is also provided on how best to use the telephone for assistance.
5. Interventions: All high-risk patients who agree to participate in this study are assigned randomly to one of the following groups:
   a. Bed rest: Patients are asked to rest for 1 hour, three times daily (morning, afternoon, and evening). A bed rest log is completed by the patient, which includes an assessment of the presence or absence of uterine contractions.
   b. Social service: Patients are assigned to a social worker who meets with her at every visit to assess

---

*Ross M, Hobel CJ, Bragonier RJ, and Bear M: Prematurity: A simplified risk scoring system. Obstet. Gynecol. In press.

social problems. Four stress management classes are provided.

c. Progestational agent: Patients receive oral Provera (medroxyprogesterone acetate) as permitted under a special protocol approved by the FDA.

d. Placebo: A number of patients equal to the number in group C are given placebo.

e. Control group: These patients receive no additional intervention other than the education program.

F. Program effectiveness: The effectiveness of this program will be determined in four ways. The outcome variable is the incidence of prematurity:

1. Incidence of prematurity in control versus study clinics.
2. Incidence of prematurity in each of the intervention groups compared to the control group (randomized) and also control clinics (without education).
3. Shifts in preterm-birth birthweight categories between study and control groups.
4. Comparison of the incidence of prematurity during the study period with the incidence of prematurity in the same population for a 5-year period before the study.

III. The French Prematurity Prevention Program*

A. Locations: Since 1971, the French have stated that reducing the incidence of prematurity is an important national goal and have developed various plans to meet this goal. One of these strategies has involved the development of a prematurity prevention program, common to three locations: Haguenau (in Eastern France), Clamart (a suburb of Paris), and Martinique (a Caribbean island under French rule).

B. Investigator responsible for the three programs: Emile Papiernik, Professor of Obstetrics and Gynecology, University of Paris-Sud, Hospital Antoine Beclere, France.

C. Funding source: French Government Social Services.

D. Dates of implementation: Haguenau, 1971; Clamart, 1972; Martinique, 1978--all to the present.

E. Program description:

1. Basic type of program: The French program is a national longitudinal one begun in 1971. It includes certain clinical components, described below, and is supported by complete work leave beginning at 34 weeks, monetary payments for early prenatal care, and free obstetric care.
2. Health care providers: In France, the program of prevention is generally understood by most obstetric care providers--obstetricians, general practitioners, and midwives--particularly since the mid 1970s, when the

*Program summary prepared by Emile Papiernik.

concepts outlined here became widely discussed in the French obstetric community. On the island of Martinique, the program was implemented more recently by midwives and is not so much the standard of care.

3. Entry into the program: Patients who seek prenatal care are assessed for risk factors by history and pelvic exam. The risk assessment system used is based on the system described by Papiernik in 1969 (Chapter 2). Some practitioners use a risk assessment "score card," while others no longer formally score patients because the notion and content of risk assessment have become a standard part of patient care. The most important parts of the Papiernik risk assessment system are the assessment of lifestyle and physical work, the patients' recognition of uterine contractions, and pelvic examinations to uncover those signs strongly indicative of the risk of preterm labor.
4. Education: The program includes education of:
   a. physicians, midwives, and associated personnel concerning
      --the correct use of risk assessment
      --the various techniques of intervention
      --the importance of individualizing and personalizing the intervention.
   b. the public (both men and women) concerning
      --the availability and importance of early and regular prenatal care
      --activities that could endanger the pregnancy (long road trips, moving, strenuous activities, and hard physical work).
   c. the patients to
      --increase their awareness of the availability of special individualized preventive care for all women and of care specific to women at high risk
      --increase their ability to detect uterine contractions early
      --elicit their cooperation in working with the obstetrical team, and to recognize and report which physical activities trigger contractions.
5. Interventions: Various specific interventions have been used in the French program, but the efficacy of only one has been studied carefully (cervical cerclage). The following interventions are used, with those employed most frequently listed first:
   a. Reduction of physical exertion accomplished by: a physician's prescription to stop work, which must be honored by employers under law and which must be accompanied by full salary or an equivalent public subsidy; a change to less strenuous work; a reduction in working hours; and/or a general emphasis on rest.

b. Household help through eliciting the support of husband, friends, and family, and/or free domestic help when needed through the local social service system.
c. System of weekly follow-up care at home by midwives for the 5 to 10 percent of patients found to be at high risk for preterm labor.
d. Oral progestins--Chlormadinone acetate was used frequently; however, its use in Clamart has been discontinued. The frequency of its use in France generally is unknown at present.
e. Cervical cerclage--the use of cerclage for classical indications and beyond was common; however, a recent randomized trial in Haguenau and Clamart indicated that its extended use did not reduce the incidence of prematurity. In fact, it was shown to increase the preterm rate in some high-risk patients. Its use is currently restricted to classical indications.

F. Program effectiveness: A November 1983 press release from the French government reported an overall drop in preterm births in France from 8.2 percent in 1973 to 5.3 percent in 1982. In the tables that follow, declining rates of preterm births are presented for a Clamart teaching hospital, the region of Haguenau, for France generally, and for the Martinique program. In the absence of a careful statistical approach to implementing the preterm prevention strategies outlined here, it is not possible to determine the cause of the declines noted.

TABLE C.2 Live Births and Percent Preterm Among Women Followed in the Prenatal Clinic of Clamart Teaching Hospital, France, 1973-1983

	1973-75	1976-78	1980-83
Births	5009	5594	8212
Percent preterm	6.46	3.37	3.76

NOTE: Preterm births are live births of less than 37 weeks gestation.

TABLE C.3 Preterm Births per 100 Live Births by Week of Gestation in Haguenau, France, 1971-1982

Week of Gestation	1971-74	1975-78	1979-82
≤32	1.8	1.3	0.8
33-34	1.2	1.0	0.8
35-36	3.1	2.4	2.5
<37	6.1	4.5	4.2

NOTE: Preterm births are live births of less than 37 weeks gestation.

TABLE C.4 Preterm Births per 100 Live Births by Week of Gestation, France, National Representative Studies

Week of Gestation	1972	1976	1981
<34	2.4	1.7	1.2
34-36	5.8	5.1	4.4
<37	8.2	6.8	5.6

NOTE: Preterm births are live births of less that 37 weeks gestation.

TABLE C.5 Live Births and Percent Preterm Among Women Followed in the Martinique Prenatal Care System

	1980	1981	1982
Births	2250	2326	2526
Percent preterm	6.0	5.0	4.4
Perinatal mortality rate[a]	16	13	12

NOTE: Preterm births are live births of less than 37 weeks gestation.

[a]For infants weighing 500 grams or more.

APPENDIX D

Notes on National Data Available to Study Low Birthweight Trends and to Monitor Related Programs

In studying the problem of low birthweight, the committee has reviewed a variety of national data sets to understand broad trends in low birthweight, its relationship to mortality and morbidity, and the extent to which certain public programs affect its incidence. Several such data sets are outlined in the section below, followed by a section noting some of the problems with these systems. The topic of data availability also is raised in other parts of the report, particularly in chapters 3 and 7.

The committee has made no detailed recommendations about how best to strengthen the data systems in this area. However, it does wish to stress how important it is for the nation to maintain and strengthen its data collection systems pertinent to low birthweight and other important health topics. Understanding, and in turn preventing, low birthweight requires fully adequate data on a broad range of factors: demographic, medical, behavioral, socioeconomic, programmatic, and others. Budgetary constraints should not be allowed to undermine existing systems. Instead, an increased commitment should be made to ensuring that adequate data are collected, analyzed, and reported in a useful and timely manner. Both state and national data systems merit support because high quality data are needed at both levels, and because many national data sets are developed from information collected by states and localities.

Data Sources

National data on the incidence of low birthweight and on other maternal/infant characteristics are available from the National Center for Health Statistics' (NCHS) Vital Statistics Registration System (VSRS), which continuously collects and compiles data from birth certificates. The VSRS provides data on the incidence of low birthweight tabulated by race, sex of infant, plurality (single births, twins, etc.), birth order of infant, and by mother's age, educational attainment, marital status, receipt of prenatal care, and interval since last birth. Data from the VSRS are published annually in an abbreviated form in the "Advance Report of Final Natality Statistics" section of the NCHS Monthly Vital Statistics Report series. More complete data are available later in another annual NCHS publication, Vital Statistics of the United States, Vol. I, Natality.

Supplemental information on the incidence of low birthweight by characteristics beyond those covered on the birth certificate is available from the National Natality Follow-back Surveys, periodically conducted by NCHS. Based on questionnaires mailed to mothers, hospitals, physicians, and other health care providers, these surveys provide birth data by characteristics such as mother's occupation and work history during pregnancy, father's occupation, source of medical care for mother and infant, family income, mother's smoking and drinking habits, and whether the baby is breast or bottle fed. To date, NCHS has conducted National Natality Surveys (NNS) from 1963 through 1969, and in 1972 and 1980. The next NNS data collection is scheduled to start in 1988. NCHS hopes to conduct subsequent National Natality Surveys at 4-year intervals. Data from the NNS are available in a variety of publications, including Vital and Health Statistics Series reports and supplements to the Monthly Vital Statistics Report. A dozen articles from the 1980 NNS have been published in Health: United States 1983[1] and in the March-April 1984 issue of Public Health Reports.[2] Public use data tapes of the follow-back surveys are also available from the National Technical Information Service.

Although they are far from current, two other sources of national low birthweight data should be noted, both special studies by NCHS: the NCHS Linked Birth/Death Certificate Study based on the 1960 birth cohort;[3] and the 1964-1966 National Natality and Infant Mortality Survey,[4] which related low birthweight to infant mortality using estimates from two separate surveys rather than linked birth/death records.

Data Needs

A major problem with national data relevant to low birthweight is the absence of data on the sequelae of low birthweight drawn from a nationally representative sample of births. At present, neither the VSRS nor the NNS provides information on morbidity or mortality associated with low birthweight. According to NCHS and the Centers for Disease Control (CDC), no national data system is currently being planned to look systematically at the relationship between low birthweight and subsequent morbidity. Efforts are being made, however, to address the need for data relating low birthweight to mortality.[5, 6]

NCHS has undertaken the "1980 National Natality Survey/National Death Index Match" project, a special supplemental study that will search and compare the 1980 and 1981 National Death Index with an NNS sample of nearly 10,000 liveborn infants. Although the numbers are small (based on the NNS oversampling of low birthweight infants, it is projected that 271 of the NNS infants will have died in their first year of life), the match will be able to report infant mortality rates by birthweight, as well as by several hundred other data items included on the NNS.[5]

In the near future, NCHS hopes to undertake a pilot program to develop a national linked birth and death certificate file for the 1982 and 1983 birth cohorts. The addition of linked files to ongoing NCHS data systems will be evaluated at the end of the pilot study. Finally, it is hoped, but not yet definite, that NCHS will conduct an Infant Mortality Follow-back Survey in 1988 to accompany the National Natality Survey.[5]

As an interim effort, CDC plans to compile linked birth and death certificate data from individual states. Current plans are to use the 1980 birth cohort. States will be asked to provide data on infant deaths by birthweight for the following characteristics: maternal age, number of previous live births, number of fetal deaths (terminations of pregnancy of 20 or more weeks gestation), level of maternal education, sex of infant, gestational age at birth, and type of delivery. The states also will be asked to provide data on cause of death by birthweight for neonatal and postneonatal deaths. Finally, CDC will request data on infant deaths by gestational age according to month prenatal care began and number of prenatal visits. All of the above information will be requested for all infants, and separately for black and for white infants. CDC plans to have the results of the study available by the spring of 1985. Once the NCHS linked birth/death certificate data collection system is under way, CDC data collection in this area probably will be phased out.[6]

A second shortcoming of the national data currently available is the considerable time lag between the end of a calendar year and publication of final national data for that year. There is a lag of approximately 2 years before publication of the rather abbreviated "Advance Report of Final Natality Statistics," and an interval of 3 to 4 years before publication of <u>Vital Statistics of the United States</u>. It is hoped that national linked birth/death certificate data for any given birth cohort will become available within 4 years or less after the year of birth. For purposes of evaluation, planning, and implementation of public policies, this relatively long lag makes it difficult to use national low birthweight data in a timely manner.

Third, national low birthweight data by income (or class, as the British use) are very limited. While the NNS does provide periodic data by income, the VSRS does not collect information by income or socioeconomic status. As a result, surrogate measures such as race or mother's education are often used, making it more difficult to determine the extent to which low birthweight is associated with poverty as distinct from other factors.

Fourth, while the NNS has collected information from married mothers on sources of family income including participation in public programs, there is no national data base that systematically and regularly links low birthweight data (incidence and outcome) to participation in public programs such as the Special Supplemental Food Program for Women, Infants and Children (WIC), Medicaid, Food Stamps, and Aid to Families with Dependent Children. This information, if linked with data on income or socioeconomic status, would be particularly useful in evaluating the impact of public policies and programs.

Finally, national data by ethnicity are less complete than they might be. The NNS does collect detailed ethnicity data, which are available on public use data tapes; however, the NNS is conducted relatively infrequently. While the VSRS currently collects data by ethnicity, reporting by states is quite uneven. National data on births of Hispanic parentage were first available from a 1978 cohort, based on reporting from 17 states.[7] By 1980, 22 states reported on this population.[8] Low birthweight data on births of Asian parentage (Chinese, Filipino, Japanese, Hawaiian, and other) were first published by NCHS in 1984, and were based on the 1980 birth cohort.[9]

References

1. National Center for Health Statistics: Health, United States, 1983, pp. 19-434. DHHS No. (PHS) 84-1232. Public Health Service. Washington, D.C.: U.S. Government Printing Office, December 1983.
2. Public Health Reports. 99:111-183, March-April 1984.
3. National Center for Health Statistics: A Study of Infant Mortality from Linked Records, by Birth Weight, Period of Gestation, and Other Variables, United States. Vital and Health Statistics, Series 20, No. 12. DHEW No. (HSM) 72-1055. Health Services and Mental Health Administration. Washington, D.C.: U.S. Government Printing Office, May 1972.
4. National Center for Health Statistics: Infant Mortality Rates: Socioeconomic Factors, United States. Prepared by B MacMahon, MG Kovar, and JJ Feldman. Vital and Health Statistics, Series 22, No. 14. DHEW No. (HSM) 72-1045. Health Services and Mental Health Administration. Washington, D.C.: U.S. Government Printing Office, March 1972.
5. Robert Israel, Deputy Director, National Center for Health Statistics, Hyattsville, Md. Personal communication, 1984.
6. Carol JR Hogue, Chief, Pregnancy Epidemiology Branch, Division of Reproductive Health, Centers for Disease Control, Atlanta, Ga. Personal Communication, 1984.
7. National Center for Health Statistics: Births of Hispanic Parentage, 1978. Prepared by S Ventura and R Heuser. Monthly Vital Statistics Report, Vol. 29, No. 12 (supplement). DHHS No. (PHS) 81-1120. Public Health Service. Washington, D.C.: U.S. Government Printing Office, March 1981.
8. National Center for Health Statistics: Births of Hispanic Parentage, 1980. Prepared by S Ventura. Monthly Vital Statistics Report, Vol. 32, No. 6 (supplement). DHHS No. (PHS) 83-1120. Public Health Service. Washington, D.C.: U.S. Government Printing Office, September 1983.
9. National Center for Health Statistics: Characteristics of Asian Births: United States, 1980. Prepared by S Taffel. Monthly Vital Statistics Report, Vol. 32, No. 10 (supplement). DHHS No. (PHS) 84-1120. Public Health Service. Washington, D.C.: U.S. Government Printing Office, February 1984.

Index

L

M

N

O

P

S

T

U

V

W